PARTIAL REMOVABLE PROSTHODONTICS

PARTIAL REMOVABLE PROSTHODONTICS

F. JAMES KRATOCHVIL, D.D.S.

Professor of Prosthodontics,
School of Dentistry,
Center for the Health Sciences,
University of California, Los Angeles

with 19 color illustrations

W. B. SAUNDERS COMPANY
A Division of Harcourt Brace & Company
Philadelphia ■ London ■ Toronto
Montreal ■ Sydney ■ Tokyo

W.B. SAUNDERS COMPANY
A Division of
Harcourt Brace & Company

The Curtis Center
Independence Square West
Philadelphia, PA 19106

Library of Congress Cataloging-in-Publication Data

Kratochvil, F. James.
Partial removable prosthodontics.

1. Partial dentures, Removable. I. Title.
[DNLM: 1. Denture, Partial, Removable. WU 515
K895p]
RK665.K73 1988 617.6'92 87-28352
ISBN 0-7216-2382-4

Listed here is the latest translated edition of this book together with the language of the translation and the publisher.

Spanish—*(1st Edition)* Nueva Editorial Interamericana, Mexico City, Mexico.

German—*(1st Edition)* Medica Verlag, Stuttgart, Germany.

Japanese—*(1st Edition)* Ishiyaku Publishers Inc, Tokyo, Japan.

Editor: Darlene Pedersen
Developmental Editor: David Kilmer
Designer: Karen O'Keefe
Production Manager: Pete Faber
Manuscript Editor: Diane Zuckerman
Illustration Coordinator: Walt Verbitski
Indexer: Ellen Murray

Partial Removable Prosthodontics ISBN 0-7216-2382-4

Last digit is the print number: 9 8 7 6 5 4

Dedicated to
my partner and wife—Kit

Preface

This book presents the basic philosophy and concepts prescribed by the author and is not intended as a reference textbook for evaluating and describing other philosophies.

Treatment for the partially edentulous patient with a removable partial prosthesis is intimately involved with all areas of dental expertise. It is not a technique but the application of a series of basic principles used in an organized treatment plan.

With this philosophy behind it, the book begins by presenting the basic principles of treatment with the idea that dentists can apply methods or techniques of their own selection if they satisfy those principles.

Following the establishment of the basic principles, later portions of the book present the application of those principles to diagnosis, treatment planning, clinical procedures, laboratory procedures, and patient considerations.

Acknowledgments

I would like to express my deepest appreciation for the help and contributions of the many individuals who provided ideas, materials, information, photos, and assistance in the assembling of this book.

I wish to offer special thanks for the patient treatment material to the prosthodontic postgraduate students at UCLA and to Dr. Ted Berg for his extensive contributions, especially in the area of laboratory procedures. Irene Petravicius of the Illustrations Section at the UCLA School of Dentistry provided outstanding drawings and diagrams as did Dr. Sameto Hobo. The photographs of procedures were ably done by the Photographic Section at Guy's Hospital, London, England and at the UCLA School of Dentistry in Los Angeles, California.

I greatly appreciate having had the excellent word processing skills of Rhoda Freeman, Barbara Mersini, and Mickey Stern at UCLA and the expertise of Mrs. Elsie Crook at Guy's Hospital Dental Department.

Finally, many thanks to Professor D.J. Neill and the staff of the Department of Prosthetic Dentistry at Guy's Hospital for their assistance.

JIM KRATOCHVIL

Contents

PARTIAL REMOVABLE PROSTHODONTICS

Plate 1

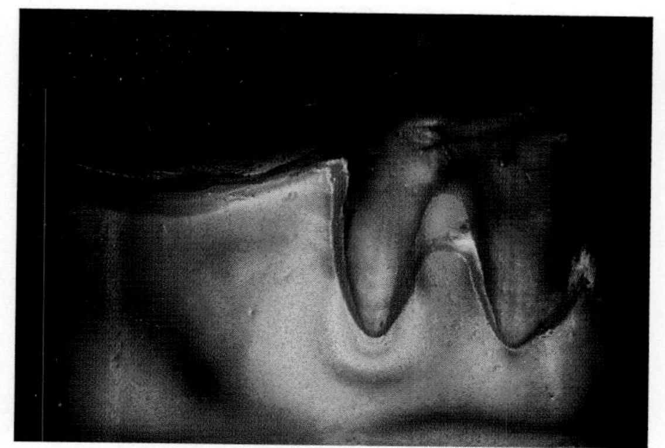

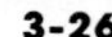
3-26

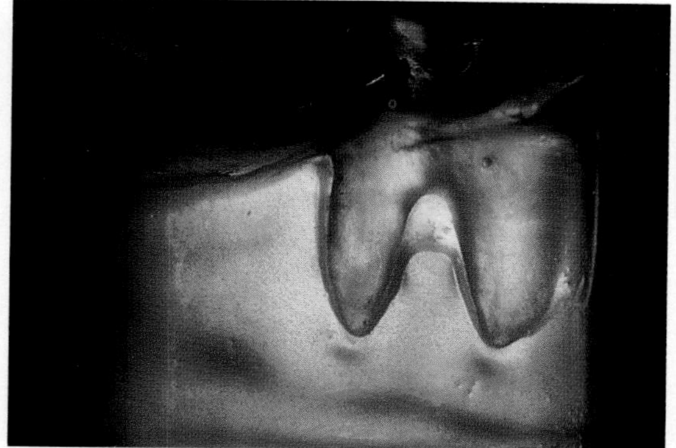

3-27

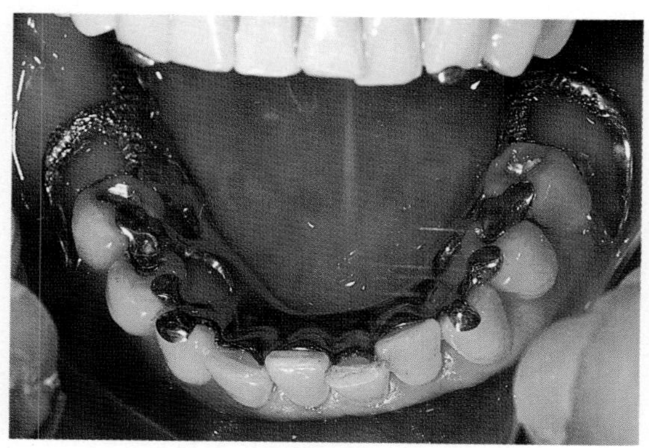

8-24

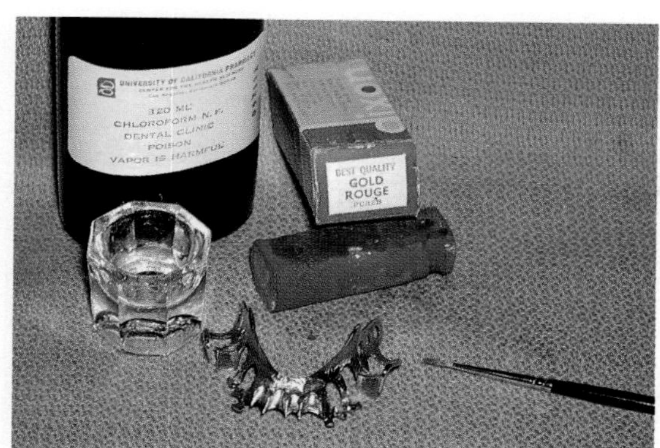

8-25

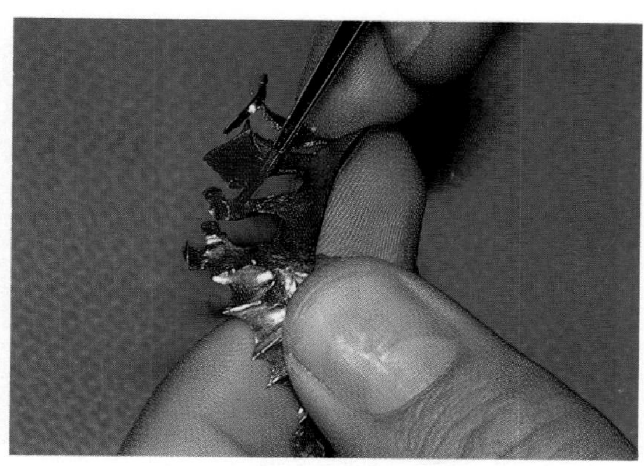

8-26

Plate 2

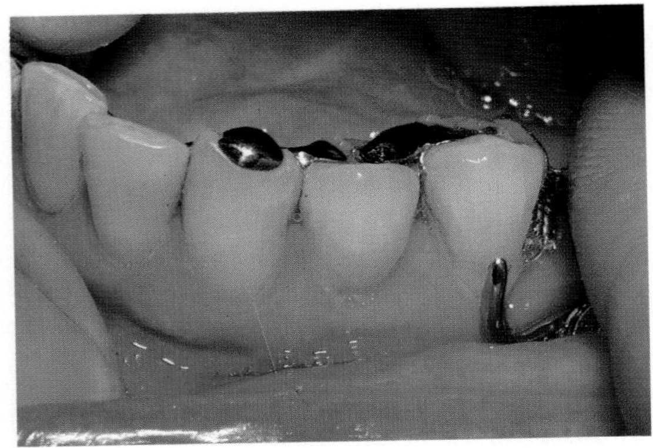

8-27

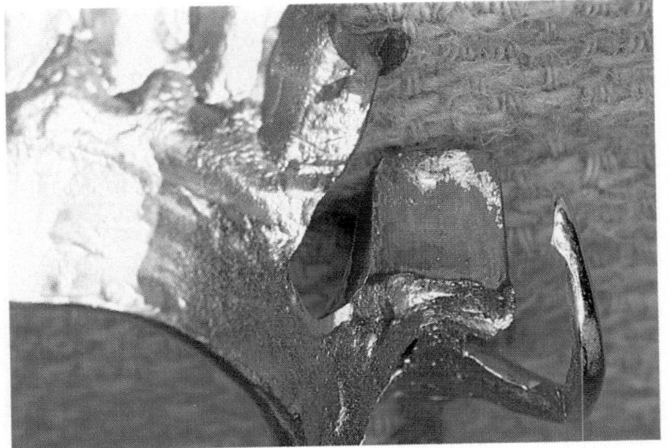

8-28

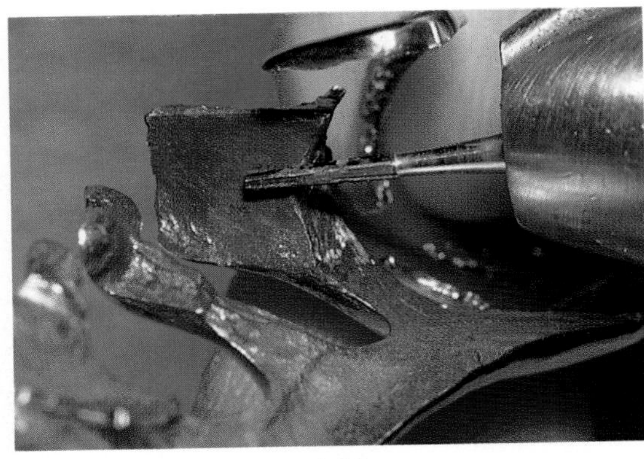

8-29

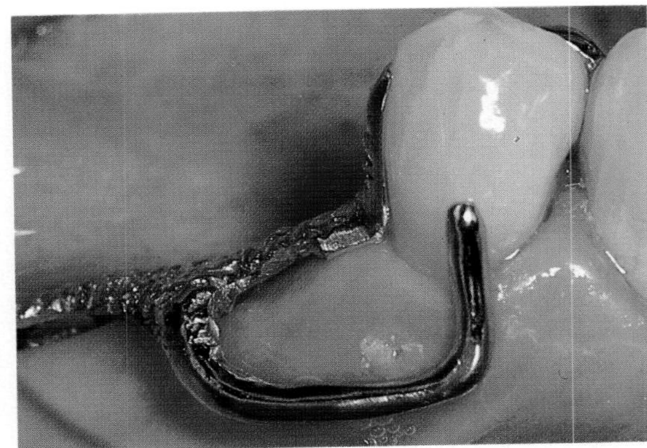

8-30

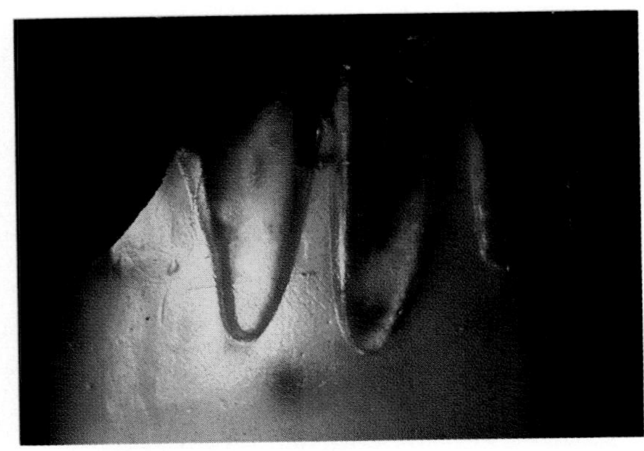

8-46

Plate 3

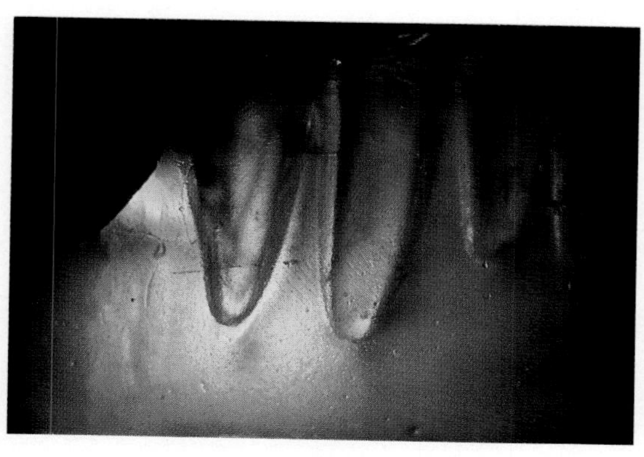

8-47

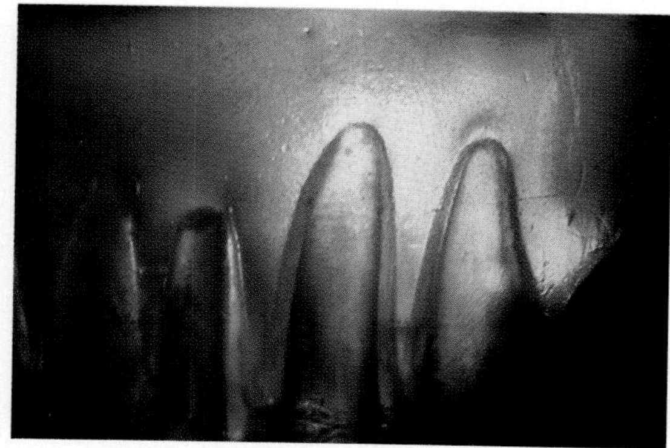

8-48

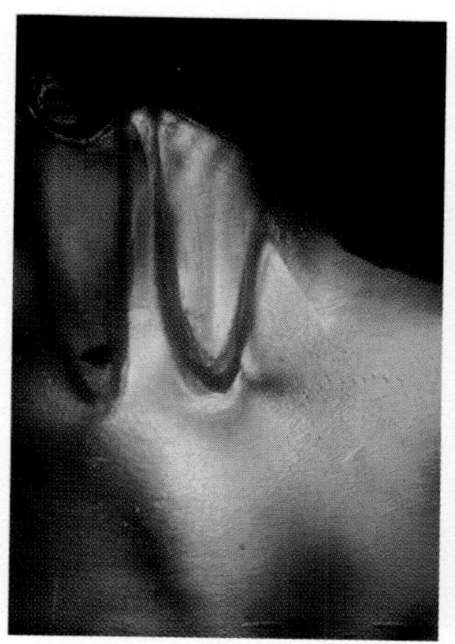

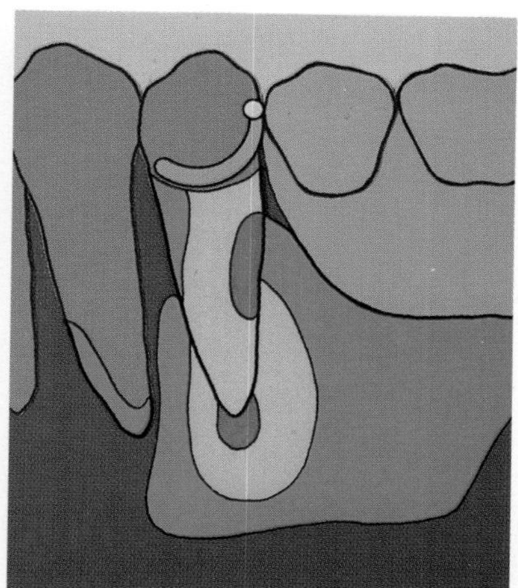

8-56

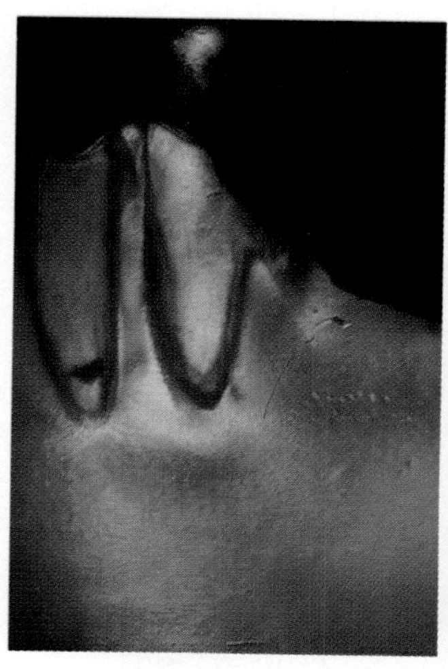

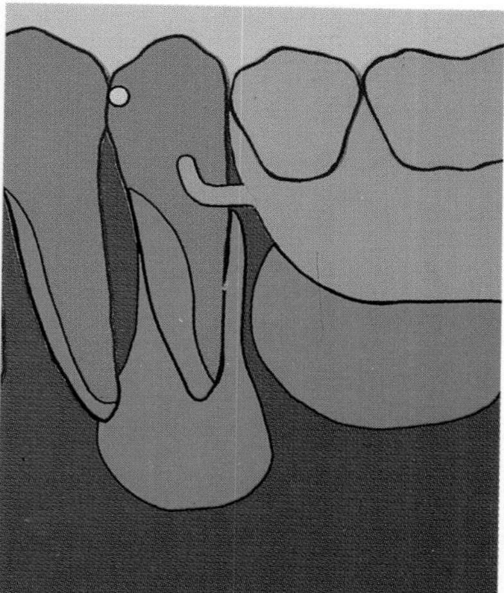

8-57

Plate 4

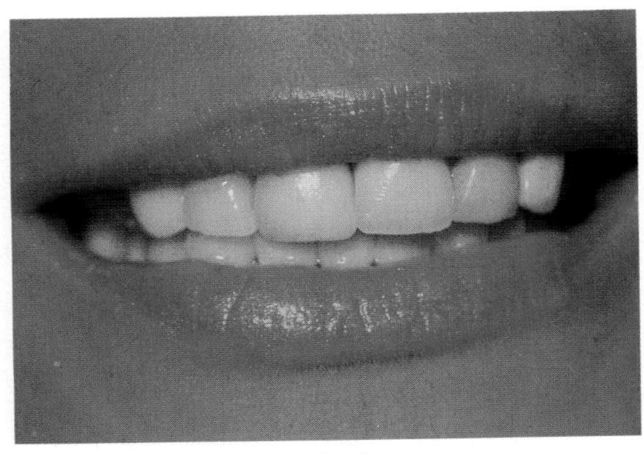

17-23

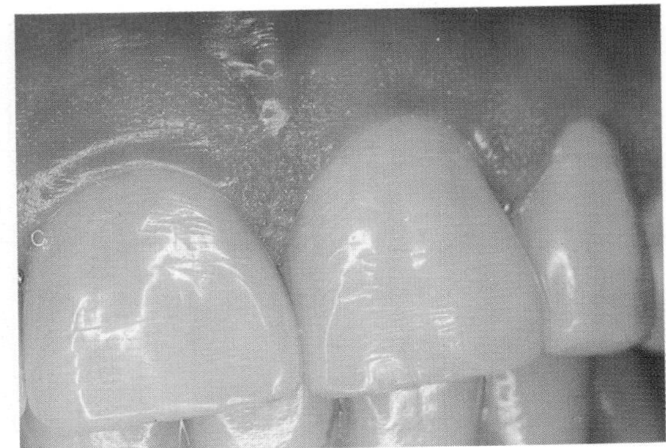

17-24

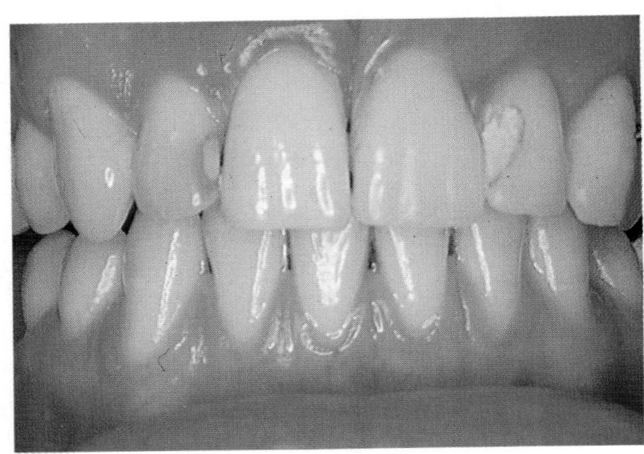

17-25

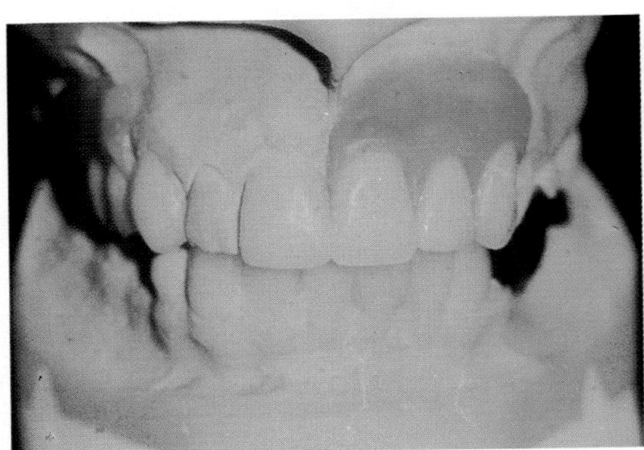

17-27

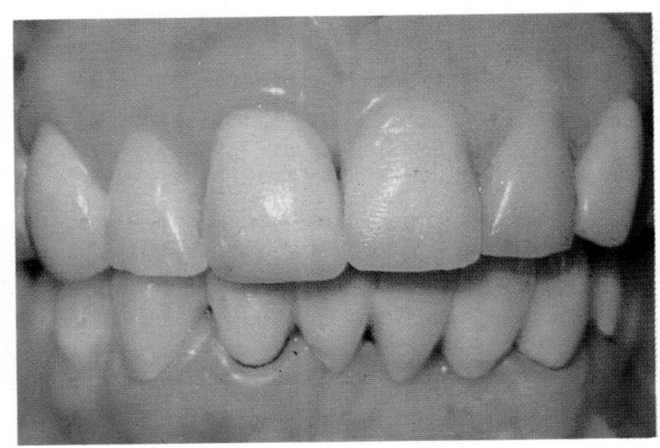

17-28

chapter 1

Principles and objectives of removable partial denture treatment

Basic principles of dental treatment for a partially edentulous arch are (1) to stabilize the individual arch and (2) to organize interarch function by control of interarch contacts. To accomplish the overall objective of stabilization of the arch requires control of the positions of all teeth in relation to each other and to their supporting structures in a given position, so that they present a united effort against functional forces. The second objective is to organize the action of the opposing arches so that they function at their optimum potential (Fig.1 – 1). This requires simultaneous interarch contacts and properly directed functional forces against supporting structures in harmony with the temporomandibular joint.

Stabilizing the Individual Arch

Teeth can move out of arch symmetry at eruption, because of loss of adjacent teeth or space irregularities (Fig. 1 – 2). If the continuity of the arch is lost, teeth may stand alone, losing the advantage of mesial-distal contact that allows them to function as a continuous unit. Loss of this unity is the first step in a cyclic progression of events that develops into arch disorganization (Fig. 1 – 3).

The eventual results of this progression may be loss of stability of individual teeth with increased mobility and lack of consistent interdigitation with teeth in the opposing arch. The mandible responds by changing position of centric occlusion to accommodate tooth movement. Individual teeth may turn from a position of optimum alignment and may tip in any direction, presenting unfavorable leverage against the periodontal ligament and bone (Fig. 1 – 4).

The basic objective of the dentist is to reorganize and stabilize the arch and to reestablish the integrity of the entire unit. Achieving these conditions requires use of all methods of dental treatment including

1. Periodontal therapy
2. Orthodontic treatment to reposition the teeth
3. Individual tooth restorations to stabilize the arch
4. Fixed partial dentures
5. Orthognathic surgery where indicated
6. Establishment and control of the occlusal plane
7. Removable partial dentures

It is imperative that the basic objective of entire arch stabilization is not lost or overshadowed by attention given to one area such as the pathologic condition of an individual tooth or local supporting structures.

Repositioning of Teeth

In some instances the ideal treatment is to return the teeth to or position them in optimal

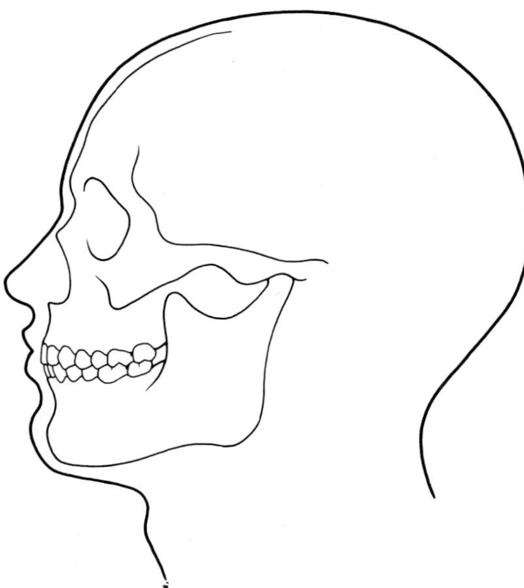

Figure 1–1 ■ The basic principles and objectives of dental treatment are (1) to restore and maintain health and control of individual dental arches, and (2) to achieve interarch control.

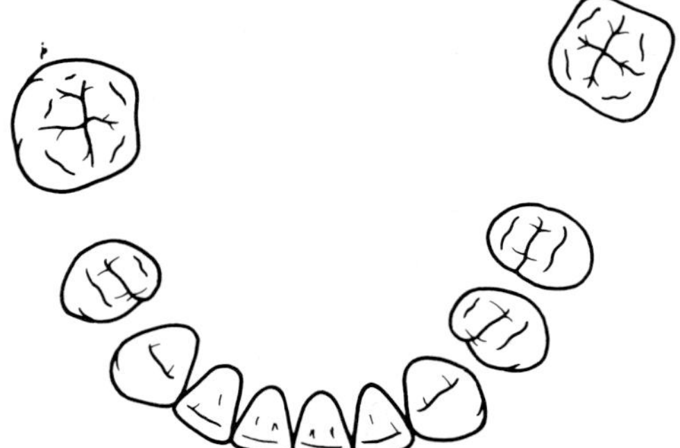

Figure 1–3 ■ Loss or absence of anterior-posterior contacts leaves teeth standing alone without stability ("divide and conquer").

locations for ideal arch form and stability. This is accomplished by orthodontic treatment (Figs. 1–5 and 1–6), which may simplify prosthetic treatment or in some instances provide the proper treatment without the need for a prosthesis.

In other instances, orthodontic treatment can improve the condition prior to treatment with a fixed or a removable prosthesis.

Stabilizing the Arch with Individual Restorations

When mesial and distal contacts between teeth are not present, the anterior-posterior continuity may be established by individual restorations if the space between the teeth is not too great and acceptable tooth-tissue contours can be developed (Figs. 1–7 and 1–8).

Establishing anterior-posterior contacts and bracing areas provides support for all remaining teeth and helps stabilize arch position and provide arch integrity.

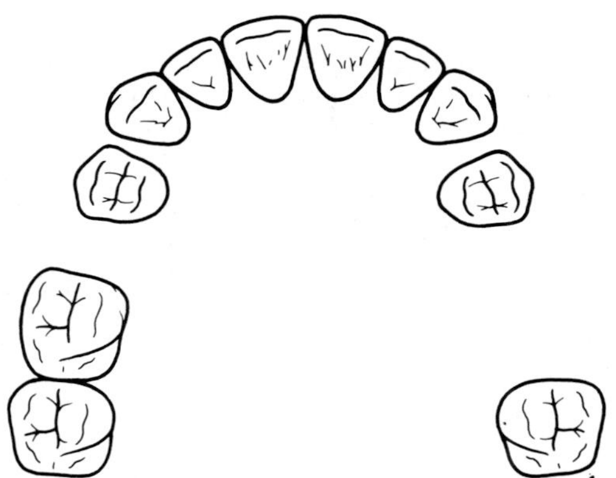

Figure 1–2 ■ Arch continuity and unity may be compromised by lack of anterior-posterior contacts, which may result in unstable occlusal contacts, mobile teeth, and fluctuating mandibular movement.

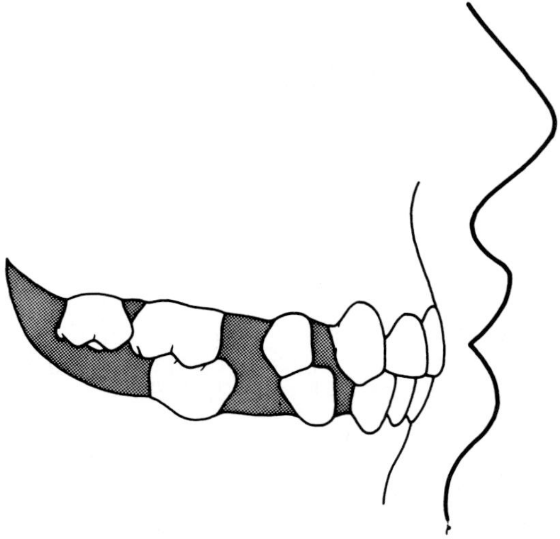

Figure 1–4 ■ Loss of arch continuity may result in tooth movement, teeth standing alone and unsupported, reduced function, unstable occlusion, a compromised occlusal plane, and disrupted mandibular function.

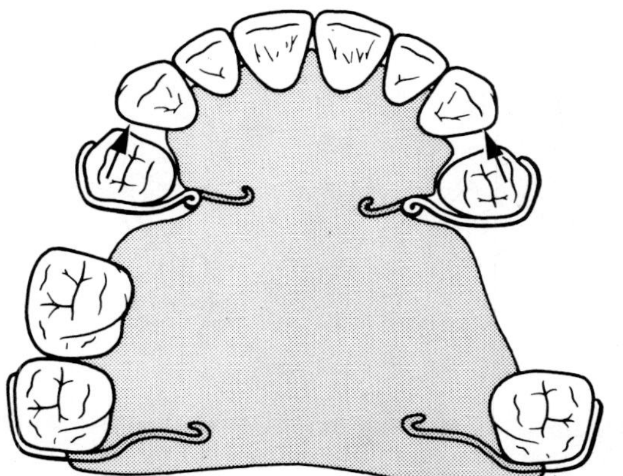

Figure 1–5 ■ A removable orthodontic prosthesis to restore premolar contact prior to prosthetic treatment.

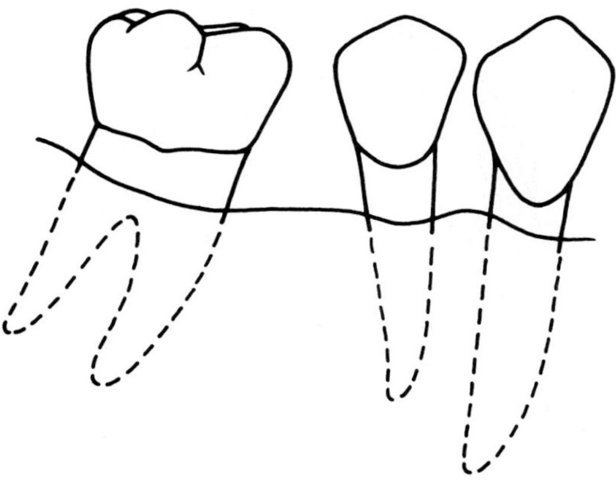

Figure 1–7 ■ Migrating teeth, resulting in disorganization of occlusion.

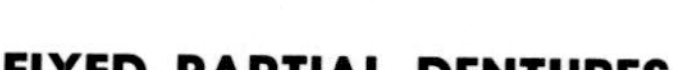

FIXED PARTIAL DENTURES

A decision may be made to restore the arch with fixed partial dentures. This procedure provides arch stabilization when properly planned (Fig. 1–9). The degree of arch stability achieved is influenced by the number of teeth involved in the restoration versus the use of cross-arch support.

When the tooth support supplied by bone and tissues is reduced, it may not be expedient to place a fixed prosthesis that depends entirely on support from one side of the arch; instead, it is necessary to join both sides of the arch for sufficient stability.

REMOVABLE PARTIAL DENTURES

In some instances, the treatment of choice is a removable prosthesis (Fig. 1–10). It can provide cross-arch support, stabilize the teeth in a given position, and unite the remaining teeth into a positive unit. It restores function and controls direction of force against remaining teeth and tissues. The removable prosthesis is rigid, bilateral, restores missing structures, and can provide excellent tooth position control, occlusion, and unity of the arch (Fig. 1–11).

This book discusses the objectives, the philosophy, and some of the procedures used when treating patients with removable partial dentures. In some instances, a combination of all treatment modalities is necessary and is recommended.

ORTHOGNATHIC SURGERY

In some patients, the basic malposition of one or both arches is caused by the location of the

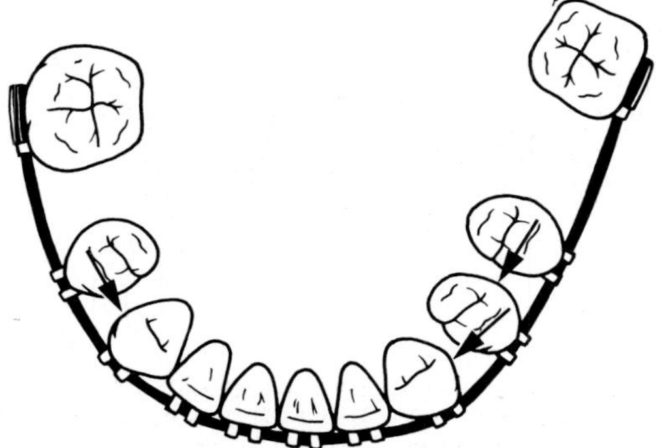

Figure 1–6 ■ Treatment by orthodontic movement to restore tooth position with bodily tooth movement.

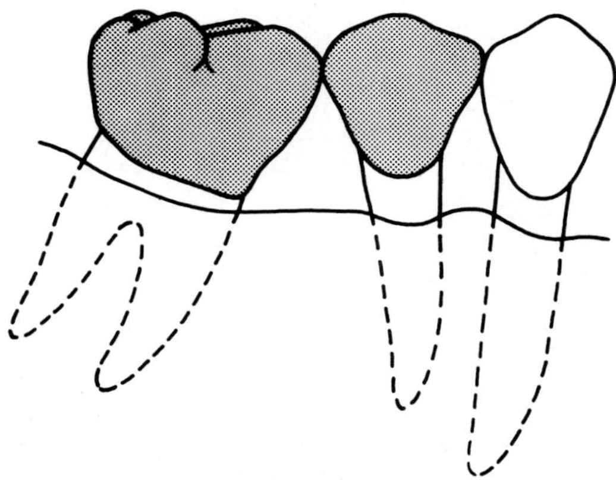

Figure 1–8 ■ Contacts, occlusion, and stability restored with overcontoured individual restorations.

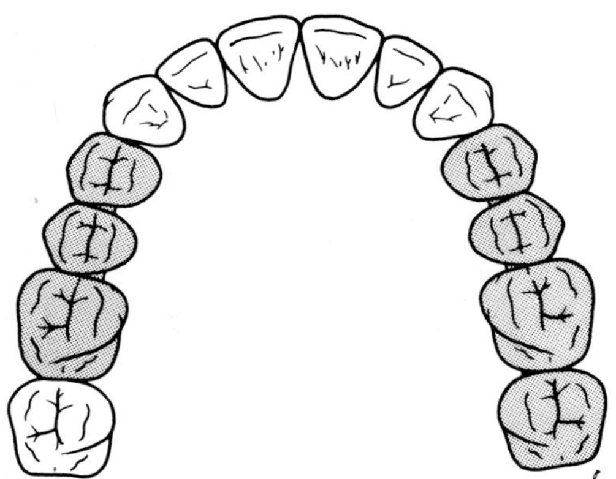

Figure 1–9 ■ Fixed partial dentures may be the treatment of choice to reestablish anterior-posterior integrity.

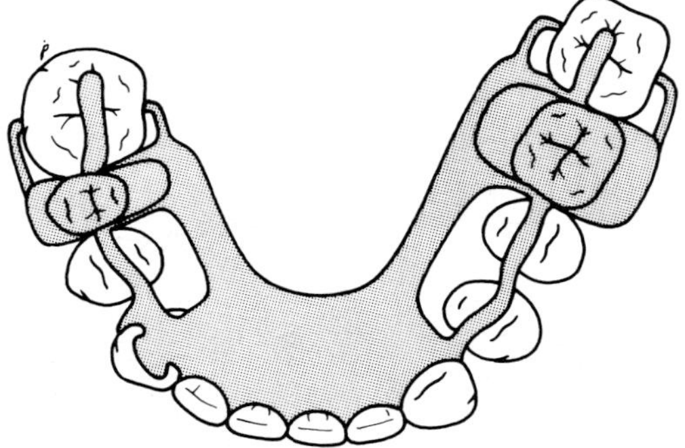

Figure 1–11 ■ A mandibular removable partial denture can unite and stabilize a compromised arch.

bone structures (Fig. 1–12). It is possible to surgically reposition one or both arches to obtain a better functional position (Fig. 1–13). The casts are repositioned in a laboratory procedure for diagnostic evaluation of potential results before a decision is made to surgically intervene. A plastic stint is fabricated on the properly repositioned diagnostic casts and is used to position and hold the mandible during the surgical procedure. The stint holds the mandible in the predetermined position during healing. Following surgery, it is usually necessary to provide additional restorative treatment in order to establish proper occlusal contacts between arches.

Supporting Structure Considerations

Of equal importance to the prosthetic treatment or restoration is evaluation of the tooth supporting structures. This includes evaluation of bone and mucosa support, and treatment of pathologic conditions, when present, to provide optimal conditions for prosthodontic treatment. Periodontal treatment may be accomplished prior to, along with, or, in some instances, after the prosthetic treatment. Abused or irritated mucosa under existing prostheses is treated immediately. The sequence may vary, depending upon individual situations, but equal emphasis on periodontal and prosthetic treatment is essential. Considerations in periodontal evaluation and treatment will be discussed in Chapter 12, under Intraoral Preparation.

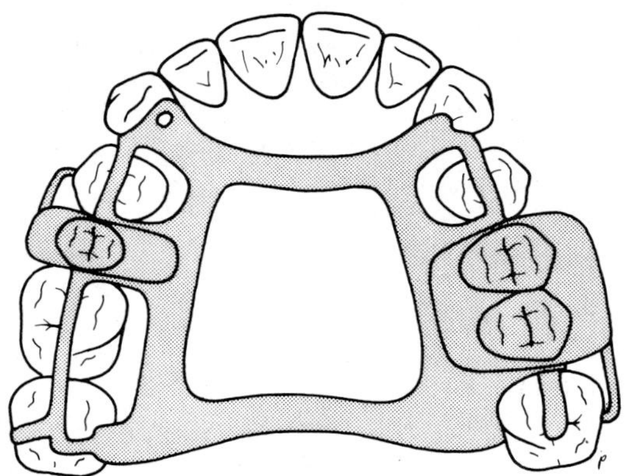

Figure 1–10 ■ A removable partial denture can provide arch stability and restore the occlusal plane with a single prosthesis.

Establishment of Proper Occlusal Plane

The malpositioned occlusal plane is a primary cause of teeth moving out of position, resulting in loss of function, and is a contributing

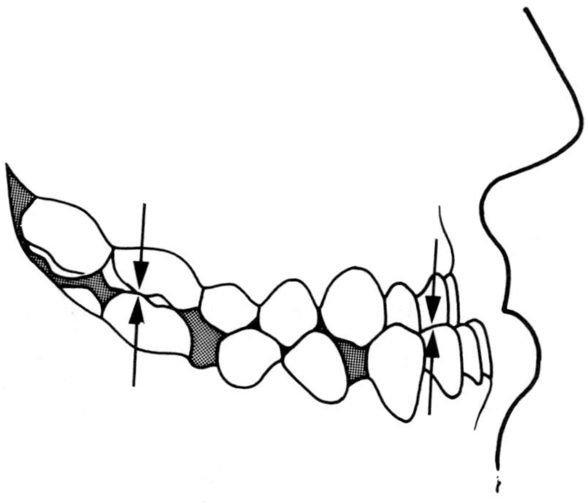

Figure 1–12 ■ Basic anatomic malposition of the mandibular arch in a prognathic position.

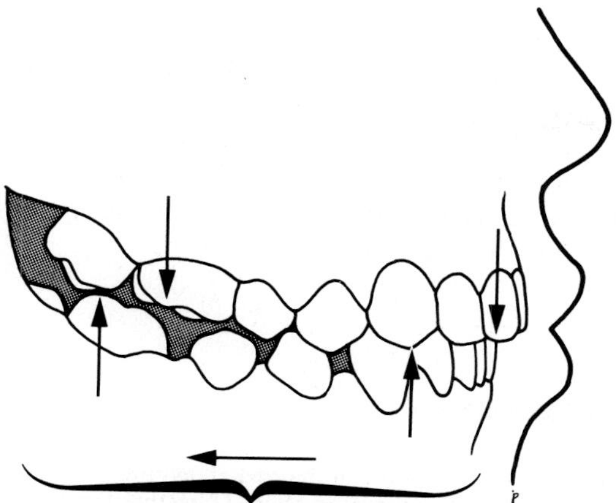

Figure 1–13 ■ A surgical procedure was done to place the mandible in a better anatomic and occlusal position. Occlusal restorations are usually necessary to maintain and restore function in addition to the surgical procedure.

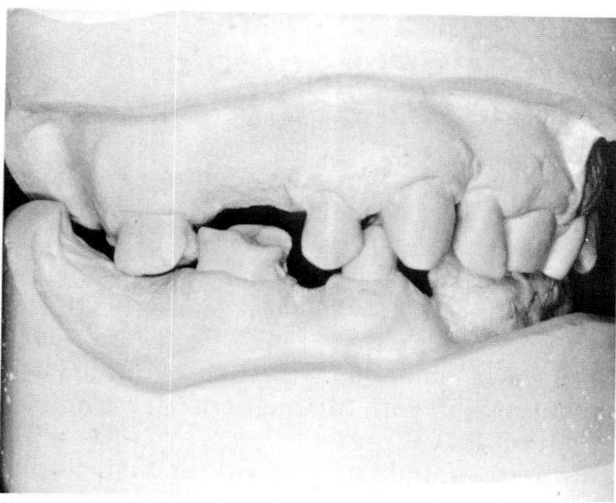

Figure 1–15 ■ Extreme occlusal plane disorganization. Extensive surgical restoration procedures are necessary for control of occlusal forces.

factor to problems involving supporting tissue and mastication, as well as esthetic and phonetic problems (Fig. 1–14). In some instances it is necessary to remove or restore teeth and supporting structures in order to obtain a properly positioned plane of occlusion (Fig. 1–15). It is essential that the occlusal plane be properly positioned and organized in order to obtain maximum functional potential.

Evaluation of the occlusal plane is the basic factor necessary for control of occlusal development and for effective functioning of natural teeth or a prosthesis. Proper position enables development of coordinated and controlled mandibular function, resulting in the best possible supporting tissue responses.

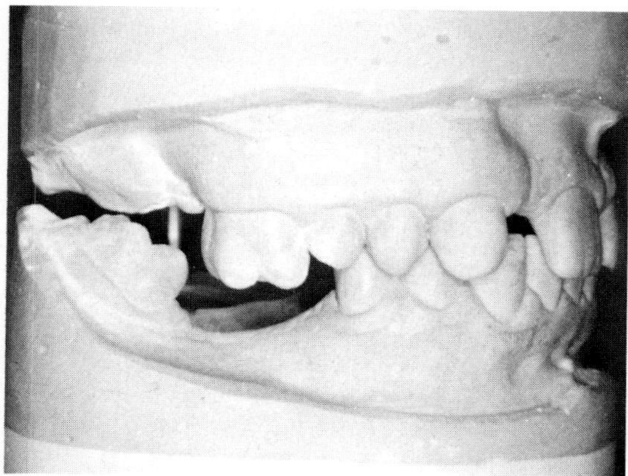

Figure 1–14 ■ Compromised occlusal plane caused by loss of teeth. Restoration at the proper position is essential for health and function.

Professional Responsibility

The dentist must realize that it is his or her professional responsibility to completely understand and develop all procedures associated with removable partial denture treatment. Properly planned partial dentures *will* restore lost portions of the oral tissues most successfully for long periods of time.

Treatment design is a critical factor when a removable partial denture is used, and it is the major factor in diagnosis and planning. Treatment decisions are entirely dependent upon the amount, type, and condition of the remaining oral anatomical structures of the patient. It is the doctor's responsibility and prerogative to make these decisions, and they cannot be ethically delegated to an individual other than a doctor.

It is seldom possible to take a treatment procedure or design in toto from one situation and apply it to another patient. The clinician must study and understand the basic principles and the rationale for removable partial denture treatment in order to prescribe the prosthesis, just as he must study and understand the basic principles of cavity preparation in order to do an amalgam restoration.

Maintenance of the Patient's Physiologic and Mental Health

When removable partial denture treatment receives proper appraisal and planning, it will be successful.

A high percentage of partially edentulous patients require removable partial dentures. It is necessary to plan treatment with regard to *preserving* and *maintaining* the tissues of the body in conjunction with treatment of the pathologic condition that is present.

Promises should not be made about restoring the teeth to their original capabilities such as may be possible with an individual tooth restoration. Do assure the patient that the best treatment will be provided to maintain the remaining oral structures. It may be possible to promise a significant improvement in esthetics, but do not stress the likelihood that the masticating ability of natural dentition will be restored. Understanding, concern, and empathy are of primary importance in treating patients.

Factors to be considered in maintaining dental health and in preserving remaining structures are as follows:

1. Bone (resorption, amount, type)
2. Periodontal factors (pocket depth, thickness of periodontal ligament and gingival attachments)
3. Mucosa (color, contour, position, health)
4. Temporomandibular joints (structure, health, support)
5. Improvement or restoration of esthetics and phonetics
6. Restoration or improvement of masticating ability
7. Restoration of remaining teeth when necessary
8. Psychological and social considerations

Each of these factors is discussed in the following chapters wherever they are involved in the treatment procedures.

REFERENCES

DeVan MM: The nature of the partial denture foundation: suggestions for its preservation. J Prosthet Dent 2:210, 1952.

Friel S: Occlusion—observations on its development from infancy to old age. Int J Orthod 13:322, 1927.

Glickman I: Role of occlusion in the etiology and treatment of periodontal disease. J Dent Res 50:199–211, 1971.

Kratochvil FJ, and Caputo A: Photoelastic analysis of pressure on teeth and bone supporting removable partial dentures. J Prosthet Dent 32:52, 1975.

Kratochvil FJ, Davidson PM, and Guijt J: Five-year survey of treatment with removable partial dentures. J Prosthet Dent 48:3, 237–244, 1982.

McLean DW: Diagnosis and correction of pathologic occlusion. J Am Dent Assoc 29:1202–1210, 1942.

Ramford SR: Indices for prevalence and incidence of periodontal disease. J Periodontol 30:51, 1959.

Sim JM: Minor Tooth Movement in Children. St Louis, CV Mosby Co, 1972.

Starshak TJ, and Sanders B: Preprosthetic Oral and Maxillofacial Surgery. St Louis, CV Mosby Co, 1980.

Wright K, Mech EM, and Yettram A: Reactive force distributions for teeth when loaded singly and when used as fixed partial denture abutments. J Prosthet Dent 42:411, 1979.

Ziebert G, and Donegan S: Tooth contacts and stability before and after occlusal adjustment. J Prosthet Dent 42:276, 1979.

chapter 2

Parts of a removable partial denture and their functions

To provide a systematic approach to partial denture treatment, it is important to identify the parts of a partial denture and their functions. Each part is presented individually in the sequence in which it is designed. The parts that receive or support the major forces are considered first.

Rests

A rest is the part of a removable partial denture that contacts a tooth; it affords primarily vertical support (Figs. 2–1 and 2–2).

Function

Positive rests control the relationship of the prosthesis to the supporting structures and are designed and placed to preserve the supporting oral structures by controlling (1) the position of the prosthesis in relation to the teeth and (2) the position of the prosthesis in relation to the periodontium and other supporting tissues.

A basic principle is that the rest must be positive and must direct functional forces in the long axis of the tooth. The greater the occlusal force, the more firmly the prosthesis should be seated in the positive rest prepared in the tooth. The most destructive situation is that in which force is placed on an inclined plane or that in which a rest produces lateral forces on supporting structures.

To provide the most ideal support position, the rest is placed as close to the center of the tooth as possible. Force delivered to the prosthesis is transferred to the supporting structures around the root of the tooth by means of the rest. These forces are best supported if they are in the long axis of the tooth, placing an equalized pull or stress on the periodontal ligament (Fig. 2–3). Lateral forces against the tooth tend to pinch the periodontal ligament between the root and the bone, producing osteoclastic activity and bone change (Fig. 2–4).

Rests are positioned, prepared, and constructed to control the direction of force delivered to the prosthesis and to supporting structures.

Major Connectors

A major connector is a rigid part of the partial denture casting that unites the rests and other parts of the prosthesis to the opposite side of the arch.

MANDIBULAR MAJOR CONNECTORS

The lingual bar or plate is a rigid major connector located lingual to the dental arch, connecting the components on one side of the arch to the components on the other side (Fig. 2–1).

MAXILLARY MAJOR CONNECTOR

This is a rigid major connector that crosses the palate and unites the components on the

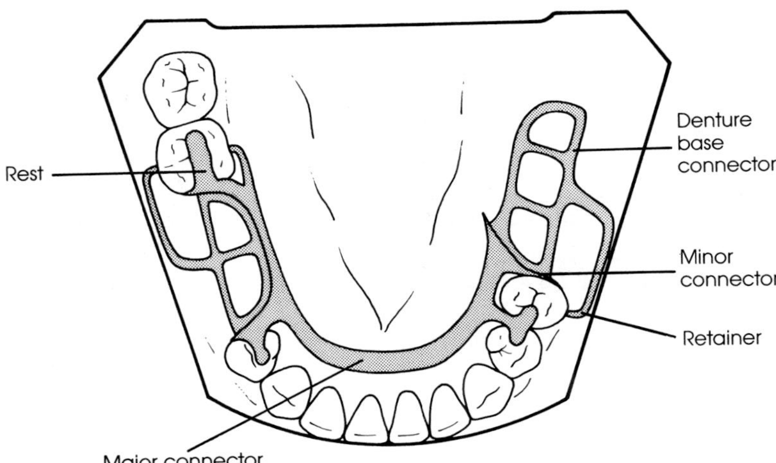

Figure 2–1 ■ The parts of a mandibular removable partial denture.

right and left sides of the arch. It may be designed in several forms (Fig. 2–2).

Function of Major Connectors

One of the primary reasons for treatment with a removable partial denture is the need to unite and stabilize the remaining teeth in the arch. To provide this support, rigid cross-arch construction design is necessary. When this stability is provided, all remaining teeth can be united to share and distribute the forces of occlusion. The design and positioning of major connectors is determined by individual patient situations and requirements. A detailed discussion is presented in the description of major connectors in Chapter 5.

Minor Connectors and Proximal Plates

Minor connectors are strong and rigid parts of a removable partial denture that connect other units, such as proximal plates and rests, with the major connector.

The proximal plate contacts the side of the tooth and extends onto the interproximal tissue (Figs. 2–1 and 2–2).

Function of Proximal Plates

1. Maintain arch integrity by anterior-posterior *bracing action.*

2. Act as retainers by frictional contact with the parallel guiding surfaces on the teeth.

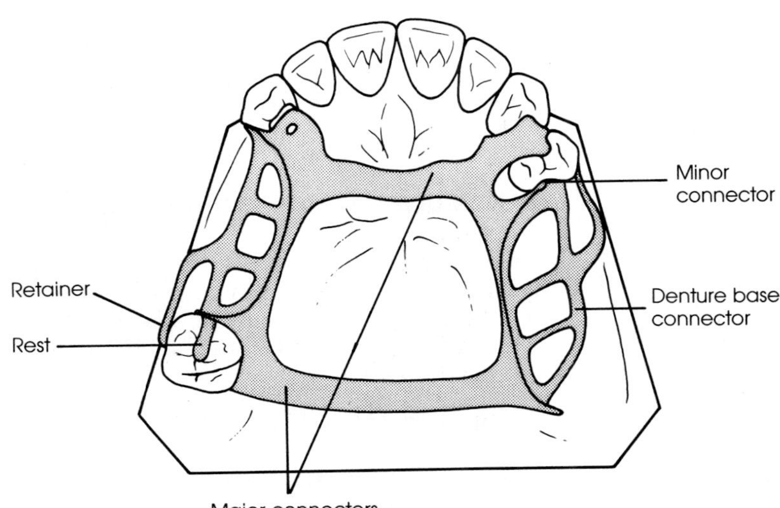

Figure 2–2 ■ The parts of a maxillary removable partial denture.

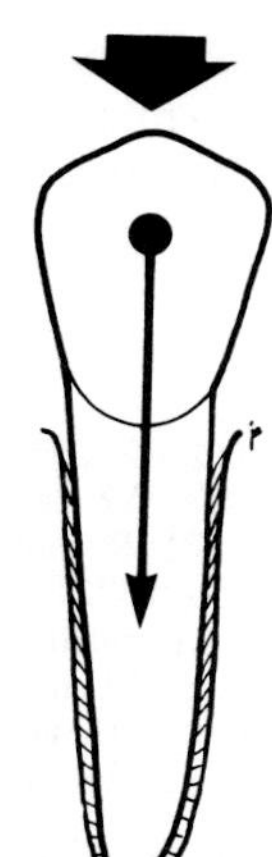

Figure 2-3 ■ The ideal location to place force on a tooth is directly in the center of the long axis of the tooth.

3. Protect against *food impaction* by adaptation of the guide plates at the tooth-tissue junction.
4. Maintain soft tissue health at the tooth-tissue junction by eliminating voids, which helps prevent tissue hypertrophy or recession.
5. Provide reciprocation action to the partial denture retainer.

Denture Base Connectors

These connectors form a structure of metal struts that engages and unites the metal casting with the resin forming the denture base (Figs. 2-1 and 2-2).

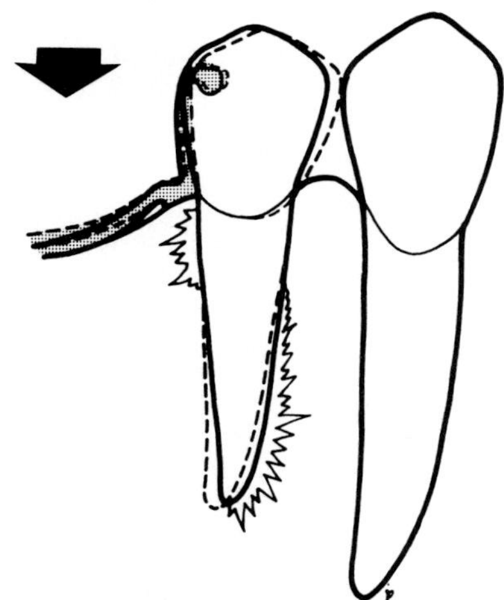

Figure 2-4 ■ Destructive lateral forces can be generated by the prosthesis.

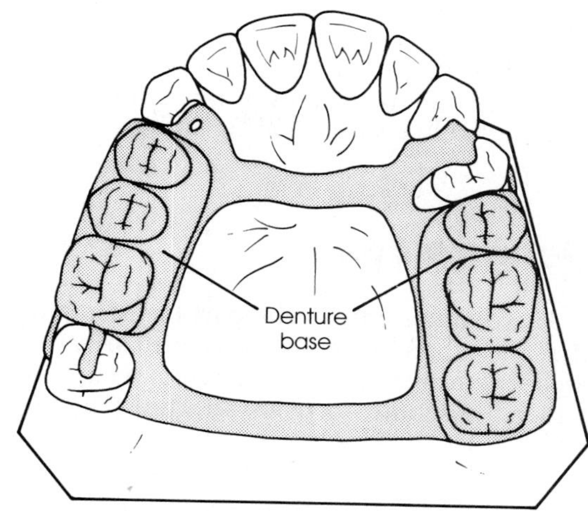

Figure 2-5 ■ Maxillary denture bases in the edentulous areas; these bases help support the prosthesis and attach the prosthetic teeth to the denture.

Function

The function of the denture base connector is to provide a strong, rigid support structure for attachment of the plastic portion of the prosthesis containing the teeth.

Retainers

A retainer is any portion of the prosthesis that contacts the teeth and helps to prevent removal of the prosthesis (Figs. 2-1 and 2-2). Rigid proximal plates provide retention as do the flexible retainer arms.

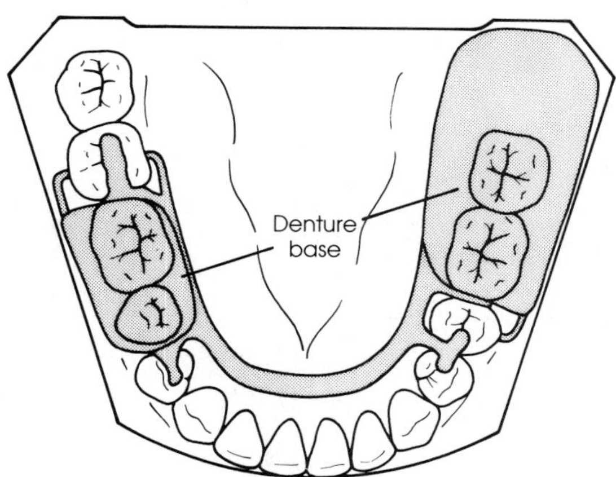

Figure 2-6 ■ Mandibular denture base areas.

Function

The function of retention is to control the position of the prosthesis in relation to the remaining teeth and supporting structures.

Denture Base

The denture base is the part of the denture that rests upon the oral mucosa, primarily in the area where the teeth have been removed, and to which the denture teeth are attached (Figs. 2–5 and 2–6).

Function

The denture base utilizes the oral mucosa in the edentulous area to its greatest potential for support, to provide attachment for prosthetic teeth, which restores mastication, and for temporomandibular joint support.

REFERENCES

Applegate OC: Essentials of Removable Partial Denture Prosthesis. Philadelphia, WB Saunders Co, 1966.

Henderson D and Steffel VL: Removable Partial Prosthesis. St Louis, CV Mosby Co, 1973.

Holmes JB: Preparation of abutment teeth for removable partial dentures. J Prosthet Dent 20:396, 1968.

Kratochvil FJ: Influence of occlusal rest position and clasp design on movement of abutment teeth. J Prosthet Dent 13:114, 1963.

Kratochvil FJ and Vig RG: Principles of Removable Partial Dentures. UCLA, Health Sciences Book Store, 1979.

Wright K, Mech EM, and Yettram A: Reactive force distribution for teeth when loaded singly and when used as fixed partial denture abutments. J Prosthet Dent 42:411, 1979.

chapter 3

The partial denture rest

Chapter 2 states that the primary function of a rest is to control the prosthesis in relationship to the teeth and supporting structures and to provide support for the partial denture by its position on the abutment teeth.

A major factor in maintaining the support structures is control of direction of the forces of movement and function so that they are in the long axis of the tooth, at right angles to the correct occlusal plane. Design and placement of rests become major factors in planning for the control of forces. A basic requirement for a rest is that it must be positive and not allow the prosthesis to slide off the tooth or allow the tooth to move out of existing relationship to other teeth as increased occlusal pressure is exerted. To this end, all rests must be positive and must provide a position or connection between prosthesis and tooth that does not allow tooth and prosthesis to separate as increasing masticatory force and functions are applied.

Positive rests preserve the remaining oral structures by

1. Controlling the position of the prosthesis in relation to the teeth.
2. Controlling the position of the prosthesis in relation to the periodontium and mucosa.
3. Controlling the amount and direction of movement of the abutment teeth.

The *rest* is the controlling factor in the triad of prosthesis-tooth-periodontium.

The anatomy of the anterior and posterior teeth requires separate consideration and design of rests if they are to function properly and transmit forces in an acceptable direction. For this reason, rests are discussed under two headings: *anterior* and *posterior* rests.

Anterior Rests

It is difficult to obtain a positive seat for rests on anterior teeth because the lingual tooth surface is sloped and without central fossae or marginal ridges. The most damaging situation is placement of the rest on an inclined surface (Fig. 3–1). Force on an inclined surface places lateral force on the tooth, which (1) causes tooth displacement and bone destruction (Fig. 3–2); (2) allows the prosthesis to move out of position and to displace tissue (Fig. 3–3); (3) disrupts and disorganizes occlusion.

It is difficult to prepare a positive anterior lingual rest in natural tooth structure because of the basic morphology of the anterior teeth, especially of mandibular anterior teeth. The enamel is quite thin near the gingiva, and an adequate rest preparation of the required depth cannot be prepared without exposure of dentin. In some instances it is possible to prepare properly contoured rest seats in maxillary canines and centrals where there is a prominent cingulum of good enamel (Fig. 3–4). However, it is usually necessary to provide a positive rest on the lingual surface of anterior teeth by means of a restorative procedure.

BASIC GENERAL REQUIREMENTS OF ANTERIOR RESTS

The anterior rest design has the basic support area as close to the center of the tooth as possible (Fig. 3–5). The ideal anterior rest fulfills the following requirements:

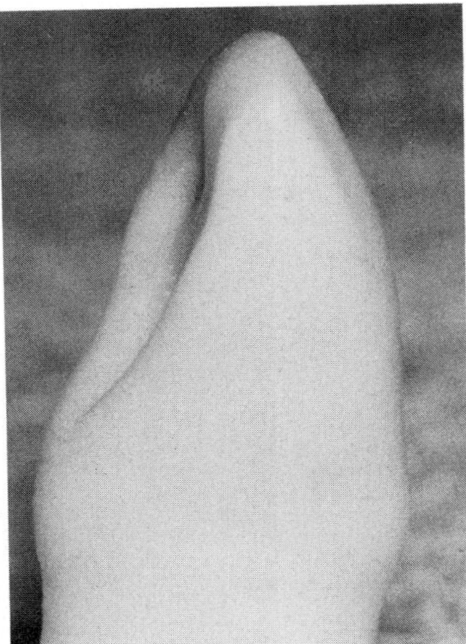

Figure 3–1 ■ The inclined surface of anterior teeth requires special consideration to provide a positive rest seat that will direct forces in the long axis of the tooth.

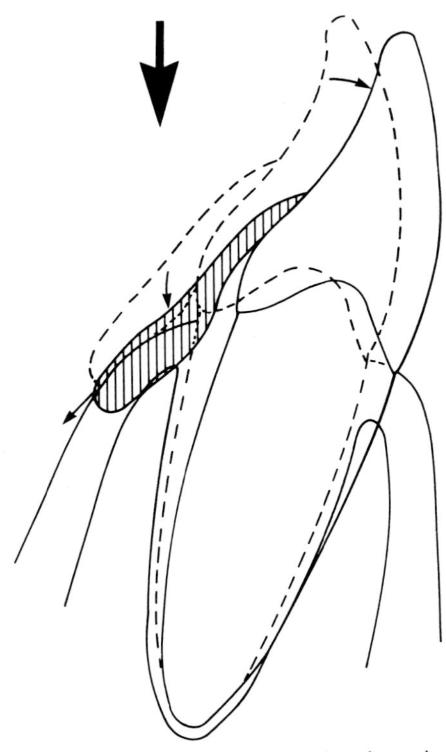

Figure 3–3 ■ Placement of partial rests on inclined surfaces displaces tooth and destroys bone.

1. The center is deeper than the surrounding rest surface.
2. It is rounded in all aspects (no sharp line angles).
3. There is easy access for impression-making and cleaning.
4. It is contoured to form a half circle (especially for extension situations).
5. There are no undercuts.
6. It is placed as close to the gingiva and bone as possible to reduce leverage.
7. There is no interference with planned occlusion.
8. It is contoured so that when increased force is applied to the prosthesis, the rest will engage more securely to prevent separation.
9. It is positioned in line with the residual ridge for an extension prosthesis (Fig. 3–6).

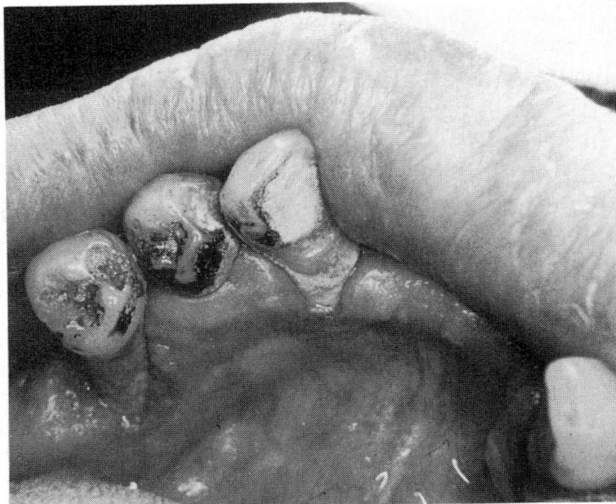

Figure 3–2 ■ Lack of positive rest seats results in destruction and displacement of teeth and supporting tissues.

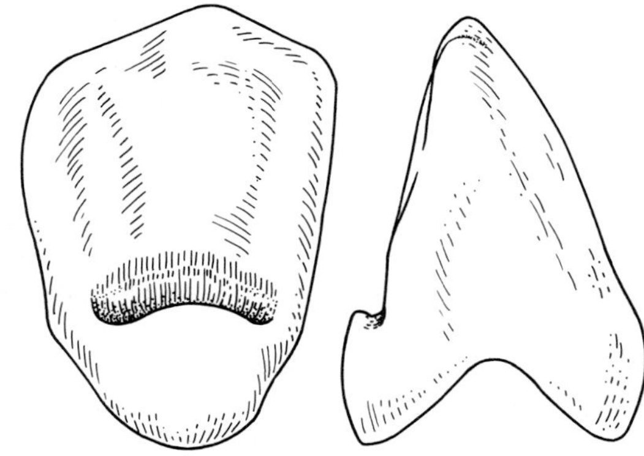

Figure 3–4 ■ It is *rare* that a properly prepared rest can be made of *enamel tooth structure*. The rest must be deeper in the center than on the periphery.

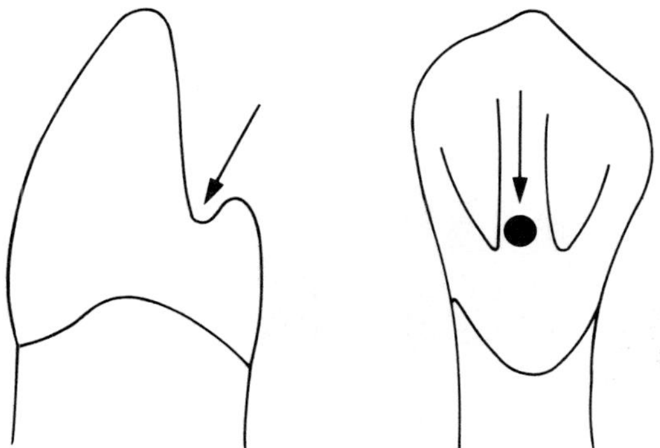

Figure 3–5 ■ The rest is positioned as close to the center of the tooth as possible, when viewed from all directions.

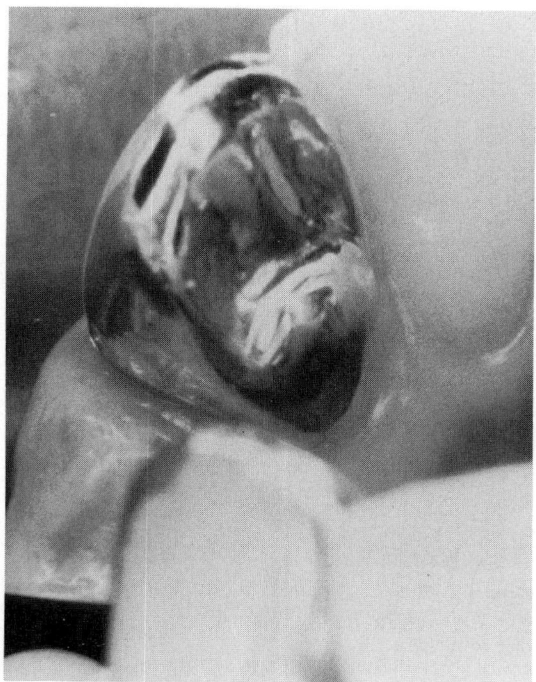

Figure 3–6 ■ The ideal rest for an extension prosthesis is positioned in line with the edentulous ridge and is circular in design.

METHODS OF PROVIDING POSITIVE ANTERIOR RESTS

Complete and Three-Quarter Crowns

When complete crowns are necessary for restoration of the entire tooth, the opportunity is available to fabricate the ideal rest (Fig. 3–7). The rest can be placed in the optimal position for support (Fig. 3–8), and all portions of the tooth topography can be planned to accommodate the partial design for ideal placement without interfering with occlusion (Fig. 3–9).

Inlays and Onlays

In many instances, a basic inlay with parallel pins can provide a positive rest when the remainder of the tooth does not require restoring (Fig. 3–10).

The advent of acid-etching and bonding has introduced a completely new, simplified, timesaving, and noninvasive procedure that shows great promise. The lingual rest can be fabricated

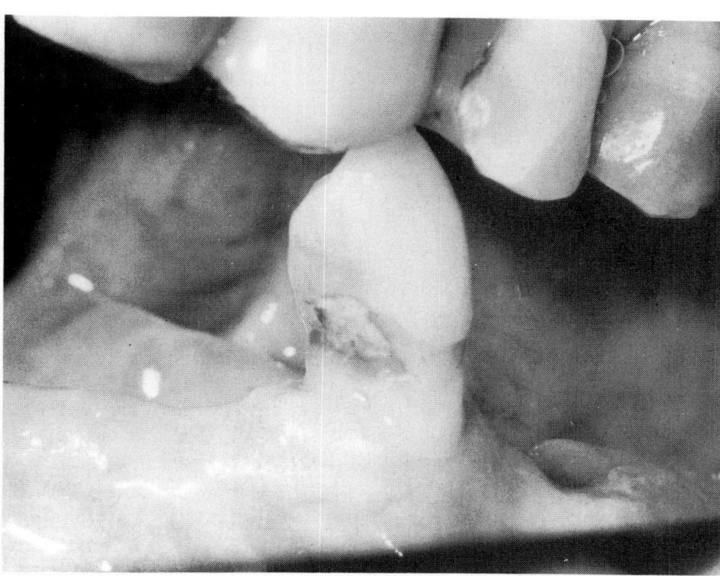

Figure 3–7 ■ When a crown is indicated, there will be an opportunity to prepare ideal contours, rests, and occlusion coordinated with the removable partial prosthesis.

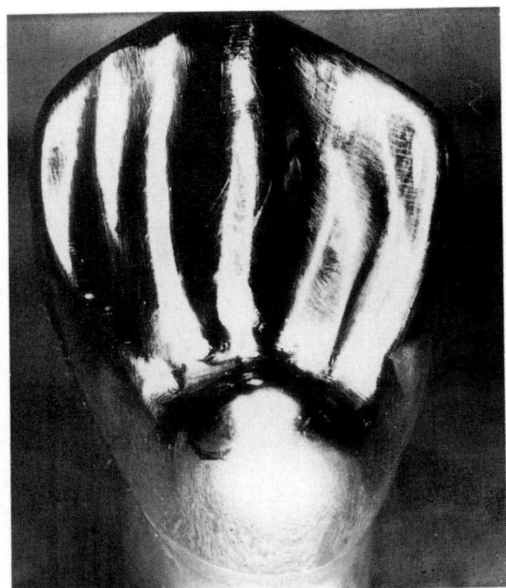

Figure 3–8 ■ Crowns are fabricated to provide *positive* rests for the prosthesis close to the gingival support area.

of metal and bonded to the enamel with minimal preparation of the tooth surface.

Composites — Light-Cured

As stated before, it is rarely possible to prepare a satisfactorily positive rest in natural tooth structures. The anatomy and thickness of the enamel do not allow sufficient depth without exposure of the dentine. However, in some instances it is possible to build up the lingual-cervical portion of the tooth with light-cured plastic to provide an adequate rest *if* the support part of the rest is contoured in enamel and *if* the plastic *only* reinforces the lateral side of the rest form (Fig. 3–11). (This procedure can be used for tooth-supported cases but not for rotation rests.)

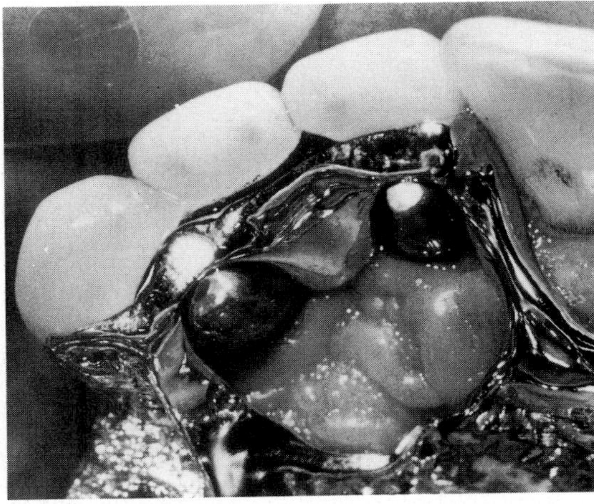

Figure 3–9 ■ Opposing occlusion influences the position of rests and can provide center contacts and anterior guidance coordinated with the removable partial denture.

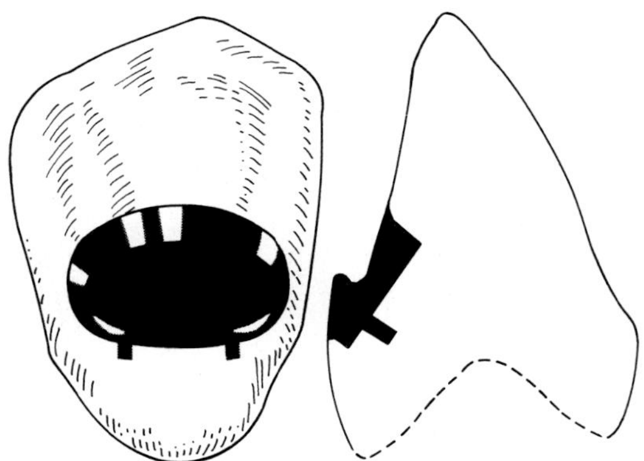

Figure 3–10 ■ An inlay with pins can provide a most positive and esthetic rest for maxillary anterior teeth.

Incisal Rests

In some situations, the incisal rest is used (Fig. 3–12). To be effective, it must restore the major

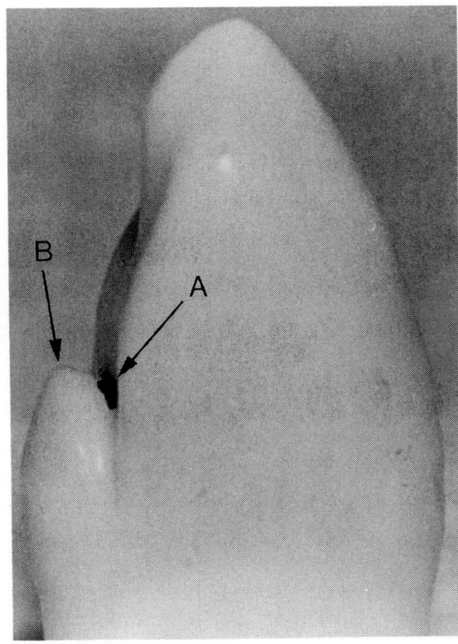

Figure 3–11 ■ Properly prepared rests in natural tooth structure usually require a restoration at the dentine-enamel junction (A). Composite may be added to the lingual portion of the tooth to provide a definite seat (B).

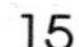

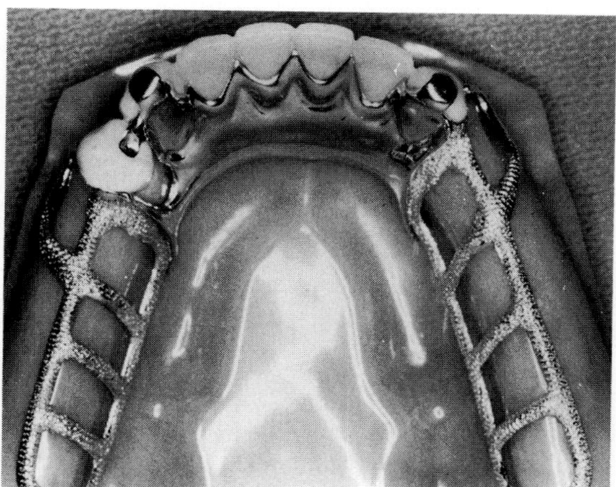

Figure 3-12 ■ The incisal rest provides a positive rest for the removable partial denture.

portion of the incisal surface to provide contact and anterior guidance to the opposing teeth in lateral and posterior excursions. This type of rest covers the incisal surface of the tooth and provides a most positive rest.

The ideal incisal rest fulfills the following requirements:

1. It provides a positive seat by extending over the incisal edge onto the labial surface of the tooth (Fig. 3-13).
2. It restores anterior anatomy as required (Fig. 3-14).
3. It stabilizes mobile teeth (Fig. 3-15).

The incisal rest is used primarily on mandibular canines and, in some instances, on the centrals and laterals. The incisal rest is rarely used on maxillary teeth because of esthetic considerations and occlusal interference with the mandibular anterior teeth.

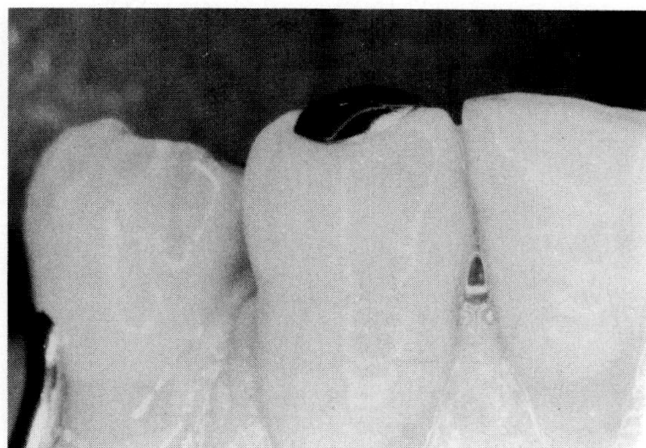

Figure 3-13 ■ The incisal rest extends onto the facial part of the tooth at an acute angle to prevent horizontal movement.

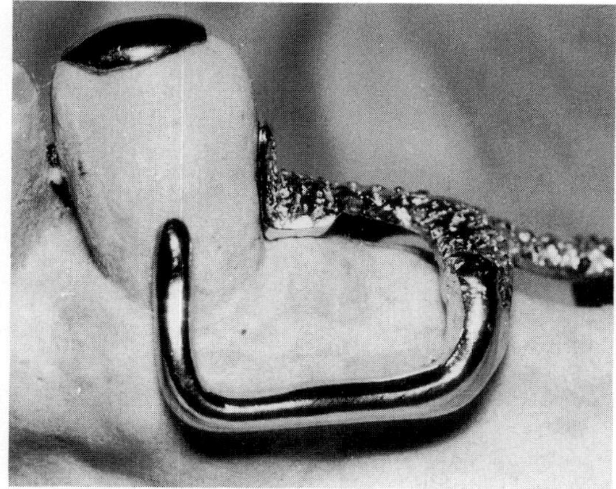

Figure 3-14 ■ The rest restores the occlusal surface to provide anterior guidance in *all* excursions. For esthetic purposes, the facial outline resembles a $\frac{3}{4}$ crown.

The indications for use of the incisal rest are

1. The need to provide a positive rest on a tooth that requires no restoration.
2. The need to restore anterior guidance.
3. The need to provide stabilization.
4. Financial limitations.
5. Geriatric considerations.

In many instances the guiding surface of the natural tooth has been abraded (Fig. 3-16), reducing the anterior guidance and allowing the posterior teeth to engage heavily in excursions. Use of the incisal rest provides positive rests and restores anterior guidance if required (Fig. 3-17).

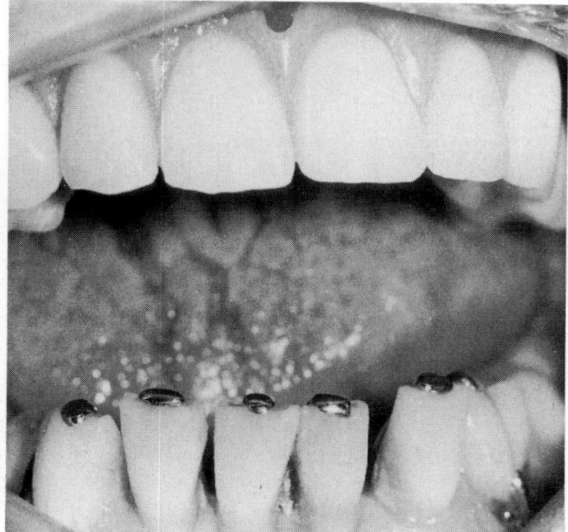

Figure 3-15 ■ Incisal rests on mobile and periodontally involved anterior teeth provide stability during treatment.

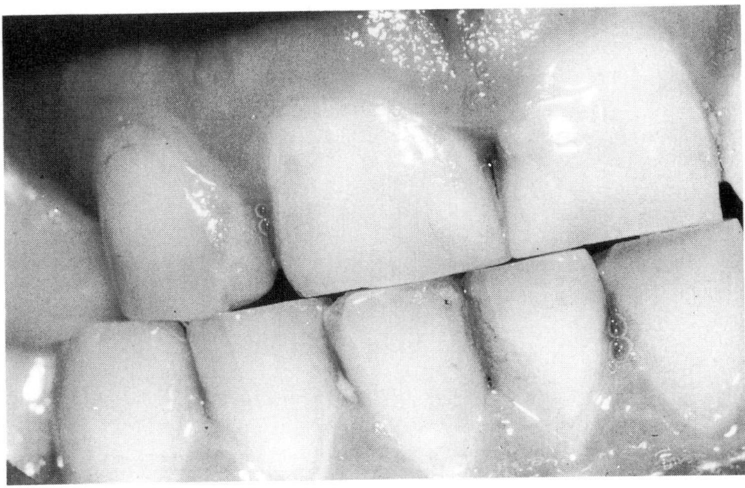

Figure 3–16 ■ Reduced anterior guidance results from loss of tooth structure. Incisal rests restore anterior guidance and help control tooth abrasion and wear.

To be effective, the rest form must provide an acute angle contour on the facial aspect of the tooth to prevent the casting from sliding off the tooth and to keep the tooth from moving away from the casting (Fig. 3–18). The incisal rest is used primarily on the mandibular rather than the maxillary arch because there are fewer esthetic considerations and interocclusal space problems in that area. Its use is usually determined by

1. Patient decisions (i.e., a request for no restorations for financial reasons or fear of trauma).
2. Geriatric considerations.
3. Health considerations.
4. Periodontal or splinting requirements.
5. Occlusal plane requirements.

The possible disadvantages of the incisal rest are (1) poorer esthetics and (2) greater leverage on the tooth because of the high attachment on the incisal rather than near the gingival area in extention partial dentures.

Concave Rests

In a few select situations, the concave rest is used. The need for its use should be carefully evaluated, since it is difficult to prepare a positive rest that provides the necessary support and bracing. Also, it is difficult to position in the center of the tooth, to keep clean, and to obtain impressions for positive placement and contact by the partial casting.

Posterior Rests

The posterior removable partial denture rests provide stabilization and support between the

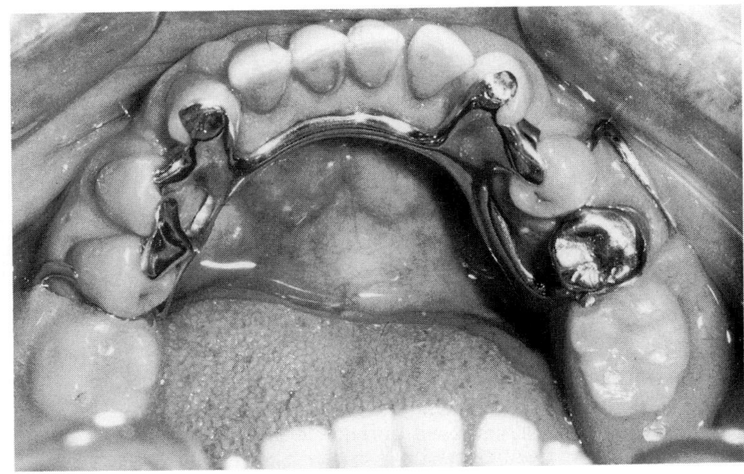

Figure 3–17 ■ Anterior rests are readily designed into overall removable partial denture planning to provide support and indirect retainers and to restore anterior guidance.

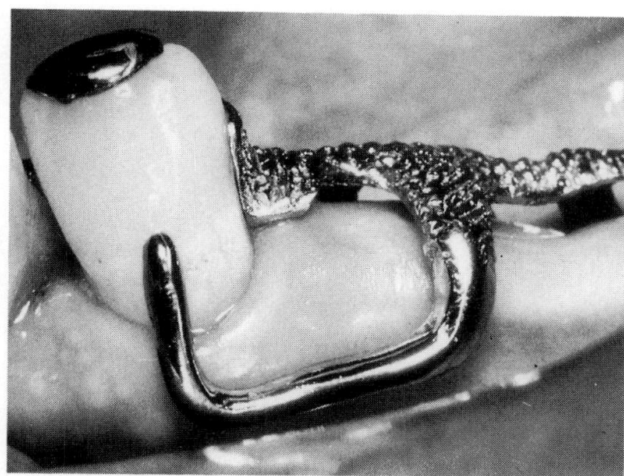

Figure 3–18 ■ Wear facets on the natural teeth provide a facial slope for rest placement to prevent facial tooth movement.

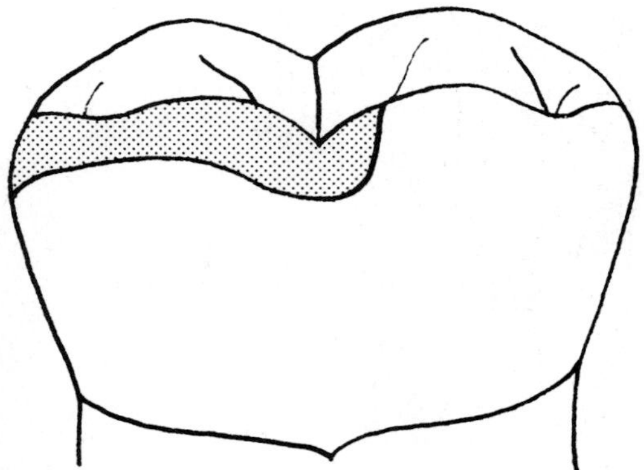

Figure 3–19 ■ The occlusal rest must be rigid, with sufficient bulk to prevent flexure.

prosthesis and the support tissues. The rest is comparable to the crowns for fixed partial dentures and must sustain the same functional forces.

Posterior rests receive the greatest force produced in the mouth during function and transmit these forces to the abutment teeth and to their supporting structures. They must receive and dispense force without moving out of position, which would change the entire denture position, and without exerting any but the most favorable direction of force on the abutment teeth. Although the greatest occlusal force is in the vertical direction, a rest transmits and must withstand forces from a horizontal direction.

FUNCTIONS

The functions of posterior rests are to

1. Provide rigid prosthetic support.
2. Restore occlusion.
3. Direct forces in the long axis of the teeth.
4. Provide reciprocation and stabilization.

Provide Rigid Support

The first consideration for the posterior rest is rigidity so that it will not flex under occlusal loads. If there is flexure, the direction of force to the abutment teeth changes, with potential danger to the supporting structures. The rest must be of sufficient dimension and strength to provide a constant, controlled relationship among tooth, prosthesis, and mucosa (Fig. 3–19).

Restore Occlusion

Rests are often extended over two or more teeth for united support and to restore the occlusal plane and the occlusal anatomy.

A most important function of the posterior rest is to restore occlusion in cases in which (1) a tooth has tipped out of proper occlusal alignment (Fig. 3–20); (2) a tooth has not erupted to proper occlusal position (Fig. 3–21); (3) there has been a loss of vertical dimension of occlusion, owing to wear or loss of teeth (Fig. 3–22).

The amount of occlusal restoration necessary is determined by the diagnostic analysis and information obtained from the mounted diagnostic casts and is discussed in detail under treatment planning (Chapter 11).

In many instances it is necessary to extend the rest over the entire mesial-distal length of the tooth to restore occlusion and the occlusal plane (Fig. 3–23).

The width of the rest is usually approxi-

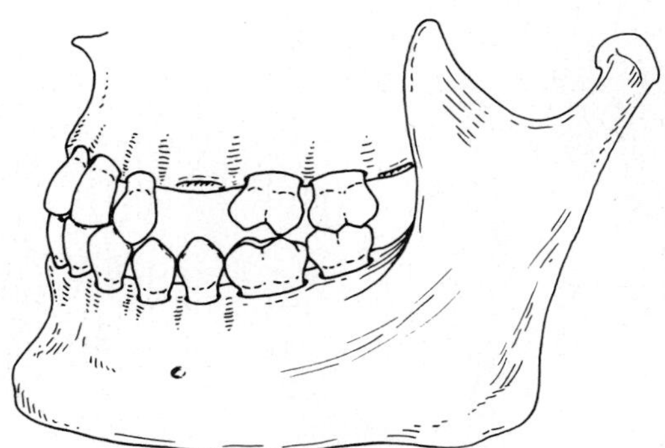

Figure 3–20 ■ When teeth have moved out of occlusal alignment, the proper occlusal plane and occlusion can be restored by the rest.

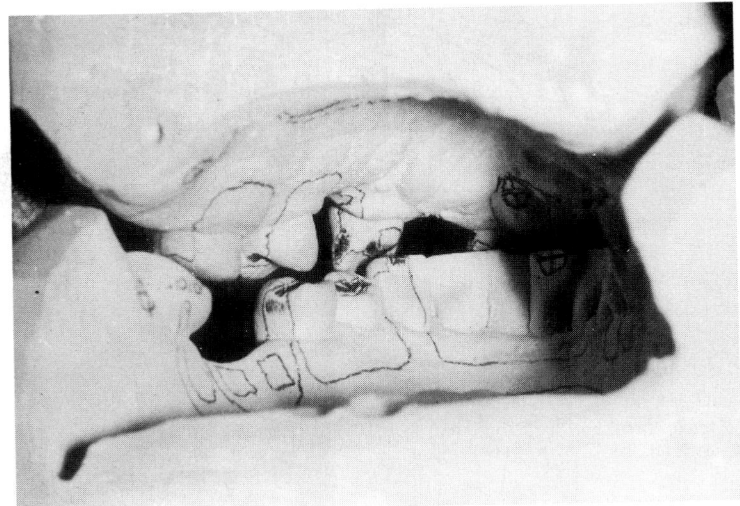

Figure 3–21 ■ Lack of occlusion can be restored by planned occlusal rests.

mately one third of the buccal lingual width of the tooth.

Direct Forces in the Long Axis of the Tooth

Preservation of remaining teeth requires that forces delivered be in the long axis of the tooth (Fig. 3–24) and in the proper direction of the periodontal ligament. To accomplish this objective in the *toothborne case,* the rest must extend at least to the center of the tooth (Fig. 3–25). If the rest is positioned only on one side of the tooth, it places a majority of the occlusal load on that side; this can result in tipping of the tooth (Fig. 3–26). By extending the rest to the middle of the tooth, force is transmitted equally to both roots and to the periodontal ligaments and from there to the bone, in the most advantageous direction (Fig. 3–27).

Provide Reciprocation and Stabilization

Rests can perform a variety of functions in addition to providing basic support and restoring occlusion. An equally important function is stabilizing the abutment teeth against torquing or twisting forces. An occlusal view of a posterior tooth (Fig. 3–28) indicates that a tooth standing alone is subject to movement in any direction, since it no longer has the positional bracing contact formerly provided by the missing teeth. The adage of "divide and conquer" is

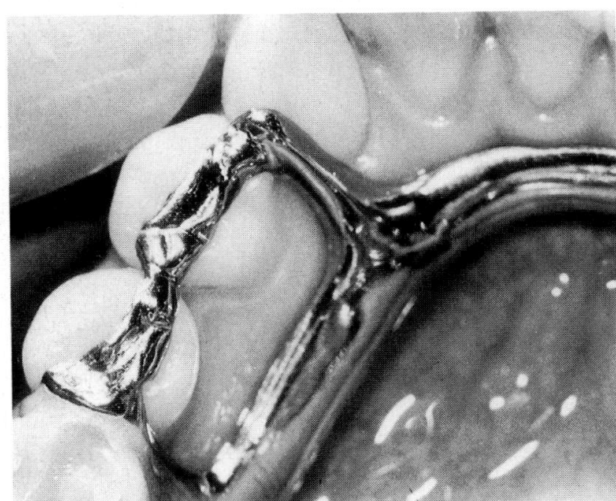

Figure 3–22 ■ The vertical dimension of occlusion is restored with a continuous rest (note the circle design, which increases strength and reduces bulk).

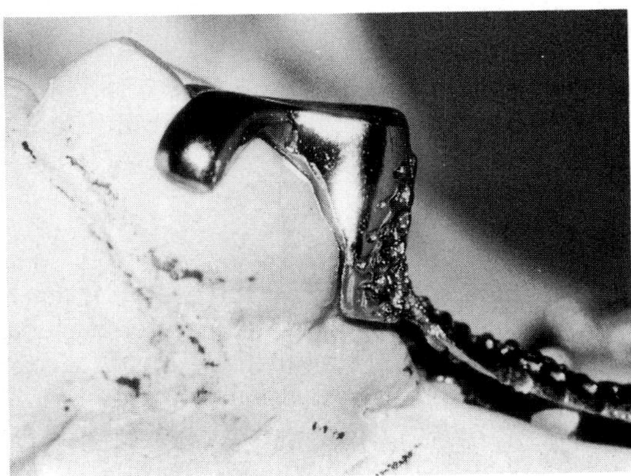

Figure 3–23 ■ Extending the rest across the occlusal surface restores the occlusal plane and prevents further tooth movement.

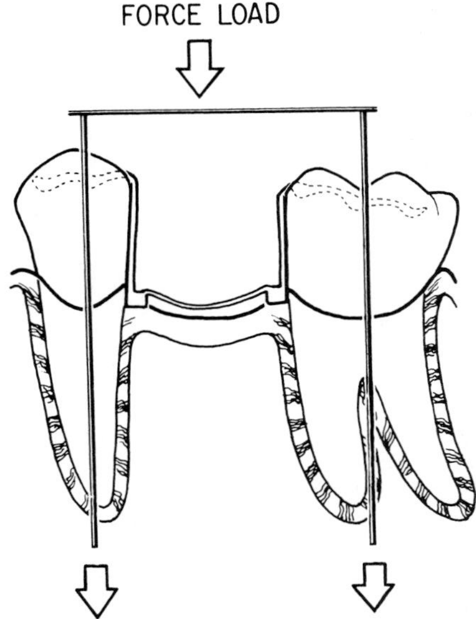

Figure 3–24 ■ Rests that extend to the center of the tooth or beyond can direct support forces in the long axis of the teeth, to the best advantage of the periodontal ligaments.

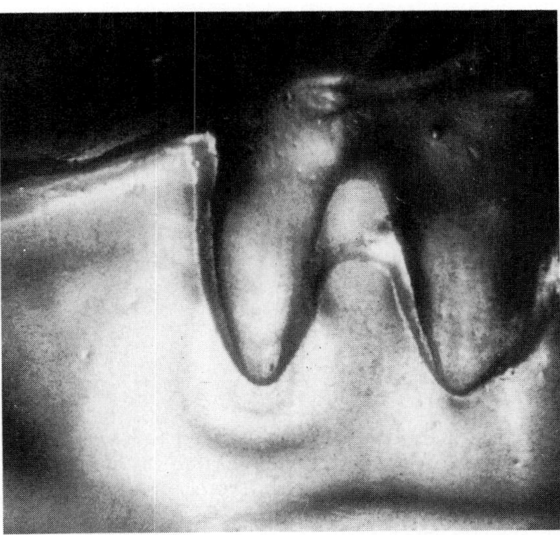

Figure 3–26 ■ A photoelastic study of a short mesial rest on a molar under load. Note that the majority of force is on the mesial root. (See also Color Plate 1, p XVII.)

most applicable to a tooth standing alone, subject to physiologic and functional forces in any direction. The rest can provide positive positional stabilization, utilizing remaining teeth in the arch; rests on remaining teeth can unify and stabilize the arch in a controlled position (Fig. 3–29).

In some situations it is advantageous to use an extension of the occlusal rest on one side of the tooth. A buccal or lingual extension prevents the tooth from moving, provides reciprocation, and interferes minimally with tooth contours and mucosa (Fig. 3–30).

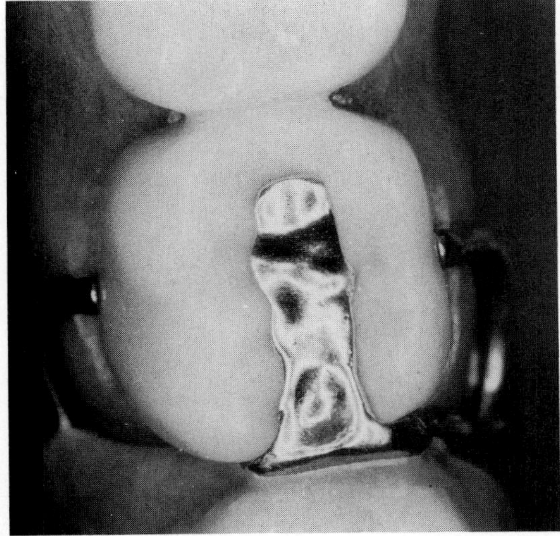

Figure 3–25 ■ The occlusal rest controls the direction of force to the tooth and provides proper occlusion. It should extend to the center of the tooth.

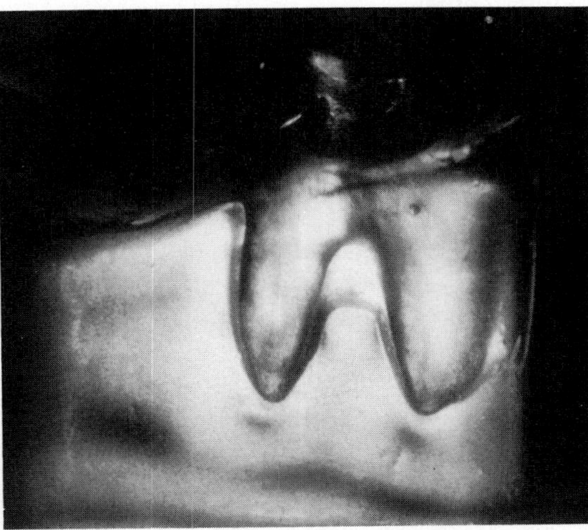

Figure 3–27 ■ A photoelastic study of a rest extended to the center of the tooth under load. Note the even distribution of force on both roots. (See also Color Plate 1, p XVII.)

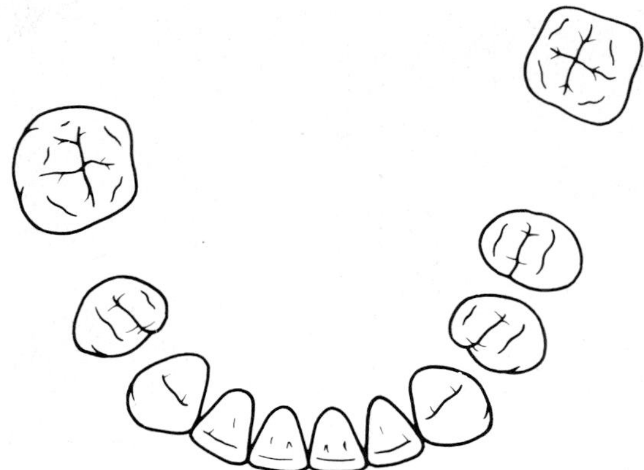

Figure 3–28 ■ Positional stability of individual teeth and of the entire arch is lost when teeth are missing. Occlusion is disorganized and compromised.

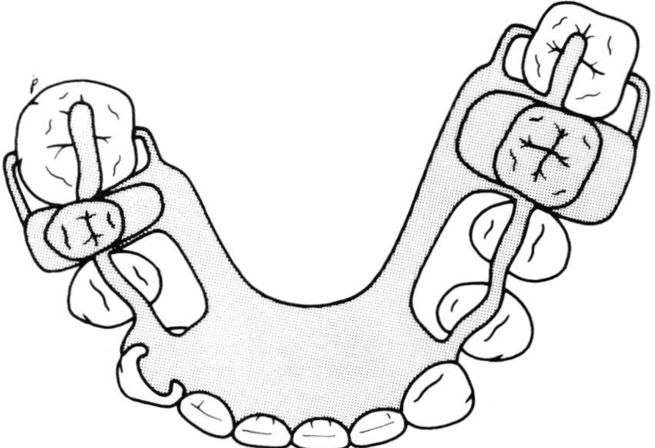

Figure 3–29 ■ A continuous rest can restore stability, control tooth position, and reorganize occlusion.

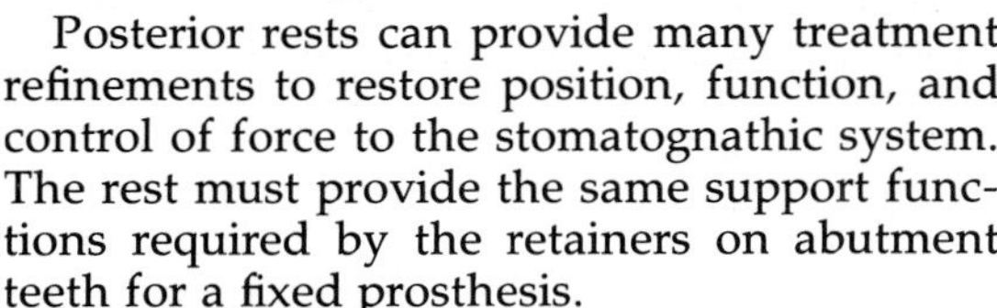

Posterior rests can provide many treatment refinements to restore position, function, and control of force to the stomatognathic system. The rest must provide the same support functions required by the retainers on abutment teeth for a fixed prosthesis.

The anatomy of posterior teeth allows for more convenient placement of positive rests in a position that enables functional forces to be directed in the long axis of the tooth.

BASIC GENERAL REQUIREMENTS OF POSTERIOR RESTS

The ideal posterior rest fulfills the following requirements:

1. It provides rigid support.
2. It extends to the center of the tooth in tooth-supported situations (Fig. 3–31).
3. All aspects are rounded, with no sharp angles (for ease of cleaning and making impressions, and to prevent tooth fracture) (Fig. 3–32).
4. The end of the rest is slightly deeper and rounded.
5. There are no undercuts in the path of insertion.
6. It is a minimum of 1 mm thick.
7. It restores the occlusal plane (Fig. 3–33).
8. It provides reciprocation (Fig. 3–34).

METHODS OF PROVIDING POSTERIOR RESTS

Natural Tooth Structure

The primary consideration is that the finished metal rest be smooth and rounded and that it lie on smooth, polished enamel or resto-

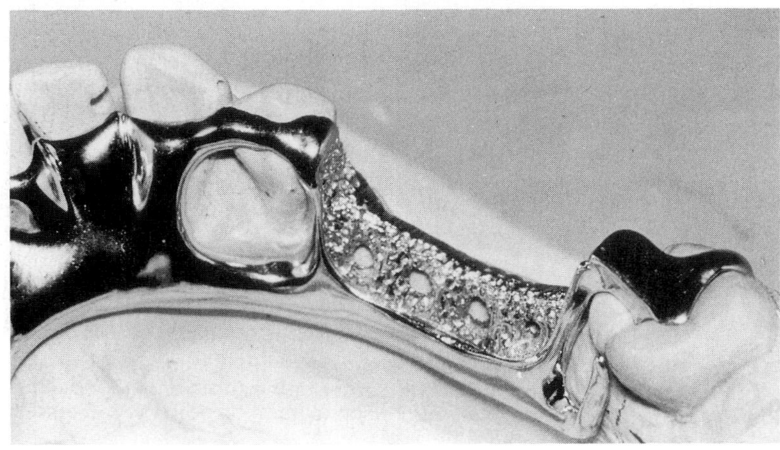

Figure 3–30 ■ A small buccal or lingual extension of the occlusal rest provides simple reciprocation for a retainer.

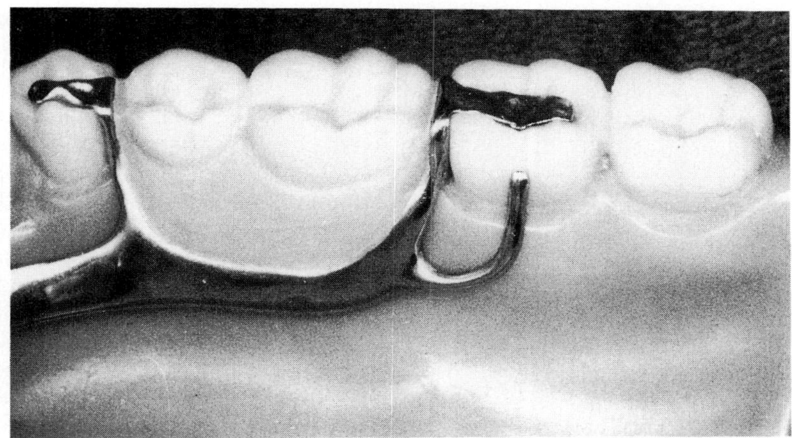

Figure 3–31 ■ Occlusal rests in tooth-supported situations extend to the center of the abutment teeth or beyond, if necessary, to provide occlusion and proper force direction to the tooth.

ration. The minimum metal thickness is 1 mm of good chrome cobalt. The rest must be placed so that it directs the force in the long axis of the tooth (see Fig. 3–24). It can be individually designed, with position determined by factors such as opposing occlusion, restoration of the occlusal plane, bracing, support, and control of direction of movement.

The width of the rest for a tooth with normal occlusal contours and position is usually equal to the width of a number 6 or 8 round bur. Special consideration is given to the contours and thickness of rests where they cross marginal ridges, since these areas are most susceptible to failure due to inadequate metal bulk.

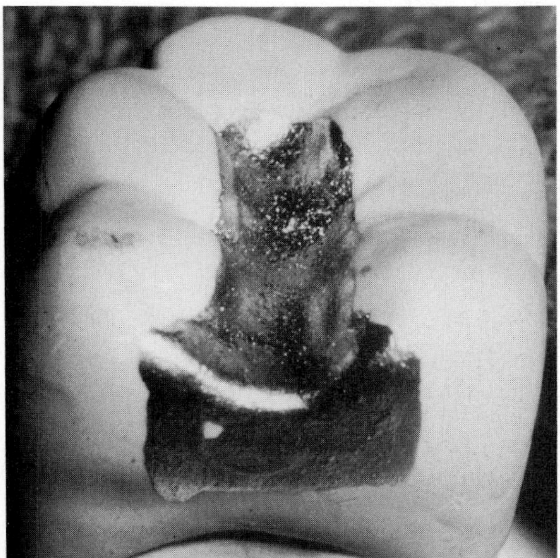

Figure 3–32 ■ The rest area is rounded in all aspects with *no* sharp angles.

Both tooth and prosthetic surfaces must be highly polished at rest area contacts for maximum tooth protection and function.

Crowns

It is often necessary to restore a tooth with a crown for a variety of reasons. When a crown is indicated, it is possible to place the removable partial denture rest in the most ideal position for contour and thickness.

Preplanning of the RPD design can influence crown preparation and tooth reduction to ensure the provision of adequate space and thickness of materials in the rest area when the crown and the RPD casting are fabricated (Fig. 3–35).

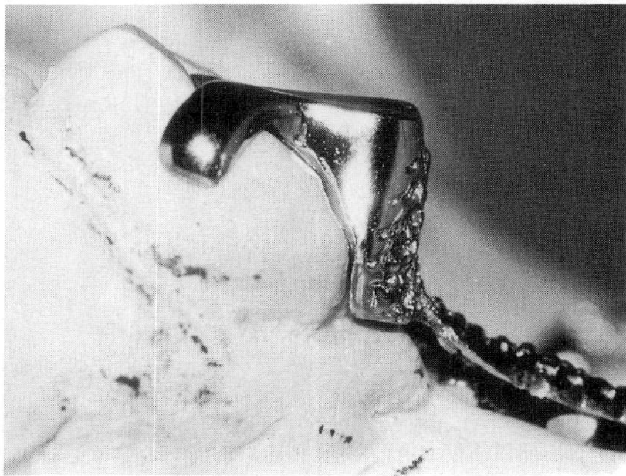

Figure 3–33 ■ A primary requirement of the occlusal rest is to restore the occlusal plane with positive occlusion.

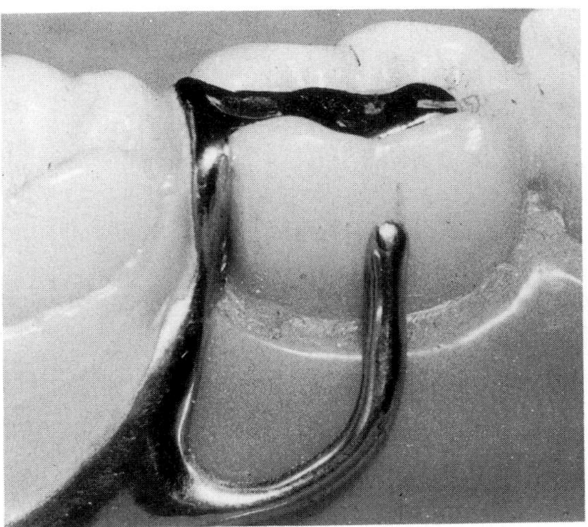

Figure 3–34 ■ The extended occlusal rest will assist in reciprocal action against the retainer by resisting turning and occlusal movement of the tooth.

Long or Continuous Rests

Splinting periodontally weakened teeth ■ Teeth often lose bone support, move to abnormal positions, and lose occlusal organization because of periodontal or systemic difficulties (Fig. 3–36). The long or continuous rest can serve as an effective stabilizing or unifying device. The rest can be designed to extend entirely across the occlusal surface of two or more teeth and, in some instances, across the entire arch (Fig. 3–37).

When occlusal force is delivered in one area, all the remaining teeth act in unison to provide support. With planning, this type of rest can restore the occlusal plane, provide support, and splint the arch.

The continuous rest is often used for a single tooth when the tooth fossa is deep and the opposing cusp is deeply recessed into the fossa,

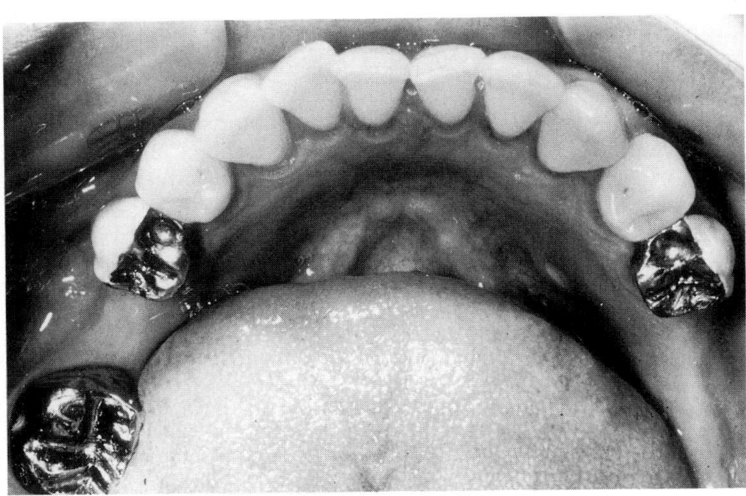

Figure 3–35 ■ Crowns are fabricated to allow for ideal placement, size, and contour of rests through treatment planning prior to crown preparation.

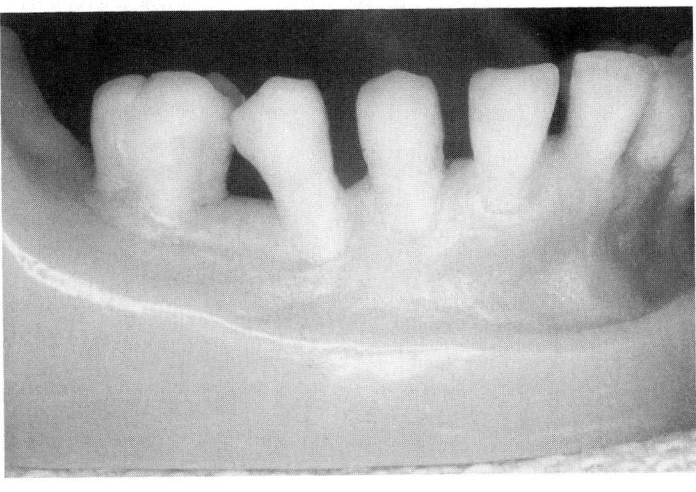

Figure 3–36 ■ Loss of tooth contacts and periodontal disease often result in tooth migration, disruption of occlusion, loss of function, and regression of supporting tissues.

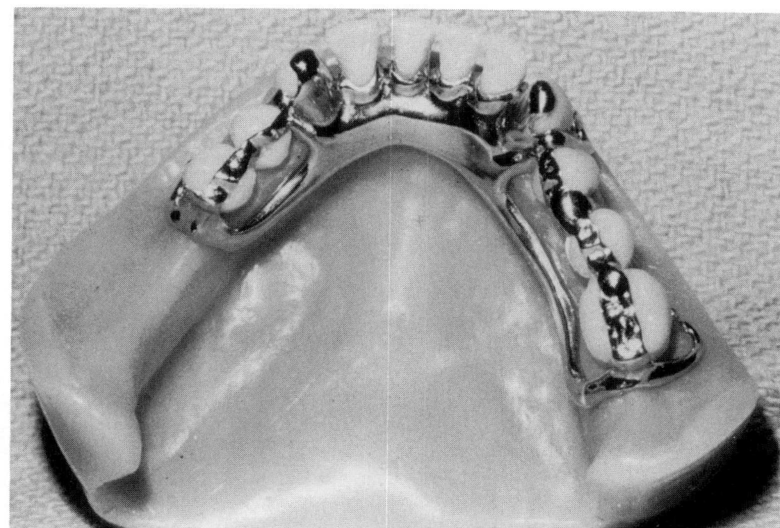

Figure 3–37 ■ A removable prosthesis can immediately restore arch unity and occlusion and can control the position of the teeth. The treatment is often confined to the remaining teeth.

causing lateral force in function beyond the capabilities of the supporting tissues. By positioning the rest to fill in the deep fossa (Fig. 3–38) and by reducing the length of the opposing cusp, a more favorable or reduced lateral force is obtained.

Positioning of the occlusal portion of the rest has two basic requirements: (1) to support the prosthesis-tooth relationship, and (2) to restore occlusion. When the occlusal plane on posterior teeth is restored, the width of the rest should not be increased beyond the normal rest width (Fig. 3–39). The inclination is to restore the entire or original occlusal topography; however, this creates complications of force and in cleaning.

A built-up rest kept to its normal width has the following advantages:

1. It has minimal tooth-metal contact, which allows easier cleaning of both tooth and casting.
2. It supplies positive occlusal contact and support in and around centric contact but

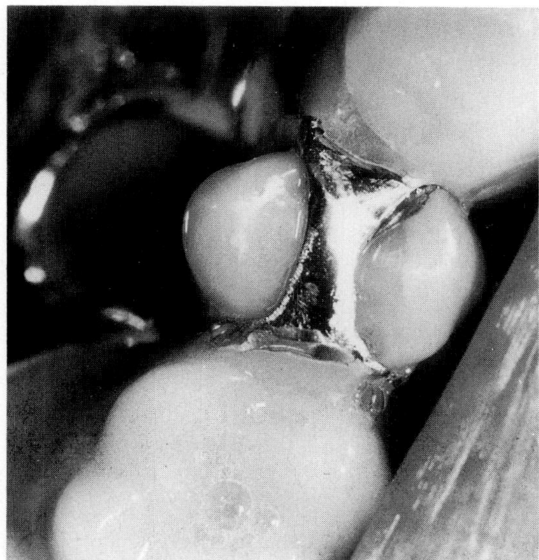

Figure 3–38 ■ The continuous rest effectively reduces a deep fossa which is causing jaw excursion difficulties from the opposing tooth cusp.

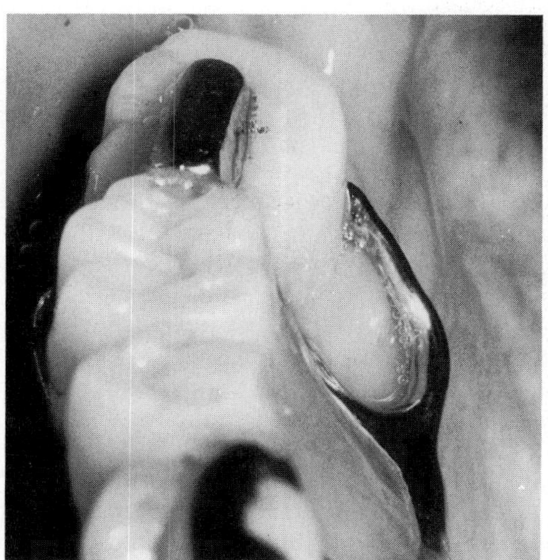

Figure 3–39 ■ The width of the occlusal rest is *not* increased when the occlusal plane is restored. Occlusal anatomy provides for contact in centric relation and for limited excursional movement.

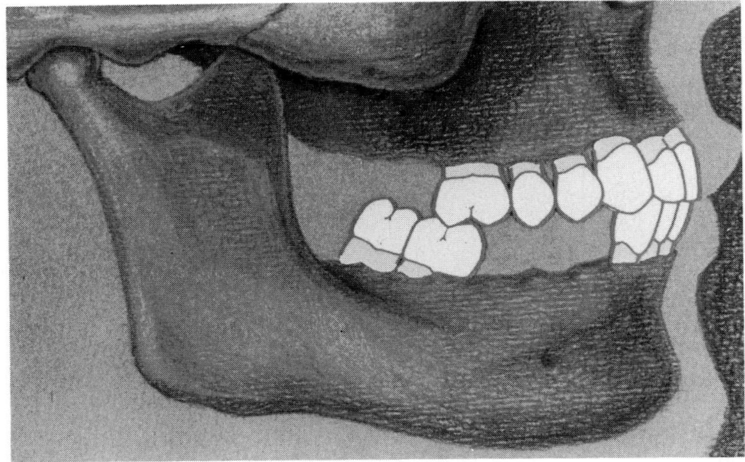

Figure 3–40 ■ Teeth move out of proper position with loss of tooth contacts and opposing occlusion.

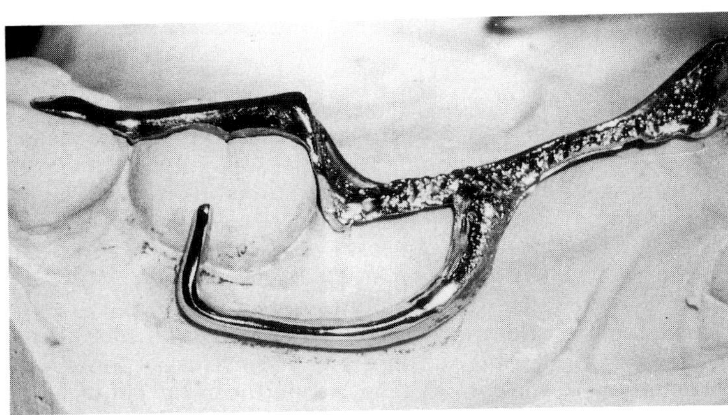

Figure 3–41 ■ The extended occlusal rest gains support from both teeth, restores occlusion, prevents the posterior molar from elongating, and eliminates the need for a maxillary prosthesis.

avoids potential lateral forces on the abutment teeth in excursions.

3. It reduces the occlusal surface area, which, in turn, reduces the force necessary to penetrate food.

4. It simplifies occlusal adjustment.

5. It simplifies adjustment of the fit of the casting to the tooth rest preparation.

6. It controls the position of unopposed teeth.

Control position of unopposed teeth ■ Many times a situation exists in which a tooth has lost its antagonist in the opposing arch but does not need a replacement for masticating functions (Fig. 3–40). Extending the rest in the partial denture planning and design not only gains support from that tooth but also holds it in position, preventing elongation (Fig. 3–41) and eliminating the necessity of a second prosthesis in the opposing arch. Elongation and tipping of such unopposed teeth can result in traumatic interference in excursions, with resultant periodontal and TM joint problems and muscle difficulties.

REFERENCES

Applegate OC: Evaluation of oral structures for removable partial dentures. J Prosthet Dent 11:882, 1961.

Cohn LA: The physiologic basis for tooth fixation in precision attached partial dentures. J Prosthet Dent 6:220, 1956.

Frechette, AR: Partial denture planning with special reference to stress distribution. J Prosthet Dent 1:710, 1951.

Frechette AR: The influence of partial design on distribution of force to abutment teeth. J Prosthet Dent 6:196–212, 1956.

Granger ER: Mechanical principles applied to partial denture construction. J Am Dent Assoc 28:12, 1941.

Kratochvil FJ: Evaluation of photoelastic stress patterns by various designs of bilateral distal extension removable partial dentures. J Prosthet Dent 38:3, 1977.

Kratochvil FJ: Influence of occlusal rest position and clasp design on movement of abutment teeth. J Prosthet Dent 13:114, 1963.

Steffel VL: Planning removable partial dentures. J Prosthet Dent 16:708, 1966.

chapter 4

Considerations at the tooth-tissue junction

An area that requires special consideration at diagnosis and treatment is the tooth-tissue junction. All specialized fields within dentistry concentrate on this area, especially those involved with periodontal and restorative treatment. Maintaining and preserving the original position and contour of teeth and mucosa as well as removing or correcting pathologic disorders are the prime objectives. Most patients treated with removable partial dentures have altered clinical crowns and supporting tissue contours that have receded or are less than ideal (Fig. 4–1). The prosthesis is placed into or against these areas, creating more difficulties in an already compromised situation.

Basic Problem

When a tooth or teeth are removed, there are contour changes in soft tissue and bone in the area. These changes usually result in extensive loss of these support structures. However, the hard structures of the teeth next to the edentulous areas may not change. This can leave a depression or undercut between the tooth and the residual tissues. When a removable prosthesis is placed, it must fit between the tooth contact area. If the tooth has its original contour, there is a space between the tooth and the prosthesis in the gingival area (Fig. 4–2). When this condition exists, it may cause the following difficulties:

1. Impaction of food into the space.
2. Hypertrophy of tissue into the space (Fig. 4–3).
3. A reduced bracing effect between the remaining teeth.
4. Increased periodontal involvement (Fig. 4–4).

Solution

The tooth-tissue junction area is treated by

1. Extending the prosthesis so that it contacts the entire interproximal surface of the tooth, *eliminating all voids* (Fig. 4–5).
2. Contacting the tooth and the tooth-tissue junction with metal.

PROXIMAL PLATES

The portion of the prosthesis that contacts this tooth-tissue area is the proximal plate, which is considered a minor connector with a specialized function. It is a thin, closely fitting metal part of the partial denture framework that covers guide surfaces of the tooth and extends onto the adjacent edentulous mucosa (Fig. 4–6). The position of the proximal plate is maintained by the positive lingual or occlusal rest.

Functions

The functions of the proximal plates are to

1. Protect against food impaction (Fig. 4–7)
2. Prevent tissue hypertrophy between tooth and prosthesis

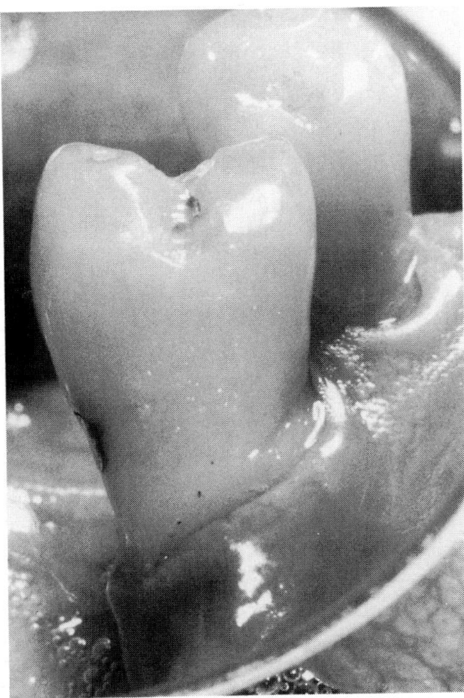

Figure 4–1 ■ When teeth are removed, the remaining mucosa and bone have abnormal topography: the exposed clinical crown is increased, requiring tooth alteration prior to partial denture treatment.

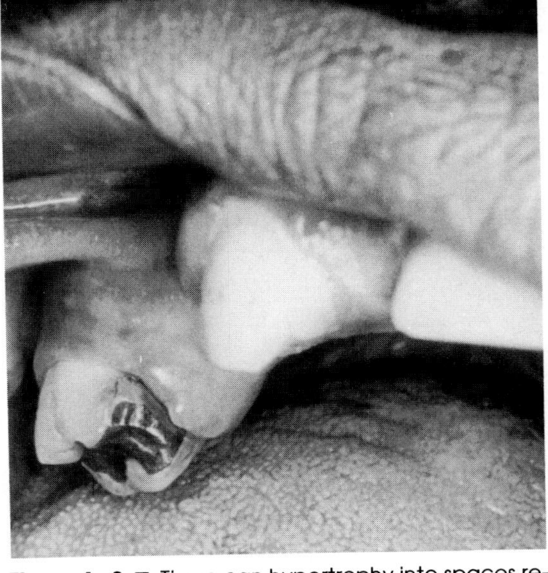

Figure 4–3 ■ Tissue can hypertrophy into spaces remaining between tooth and prosthesis.

3. Resist dislodgement of the prosthesis by frictional contact with the teeth (retention)
4. Maintain arch integrity by anterior-posterior bracing action, which controls tooth movement (Fig. 4–8)
5. Act with other connectors in reciprocation opposite retainers (Fig. 4–9A and B)

Contouring of the tooth surface as a preparation procedure forms a "guide surface" (Fig. 4–10) that allows the prosthesis to slide into position, eliminating all voids and restoring and replacing tissues that have been lost. The guide surfaces that extend along the entire length of the clinical crown provide positive bracing for the remaining teeth; they extend vertically from the occlusal surface to the gingival surface contact (Fig. 4–11). The prepared tooth surface usually has a rounded, contoured topography, allowing the prosthesis to obliterate the void.

Metal is the material of choice for tooth and tissue contact. The metal can be precisely cast to fit tooth contour and is not readily abraded or distorted during fabrication or function. It is most compatible with the tissues and can be easily cleaned. The metal is designed to cover

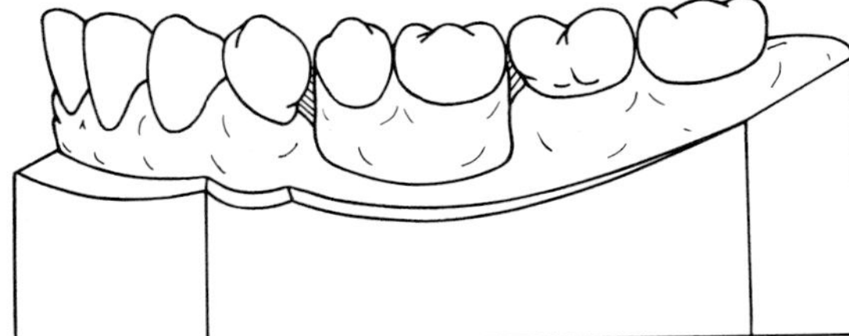

Figure 4–2 ■ When teeth are removed, mucosa and bone are lost, but remaining tooth contours are the same. If a prosthesis is placed between the unaltered tooth contacts, a space will remain at the gingival area.

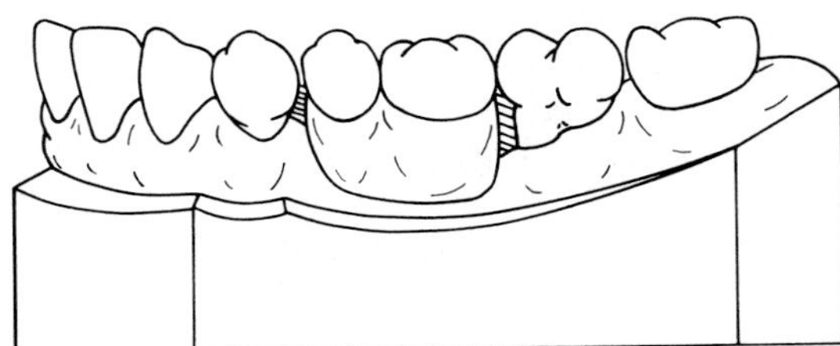

Figure 4–4 ■ When space is left between prosthesis and tooth, increased periodontal difficulties and recession from food impaction can result.

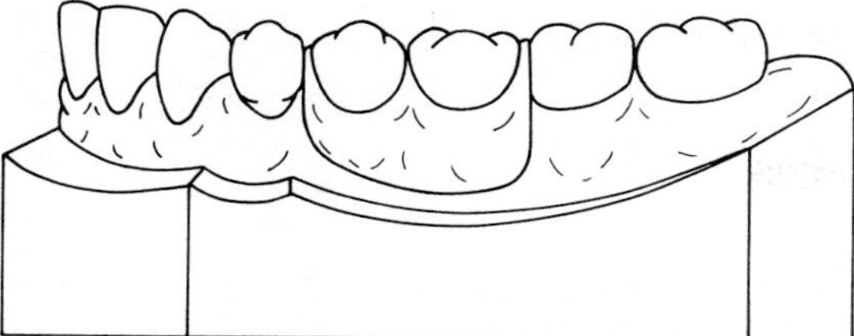

Figure 4–5 ■ Tooth alteration will permit the design of a prosthesis that can eliminate all spaces and voids and prosthetically restore original contours.

cervical soft tissue for at least 2 mm beyond the tooth-mucosa junction. The termination of the metal "interproximal plate" is shaped to form a right angle, so that the plastic material of the prosthesis can make a butt joint against the metal for strength (Fig. 4–12). If the plastic forms a thin or tapered junction, it distorts or fractures, resulting in the accumulation of debris, which is detrimental to the gingival sulcus. The junction of all metal and plastic portions of the prosthesis must have bulk and a definite finish margin.

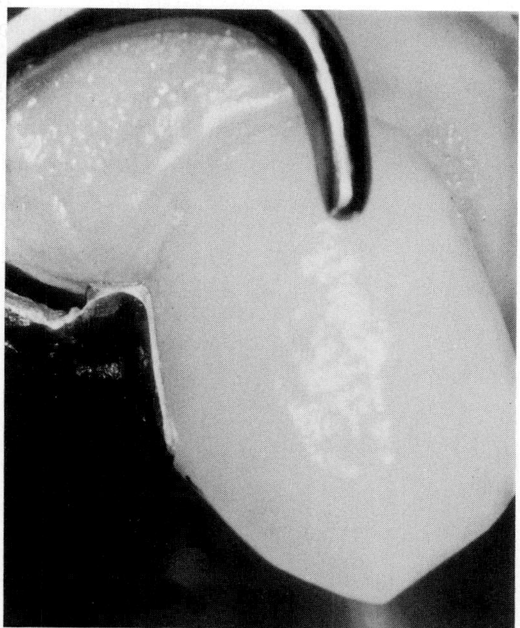

Figure 4–6 ■ The proximal plate of metal contacts the tooth and mucosa with no space between prosthesis and tissue. The metal is clean, strong, and durable and controlled in position by the positive lingual rest.

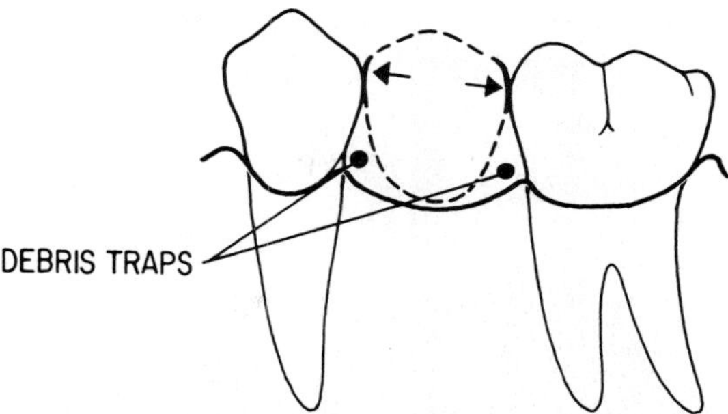

Figure 4–7 ■ Hygiene is a problem at the interproximal area with fixed partial dentures and the space between pontic and tooth must be opened wide for cleansing.

The placement of plastic material at the tooth-gingival area can be most detrimental. Plastic is quite porous and can retain and discharge toxins into the tooth-tissue junction area, causing periodontal problems and tooth deterioration.

The ideal prosthesis restores the lost tissues to the contour that was present when the natural structures were intact (Fig. 4–5). When there is extensive support structure loss, including bone and mucosa, there is exposure of more of the clinical crown and root structure of the tooth. The greater the recession, the greater the loss of stability and support, and there can also be greater difficulty in contouring the clinical crown to eliminate spaces and voids. In these circumstances, it may be necessary to place crowns or onlays to provide guiding surfaces all

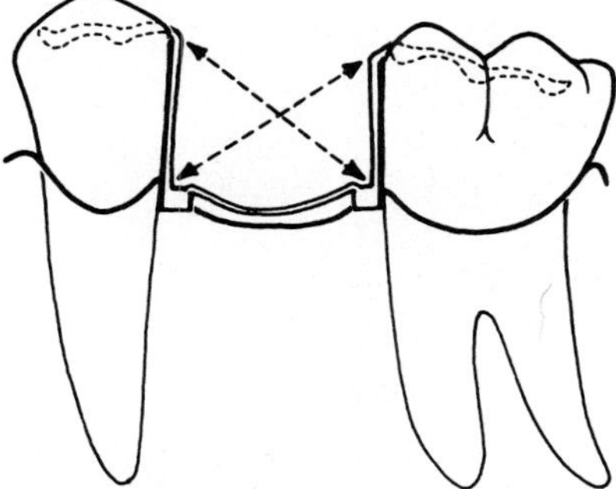

Figure 4–8 ■ Well-fitting proximal plates, in conjunction with occlusal rests, provide stability and support for the remaining teeth by their buttressing action.

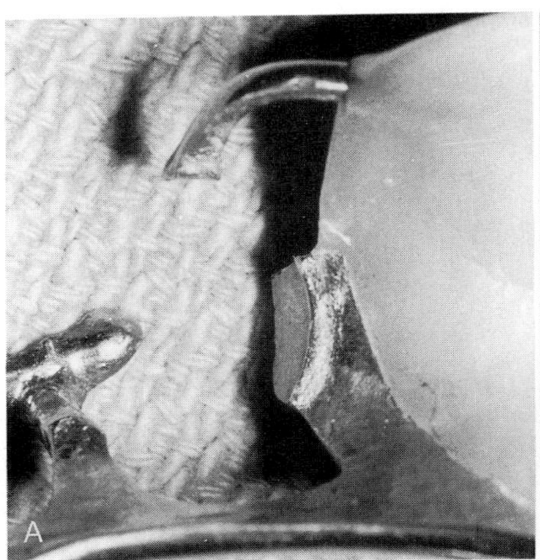

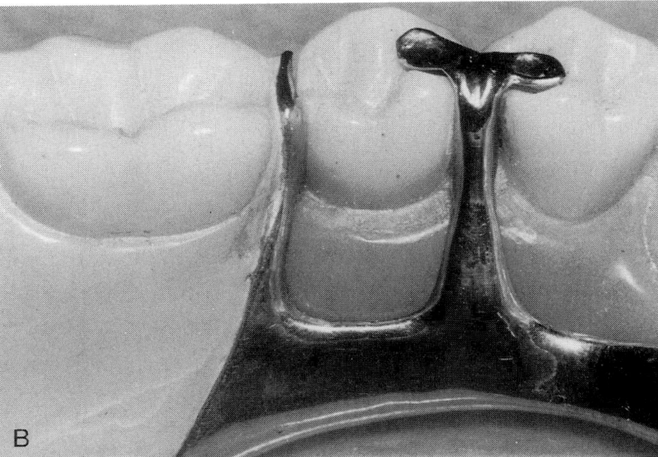

Figure 4–9 ■ *A* and *B*, The lingual portion of the distal proximal plate, in conjunction with the mesial strut and rest, provides reciprocation against possible lingual movement of the tooth by the retainer.

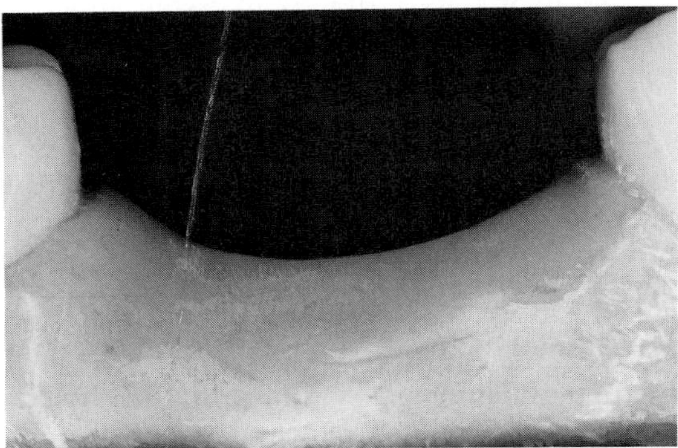

Figure 4–10 ■ The mesial and distal surfaces of the teeth are prepared parallel to each other and to other teeth in the arch that are used as guiding surfaces.

the way to the gingiva, since these weak teeth are most in need of protection and support for continued survival.

The width of the guiding plane is determined by the tissue contour of the gingiva at the edentulous area. If the residual ridge topography is high and well rounded when viewed from the facial-lingual aspect, the metal guide surface need not be too wide, extending only to a self-cleansing area on the facial and lingual side (Fig. 4–13). If the tissue is quite receded and depressed, the interproximal plate must be wide enough to cover and protect the invagination and must extend to a self-cleansing area.

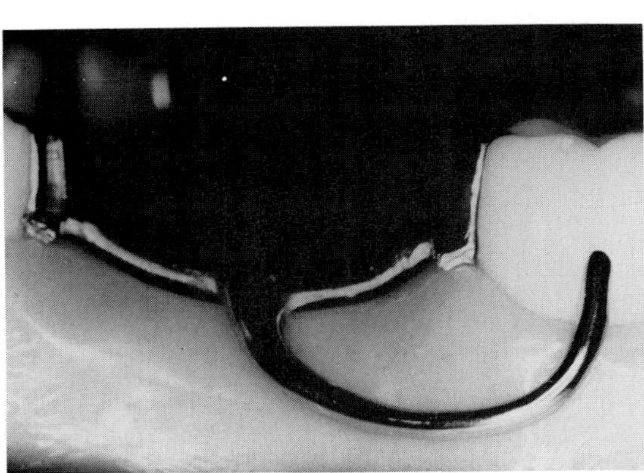

Figure 4–11 ■ Preparation of the abutment teeth permits the metal guide plate to contact the tooth to the gingiva.

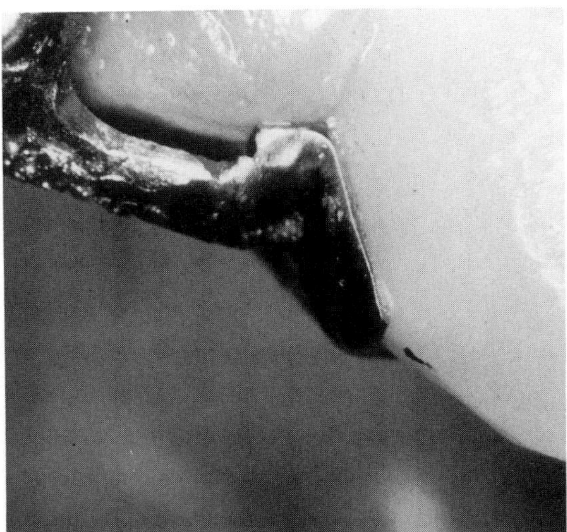

Figure 4–12 ■ The mucosal portion of the metal is constructed to form a sharp right angle for a strong union with the plastic of the denture base.

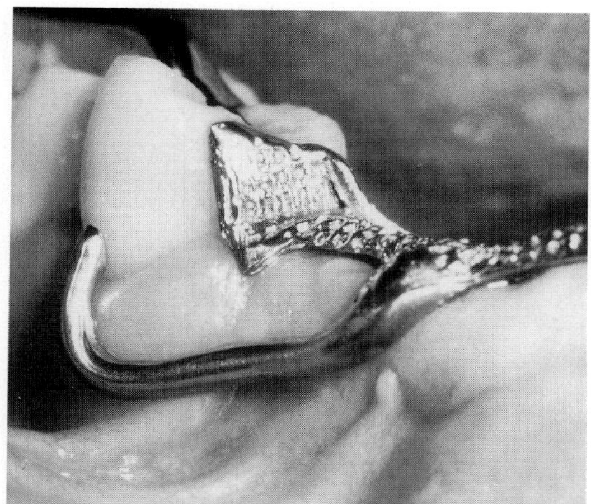

Figure 4–13 ■ Facial-lingual width of the proximal plate is determined by the topography of the mucosa. The facial extension must continue to a self-cleansing area.

REFERENCES

Applegate OC: The interdependence of periodontics and removable denture prosthesis. J Prosthet Dent 8:269, 1958.

Kratochvil, FJ: Influence of occlusal rest position and clasp design on movement of abutment teeth. J Prosthet Dent 13:114, 1963.

Kratochvil FJ: Maintaining supporting structures with a removable partial denture prosthesis. J Prosthet Dent 25:167, 1971.

Kratochvil FJ: Principles of removable partial dentures. RGVG, UCLA. Syllabus, 1968.

Stewart KL and Rudd KD: Stabilizing periodontally weakened teeth with removable partial dentures. J Prosthet Dent 19:475, 1968.

Thayer H and Kratochvil FJ: Periodontal considerations with removable partial dentures. Dent Clin North Am 24:357, 1980.

Wearhang J: Justification for splinting in periodontal therapy. J Prosthet Dent 22:201, 1964.

chapter 5

Major connectors

By definition, the function of the major connector is to provide a rigid union of all portions of the prosthesis. Rigidity is necessary to

1. Control the relationship of remaining teeth to each other.

2. Control the direction of force against all remaining support structures and opposing occlusion.

3 Utilize and unite all remaining structures of the arch to provide the greatest potential to control functional forces.

Occlusal pressures or forces delivered to the prosthesis are transmitted through (A) the *occlusal surfaces* of the prosthesis to (B) the *rests* and then through (C) the *major connectors* to be distributed to (D) the remaining *natural teeth* and (E) the *edentulous mucosa* (in extension situations).

Failure to provide rigid connection can result in uncontrolled and destructive forces on abutment teeth, mucosa, and bone.

Maxillary Major Connectors

ANTERIOR-POSTERIOR CONNECTORS

Circular maxillary major connectors (Fig. 5–1) provide optimal rigidity. This design, referred to as the *anterior-posterior palatal design,* has the physical properties to provide maximum resistance to flexure and distortion when the forces of mastication occur. Most maxillary prostheses are designed in this manner. If the anterior palatal connector is used without the posterior component, it requires a great increase in bulk and area coverage to ensure the required rigidity.

The posterior palatal metal connector should not extend beyond the vibrating line of the palate and, in many instances, can be positioned forward of that landmark. It is imperative that the connector be in intimate contact with the tissues, since any space between them can accumulate debris and cause discomfort to the patient. A light post-dam is designed at the anterior and posterior tissue surfaces of the posterior connector to provide a seal to prevent accumulation of debris (Fig. 5–2).

The anterior portion of the connector is positioned according to diagnostic and treatment decisions, as follows:

1. If anterior teeth are to be replaced by the prosthesis, the connector will extend into the replacement area (Fig. 5–3).

2. The connector will extend onto the anterior teeth for bracing and lateral stabilization.

3. The connector will provide an indirect rest to resist removal.

4. The connector will stabilize a mobile tooth (Fig. 5–4).

If anterior lingual coverage is not required, the connector is designed well away from the teeth (Fig. 5–5). The borders of the connector terminate in the valley of the rugae to minimize the junction and provide a smooth transition from metal to mucosa.

The contour of the palatal connector is thickest in the central portion of the casting and

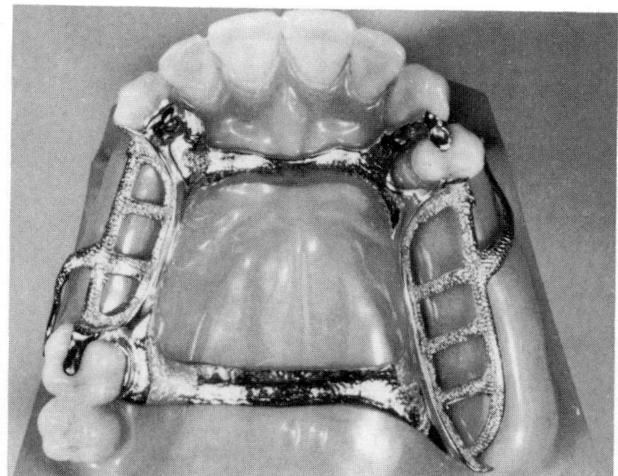

Figure 5-1 ■ The circular design of the maxillary casting provides maximum rigidity and strength, with minimum bulk.

tapers to blend smoothly into the mucosa at the margins (Fig. 5-6). This design with a thickened central portion provides an I-beam design for rigidity.

The contour of all parts of the prosthesis should be a smooth blending of existing tissues to the prosthesis, and ideally reproduces the contours of the missing natural structures.

CENTRAL PALATAL CONNECTOR

A replacement for one or two teeth unilaterally (Fig. 5-7) can be designed with a central palatal connector. The connector width is increased to provide the necessary rigidity, cross-arch support, and control of the prosthesis.

Mandibular Major Connectors

Because of patient anatomy—particularly tongue position—mandibular major connectors cannot be circular in design. This factor complicates construction of a rigid casting. Rigidity of the entire prosthesis is further diminished by the smaller edentulous support area in comparison with that of the maxillary arch. It is necessary to increase the bulk of the major connector to provide rigidity. A design that reproduces natural contours and topography of tissues provides the most ideal prosthesis and better patient acceptance.

Two types of mandibular major connectors are

(1) The lingual bar.
(2) Lingual tooth coverage (lingual plate).

LINGUAL BAR

The lingual bar is the design of choice because of its simplicity and minimal tissue coverage (Fig. 5-8). The decision to use a lingual bar is determined by two factors:

(A) The anatomic space available.
(B) The periodontal situation of the remaining teeth.

Anatomic Space Considerations

1. Sufficient space must be available between the floor of the mouth and the crest of the gingiva to allow placement of a rigid major connector.

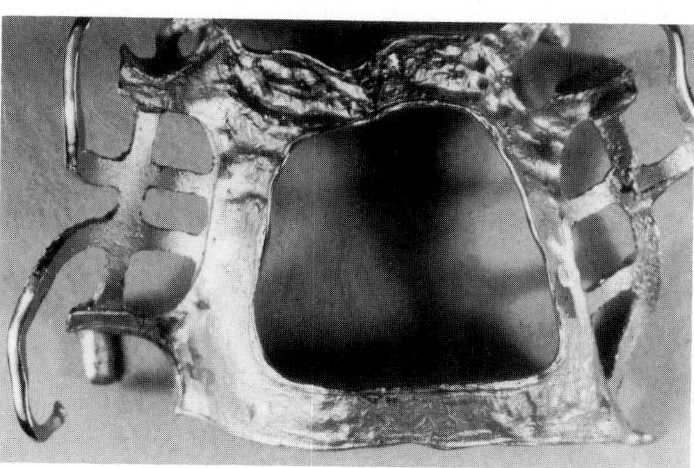

Figure 5-2 ■ A light V-shaped postdam at the borders of the major maxillary connector provides a dam, which helps prevent accumulation of debris under the prosthesis.

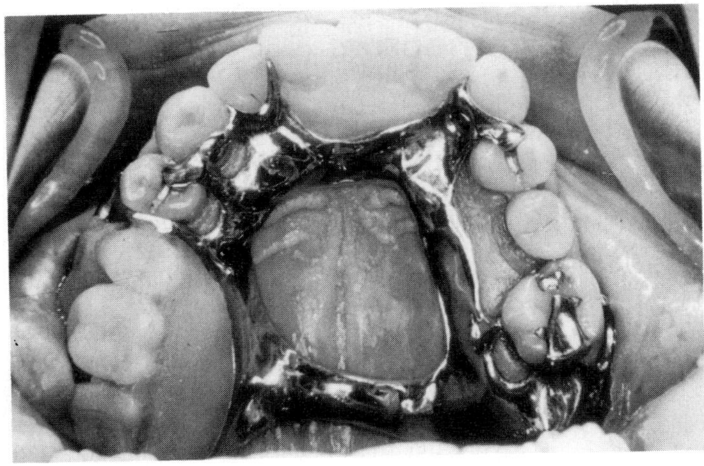

Figure 5-3 ■ The replacement of anterior teeth, such as the centrals and the lateral in this situation, requires design of the denture base connectors and the interproximal plates for attachment of prosthetic teeth.

2. Placement of the lingual bar must not interfere with the function of the lingual frenum or with tongue activity.

It is desirable to design the entire prosthesis, including the major connector, to be as simple and as neat as possible, while still providing the required properties and satisfying the objectives and specifications.

The superior portion of the bar is positioned well below or away from the gingival crest tissues (Fig. 5-9). If positioned too close, it may cause

1. Hypertrophy of tissue over the bar (Fig. 5-10).
2. Food impaction and tissue irritation between bar and tissue.

The lingual bar should be placed on unattached tissue. The location of this tissue is determined intraorally and the measurements recorded. When the bar is placed over unattached tissue, it can be relieved or a space can be left between bar and mucosa without concern that tissue might hypertrophy into the space.

Alveolar or attached tissue has a tendency to hypertrophy to fill the space between prosthesis and tissue. The basic idea is to design the casting to contact attached alveolar tissues. On these tissues, the casting is not relieved, except as necessary where physical undercuts would prevent placement of the prosthesis (Fig. 5-11).

The location of the junction of attached and unattached gingiva *cannot* be determined by inspection of a cast and must be located by intraoral examination. A method of measurement is to use a periodontal probe that has millimeter

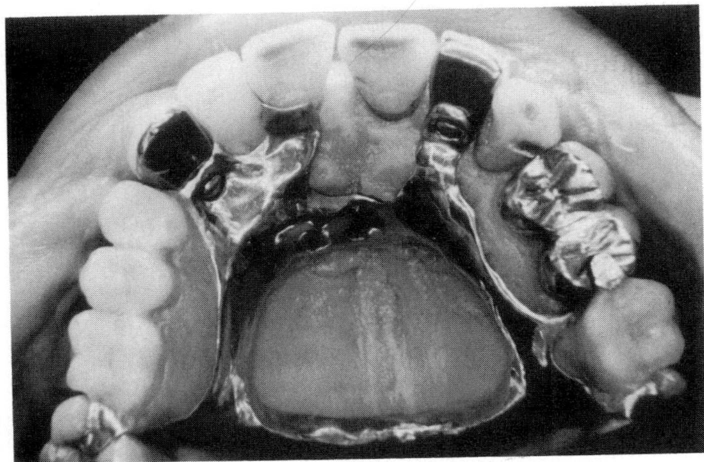

Figure 5-4 ■ Individual teeth with periodontal involvement and mobility can be stabilized by the partial denture rest attached to the major connector.

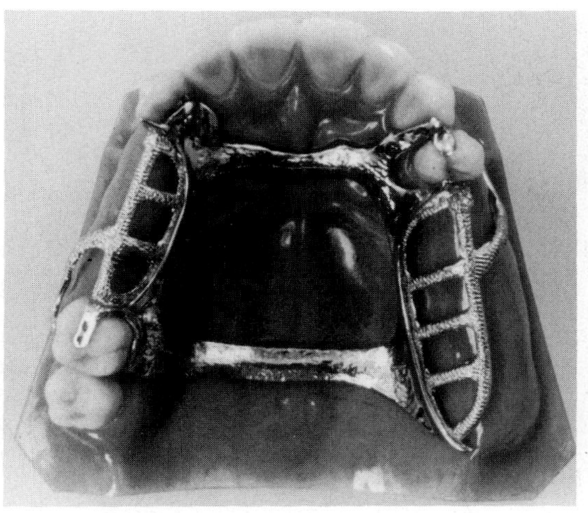

Figure 5–5 ■ When anterior tooth involvement is *not* required, the prosthesis is designed well away from the anterior lingual palate area. This minimizes interference with tongue action in phonetics and in other functions.

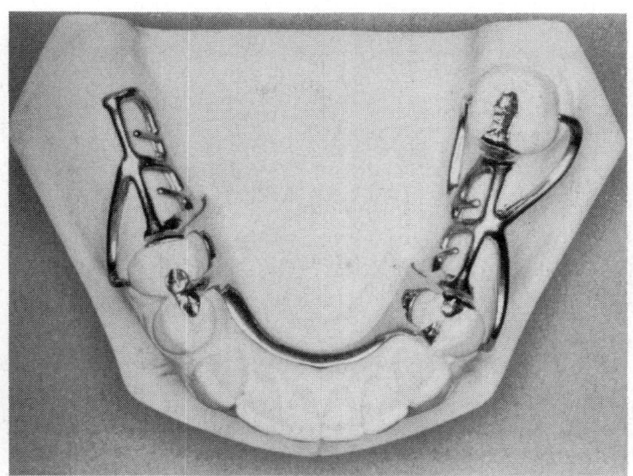

Figure 5–8 ■ The basic lingual bar is the design of choice, when space and periodontal conditions permit.

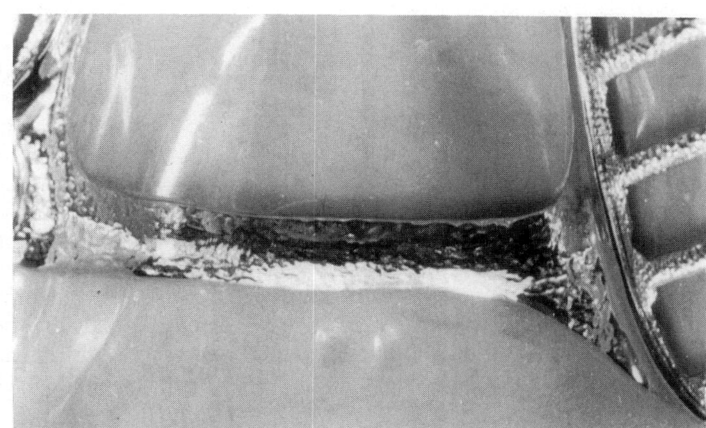

Figure 5–6 ■ A central ridge in the palatal connector provides maximum strength and rigidity with minimum oral interference and tapers to a thin border.

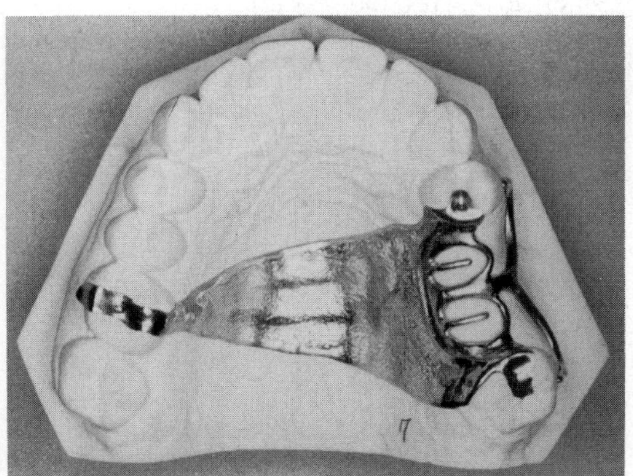

Figure 5–7 ■ Unilateral tooth replacements without complications can sometimes provide the necessary cross-arch support with a central palatal connector. The anterior-posterior width is increased.

markings. Measure from the gingival crest to the alveolar junction in the mouth (Fig. 5–12) and transfer the measurement of that position to the dental cast (Fig. 5–13) and to the patient record.

Periodontal Considerations

The lingual bar is the design of choice whenever possible because of simplicity and minimal tooth-mucosa contact. Simplicity of design

1. Reduces interference with mouth functions.
2. Reduces food and plaque accumulation.
3. Simplifies fabrication procedures.

When there is periodontal involvement of remaining teeth with mobility and need of stabili-

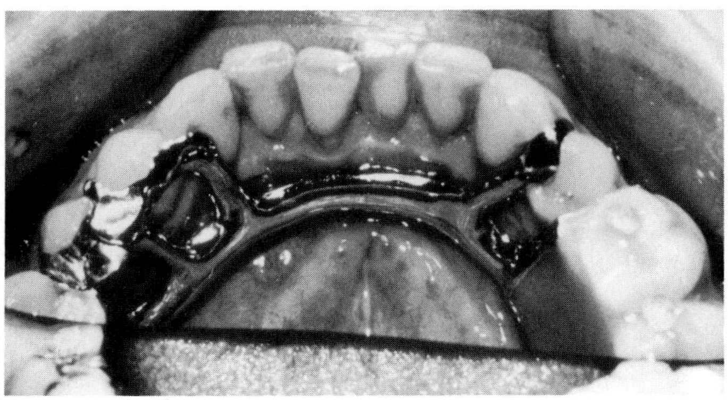

Figure 5–9 ■ When the lingual bar is used, the superior surface must be positioned well away from the crest of the gingival tissues.

zation, the lingual bar may not be indicated, since it would not fulfill support and stabilization requirements.

LINGUAL COVERAGE (LINGUAL PLATE)

The decision to use lingual coverage is determined by diagnostic findings concerning

(A) The anatomic space available.
(B) The periodontal situation.

Anatomic Space Considerations

Clinical examination of the patient can reveal high lingual frenum and floor of mouth attachments, with insufficient space to place a lingual bar that would provide rigidity. In these situations, lingual coverage provides the necessary bulk and strength, without causing undue functional interference (Fig. 5–14).

Periodontal Considerations

Lingual coverage is considered the necessary treatment when the following factors are present:

1. Mobility of anterior teeth.
2. Recession of supporting tissues.
3. Extensive deposits of calculus and stains on the teeth.

Mobile anterior teeth ■ Mobility of mandibular anterior teeth can be caused by periodontal difficulties such as tissue and bone recession resulting from calculus deposition on the lingual surface of the teeth opposite the saliva ducts. Anterior hyperocclusion can contribute to mobility in conjunction with periodontal difficulties.

Placement of lingual coverage can provide stabilization for the teeth and can buttress them against lateral and distal forces, since the lingual surfaces of the maxillary anterior teeth

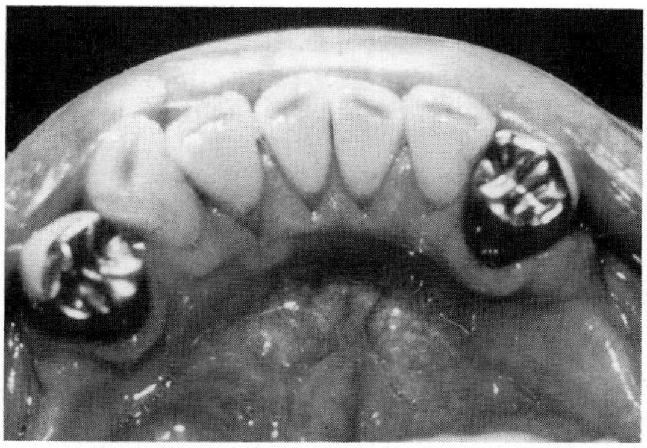

Figure 5–10 ■ Small spaces left in between attached mucosa and prosthesis result in tissue hypertrophy. Design the prosthesis *well away* from the mucosa, or *contact* and *cover* the attached mucosa in its entirety with no space left in between.

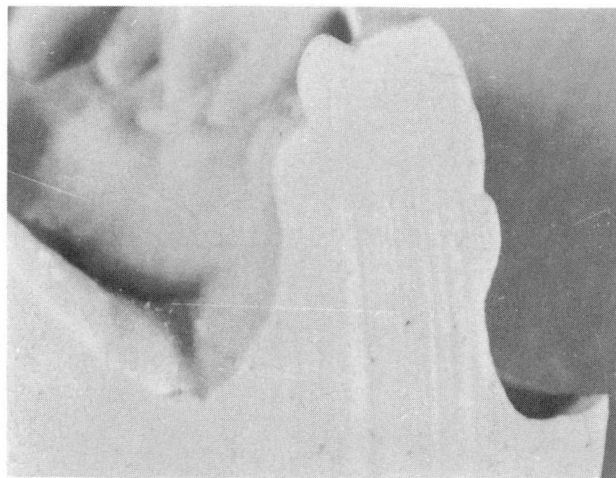

Figure 5–11 ■ Physical tissue undercuts require a space between metal casting and tissues to permit physical placement of the prosthesis.

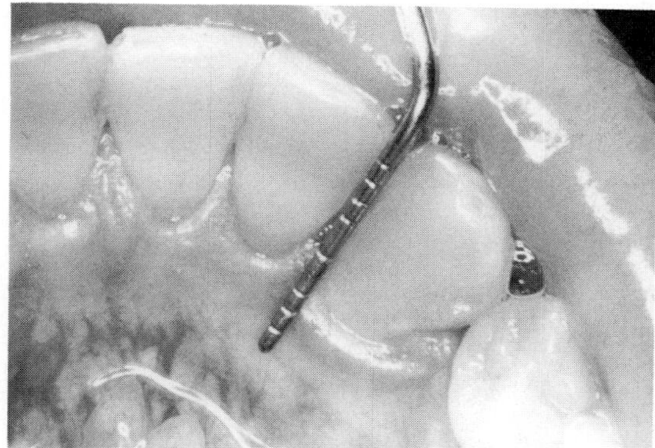

Figure 5–12 ■ The location of the extension of attached mucosa can be quickly measured with a periodontal probe and recorded.

contact the mandibular anterior teeth in protrusive and lateral excursions (Fig. 5–15).

Recession of supporting tissues ■ When the support tissues on the lingual side of the anterior teeth recede, a flat surface or plateau is often formed (Fig. 5–16). This type of tissue topography results in additional difficulties, since debris accumulates in that area and contributes to further recession.

It is possible to restore the contour of the missing tissues with lingual coverage by contouring the casting to reproduce the anatomical topography of the missing tissues. This does not invade the tongue space but will help prevent food impaction. The metal of the casting is in intimate contact with the attached mucosa, including as much of the interdental papillae as possible (Fig. 5–17A). The lingual anatomy of the anterior teeth presents minimal tooth undercuts (Fig. 5–17B).

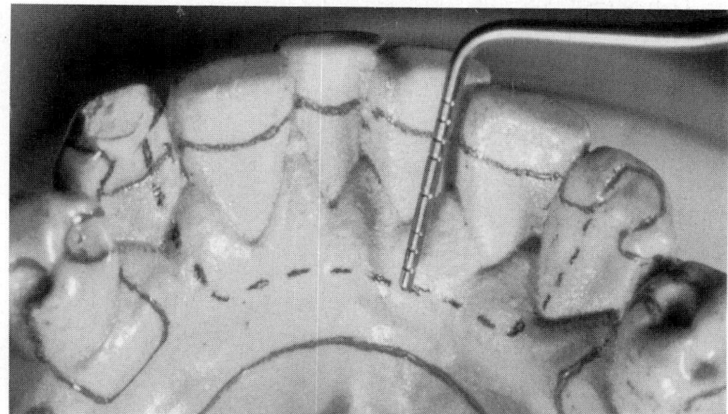

Figure 5–13 ■ The measurement of the position of the attached mucosa is transferred to the diagnostic and working cast for location of the lingual bar.

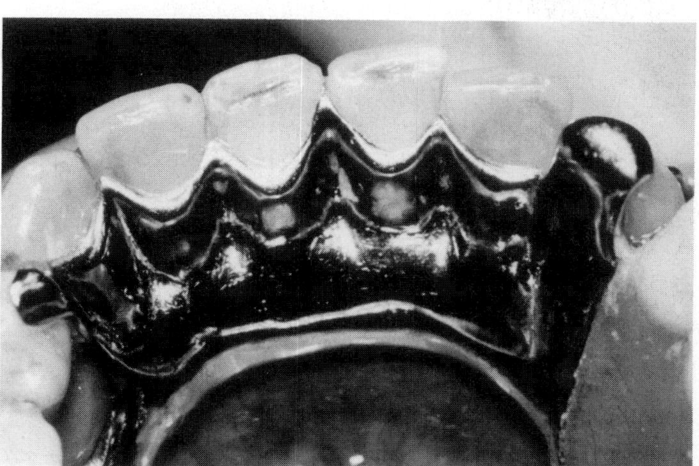

Figure 5–14 ■ Lingual coverage can duplicate normal lingual contours and provide strength with minimal function interference.

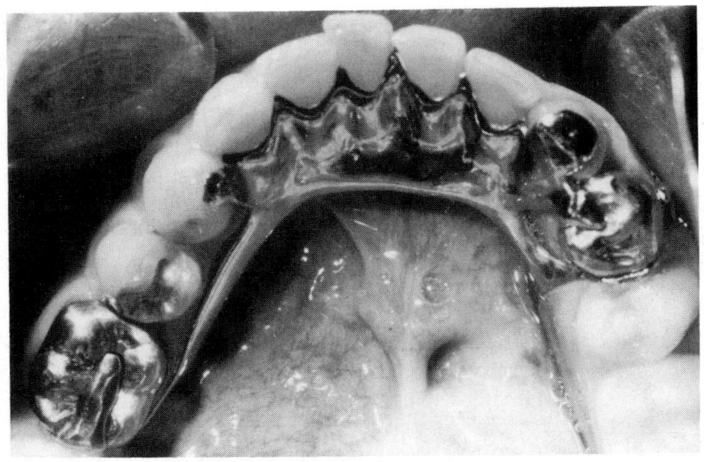

Figure 5–15 ■ Lingual coverage provides excellent lingual and lateral stabilization for mobile teeth.

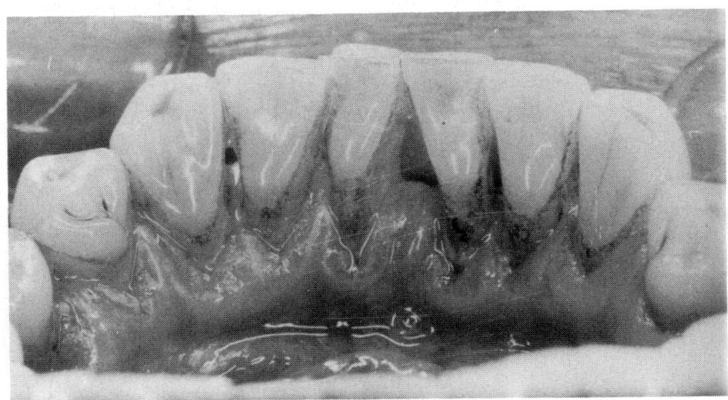

Figure 5–16 ■ Recession results in flat tissue topography, with potential for food and debris impaction.

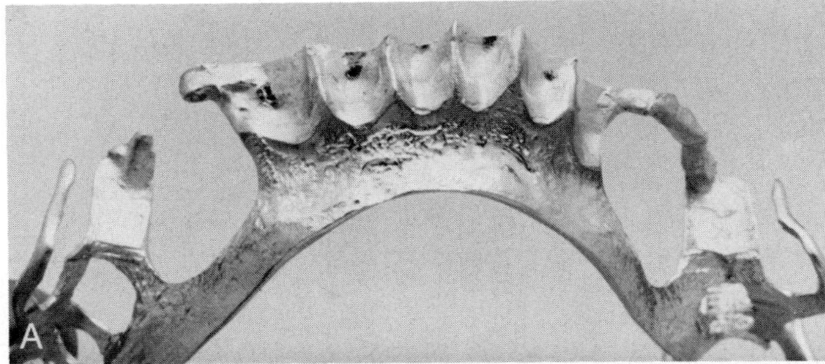

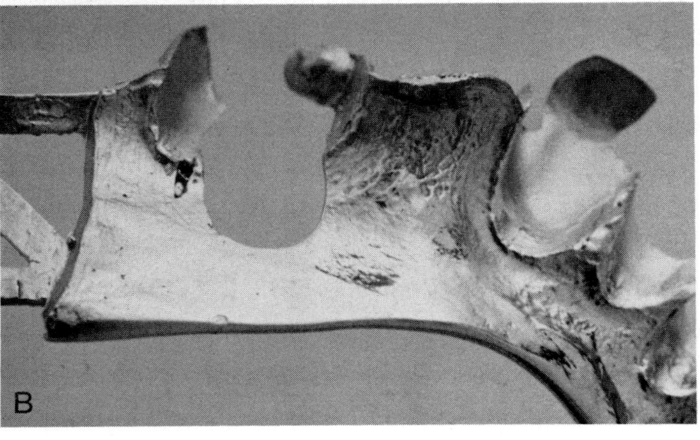

Figure 5–17 ■ *A*, The tissue surface of the casting is fabricated to *contact* all possible areas of attached mucosa. *B*, The casting duplicates tissue details, with no space between casting and tissue, where contacting attached mucosa.

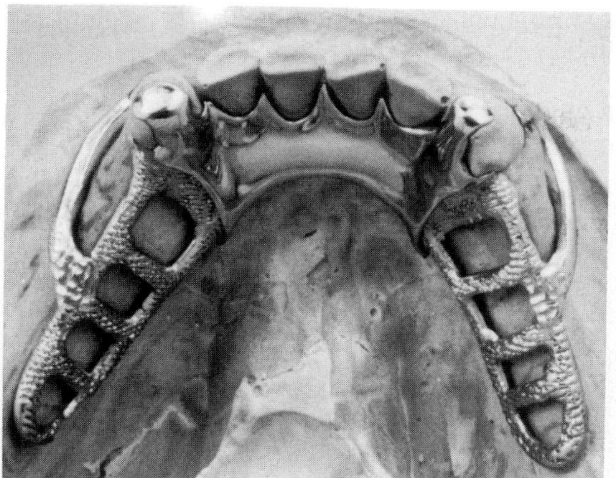

Figure 5–18 ■ Lingual coverage acts as an indirect retainer when few anterior teeth remain.

Indirect Rest

Incorporation of lingual coverage can provide an indirect rest to assist in keeping a prosthesis in place against removal forces and during fabrication procedures.

The lingual coverage is usually used as an indirect rest when six or fewer anterior teeth remain (Fig. 5–18).

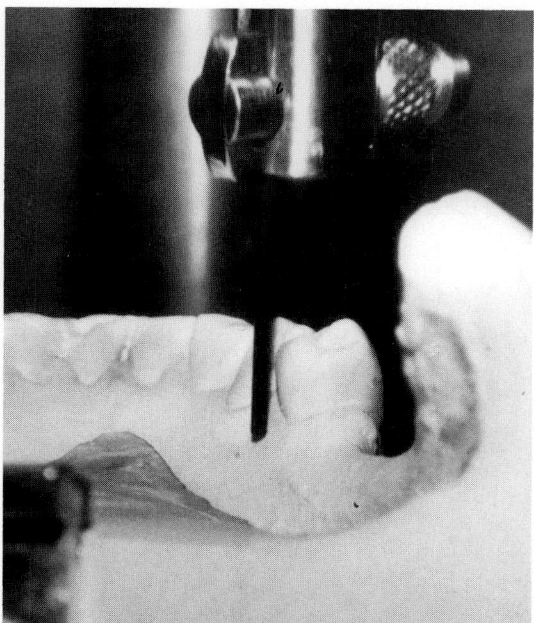

Figure 5–19 ■ Lingual contours of posterior teeth often present undercuts at the tissue junction. Lingual coverage of posterior teeth is difficult *without* leaving *space* between casting and tissue.

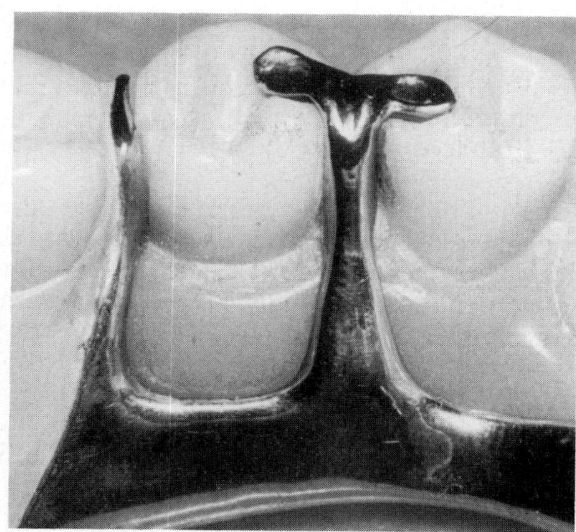

Figure 5–20 ■ The lingual surfaces of tissue will retain natural contours when the prosthesis is designed well away from the tooth-tissue junction.

Lingual Contours of Posterior Teeth — Undercuts

An area for special consideration in design and placement of the mandibular major connector is the lingual side of the posterior teeth.

Anatomy of the lingual suface of these teeth includes an *undercut* at the tooth-tissue junction, which produces a void or space in that area in most instances (Fig. 5–19). When this space exists between prosthesis and tissue, there can be hypertrophy of tissue and accumulation of

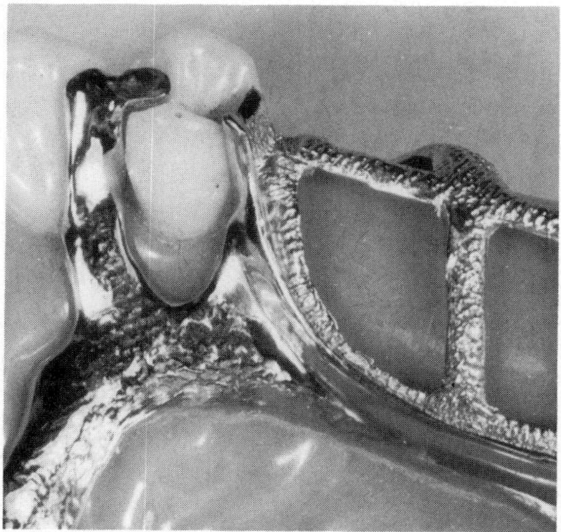

Figure 5–21 ■ When possible, the casting is designed to cross the tooth-tissue junction at *right* angles and in the center of the tooth to help reduce food impaction.

debris. This situation can be treated in two ways:

1. Design the casting away from the gingival crest in an inferior direction.

2. Reshape or restore the teeth to remove the undercuts.

Casting design ■ Designing away from the gingival crest is an effective method that causes minimal interference with the tooth and tissue contours; the casting should be well away from the crestal tissues (Fig. 5–20). If possible, the horizontal portion of the lingual bar is positioned on the unattached gingiva. When the lingual connector is placed in this position, it

1. Does not interfere with normal tooth and tissue contours.
2. Helps prevent tissue hypertrophy.
3. Provides a more normal self-cleansing situation.
4. Reduces the potential for lateral force on these teeth in extension situations.

Reshape, restore, or reposition teeth ■ Posterior teeth can be *reshaped* to reduce or eliminate undercuts.

Placement of *restorations* such as crowns will also remove the undercuts.

Realignment of malpositioned teeth to proper position with orthodontic procedures is often the treatment to consider.

BASIC CONCEPTS FOR LINGUAL CONTOURS OF MAJOR CONNECTORS

1. Shape lingual contours to reproduce the original tissues.
2. Cross the tooth-tissue junction at a right angle to the tooth (Fig. 5–20).
3. Design the casting to cross the tooth-tissue junction in the center of the anterior teeth when possible (Fig. 5–21). This will help to reduce food impaction.

REFERENCES

Academy of Prosthodontics: Glossary of Prosthetic Terms. St Louis, CV Mosby Co, 1987.

Frechette AR: The influence of partial design on distribution of force to abutment teeth. J Prosthet Dent 6:195, 1956.

McCracken WL: Contemporary partial denture designs. J Prosthet Dent 8:71, 1958.

Schmidt AH: Planning and designing removable partial dentures. J Prosthet Dent 3:783–806, 1953.

Steffle VL: Simplified clasp partial dentures designed for maximum function. J Am Dent Assoc 32:1093–1100, 1945.

chapter 6

Design for denture base connectors

Functions

The functions of the denture base connectors are to

1. Provide a framework for the attachment of the plastic portion of the prosthesis to the metal casting.
2. Provide the necessary strength to maintain rigidity throughout the prosthesis.
3. Establish a positive finish line at the junction between the plastic of the denture base and the metal parts of the prosthesis.

Attachment for Casting and Denture Base

This is a mechanical merging and requires that the plastic portion of the denture base surround the metal to form a good union. For strength, the metal of the denture base connector must be embedded at least 1 mm within the plastic of the denture base. The connector is fabricated to allow for this thickness of plastic in the denture base portion of the prosthesis (Fig. 6–1). If adequate thickness of the plastic material is not provided, it can break under the stress and pressure of function.

Placement of the connectors is influenced by (1) the amount of space between the opposing arches and (2) the placement of the denture teeth.

In the mandibular posterior arch, the connectors are positioned on the crest of the residual ridge and on the lingual surface of the ridge (Fig. 6–2). This leaves the facial portion of the ridge clear for positioning of the prosthetic denture teeth without removing or shortening the facial part of the tooth, which can affect esthetics and the tooth retention areas.

There is often very little space between the tuberosity of the maxillary arch and the retromolar pad area of the opposing arch. The denture base connector is designed well away from this area to prevent space problems and undue thinness of plastic over metal (Fig. 6–3). The connectors are not positioned on the facial portion of the arch, where they may interfere with placement of the denture teeth.

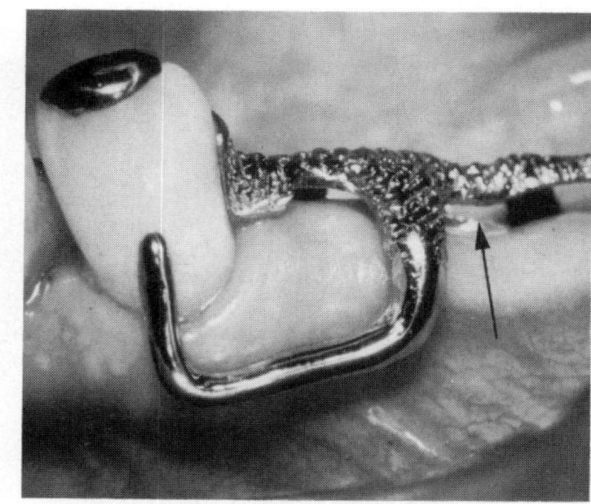

Figure 6–1 ■ Adequate space of a minimum of 1 mm is provided between the mucosa and the denture base connectors for sufficient bulk of plastic to provide strength.

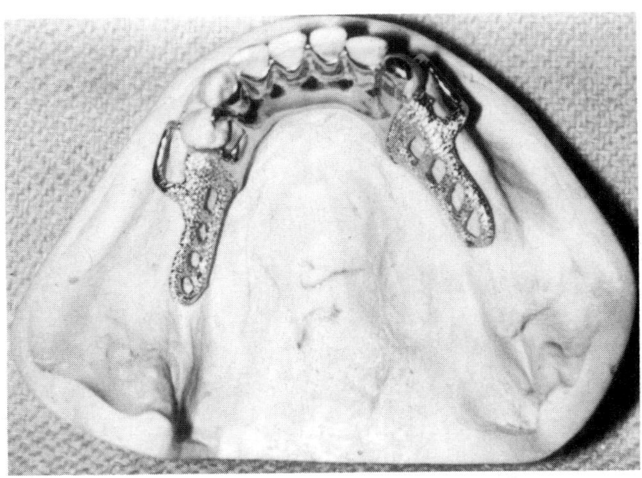

Figure 6–2 ■ The metal of the denture base connectors is positioned on the crest of the ridge and on the lingual surface. The facial portion of the ridge is unobstructed for placement of prosthetic teeth.

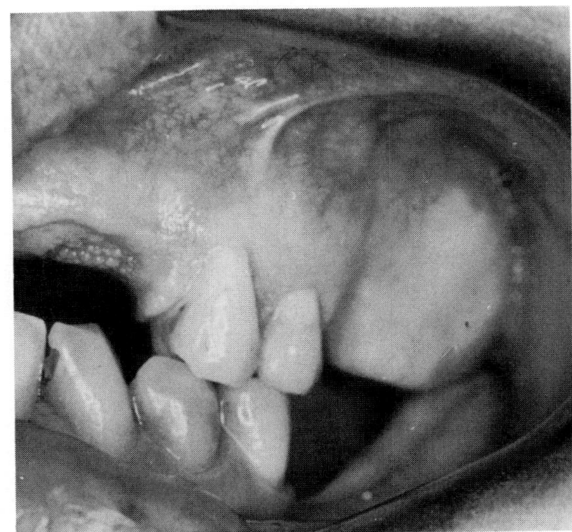

Figure 6–3 ■ The maxillary denture base casting is positioned well away from the tuberosity area, where there is minimal space.

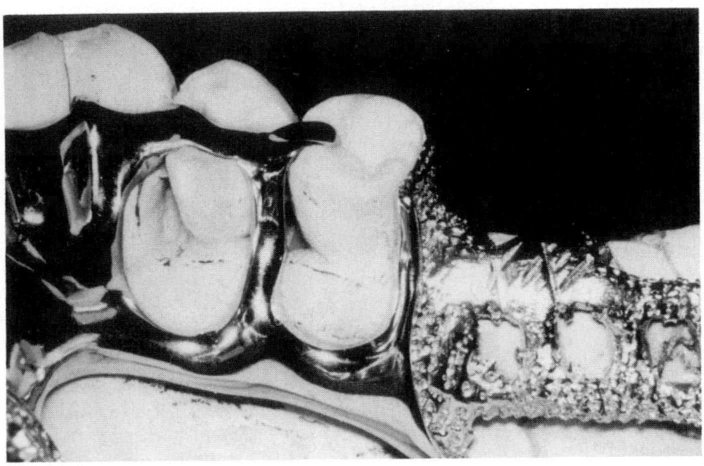

Figure 6–4 ■ The junction area between the major connector and the denture base connector must have sufficient bulk for strength. This is an area of frequent flexure and breakage.

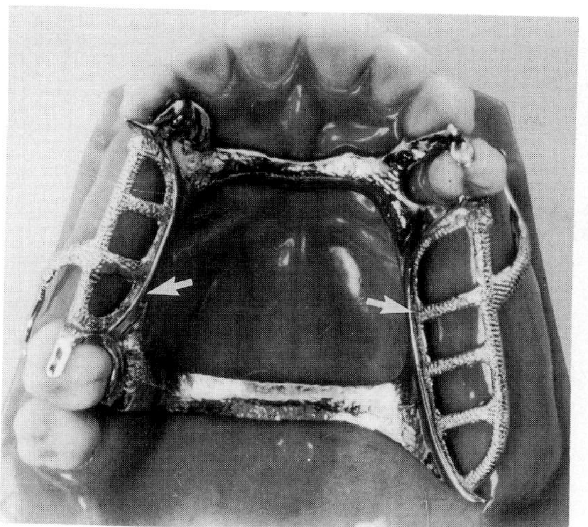

Figure 6–5 ■ The metal finish line for juncture with the plastic on the tongue side of the prosthesis is at right angles to provide bulk and strength for both metal and plastic.

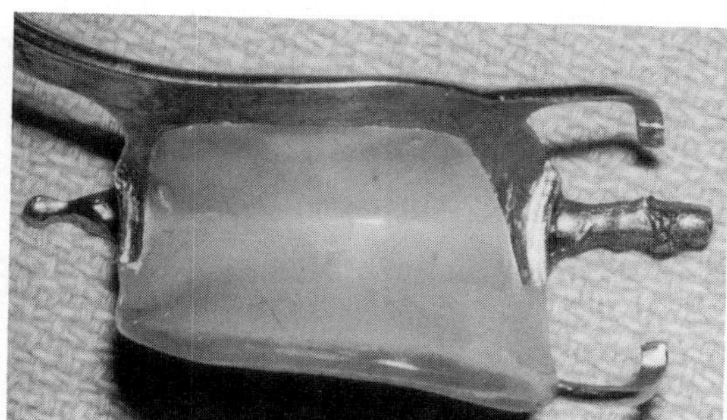

Figure 6–6 ■ A metal finish line is provided on the tissue side of the prosthesis for the metal-plastic junction. Note that the plastic is well away from tooth-tissue junction.

Strength and Rigidity

The junction of the denture base connector and the major connector can be a weak area. Sufficient bulk and proper design for strength and rigidity are required. The connector should be fan-shaped in the junction area, with increased bulk to provide strength (Fig. 6–4).

Finish Lines

Junctions of plastic with metal casting require bulk and must be made at a 90 degree angle. If the plastic is thin or forms a tapered union, it can break or curl away from the metal; this allows debris to collect, causing discoloration, stain, odor, and formation of toxins.

A finish line is provided on the tongue or facial side of the prosthesis as well as on the ridge or support side (Fig. 6–5 and 6–6). The finish line should be positioned *at least* 2 mm away from the tooth gingival junction area.

REFERENCES

Academy of Prosthodontics: Glossary of Prosthetic Terms. St Louis, CV Mosby Co, 1968.

Kratochvil FJ: Principles of Removable Partial Dentures. RGVG, UCLA, 1968.

chapter 7

Retainers: their design and position

A removable partial denture retainer has previously been defined as "any portion of the prosthesis that contacts the teeth and helps to prevent removal of the prosthesis." The interproximal plate portions of the major connectors thus contribute to retention by parallelism of the proximal plates to each other and by the frictional contact of metal to tooth. The *direct retainers* are flexible parts of the casting that are deliberately designed to enter undercuts on abutment teeth to resist removal of the prosthesis and to help prevent dislodgement.

There are two basic types of direct retainers, as classified by DeVan. They are

1. Infrabulge retainers.
2. Suprabulge retainers.

This classification is based on the origin of the retainer from an occlusal or gingival location.

Infrabulge Retainers

An infrabulge retainer is a direct retainer that approaches the crown of the tooth from an apical direction and does not cross the survey line of the tooth, when the prosthesis is in a seated position. The I bar is an infrabulge retainer (Fig. 7–1). The advantages of the I bar are that it allows

1. Minimal tooth contact.
2. Exact placement of retention contact.
3. Minimal interference with natural tooth contour.
4. Maximum natural cleansing action.
5. Passive functional movement of an extension prosthesis.
6. Reduced display of metal, for better esthetics.

I bars are designed to cross the tooth-tissue junction at right angles or in the long axis of the tooth (Fig. 7–2). From the point of retention contact, the retainer extends in a straight line to the unattached tissues (Fig. 7–3). This positioning minimizes the amount of debris that collects on the abutment tooth. The size of the retention undercut used is 0.010 in or 0.25 mm. The part of the retainer that contacts the tooth is circular or oval in shape. Placement of the 0.010-in retention contact is determined with the undercut gauge to ensure the exact amount

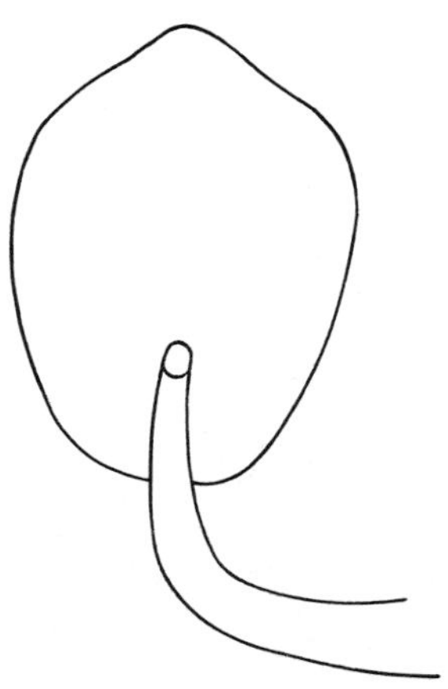

Figure 7–1 ■ The infrabulge retainer—commonly called an I-bar retainer. The retainer approaches the tooth in a straight line from an apical or mucosal direction.

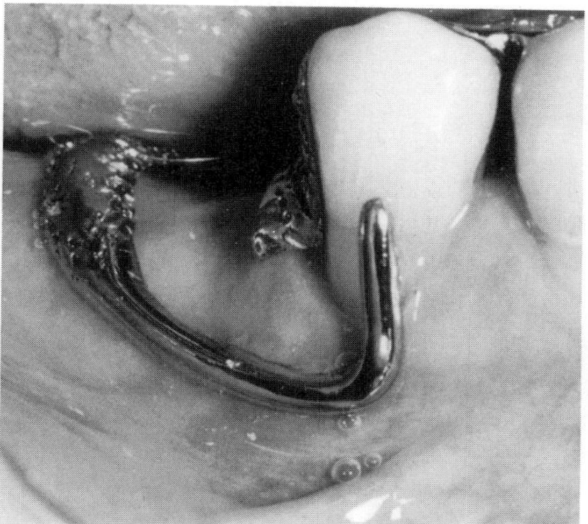

Figure 7–2 ■ The infrabulge retainer crosses the tooth-tissue junction at right angles and in a straight line, until it reaches the unattached mucosa, where it turns to a horizontal position.

of retention. The undercut gauge is placed in the arm of the survey instrument (Fig. 7–4). The procedure is described in detail in Chapters 9 and 10 under Design Principles and Use of the Surveyor. The horizontal portion of the retainer is placed on unattached tissue whenever possible. Junction of the retainer with the prosthesis is at the interproximal area between the denture teeth, so as not to interfere with their placement or cause an esthetic problem due to short teeth (Fig. 7–5). The portion of the retainer that is seated over the mucosa must be relieved from

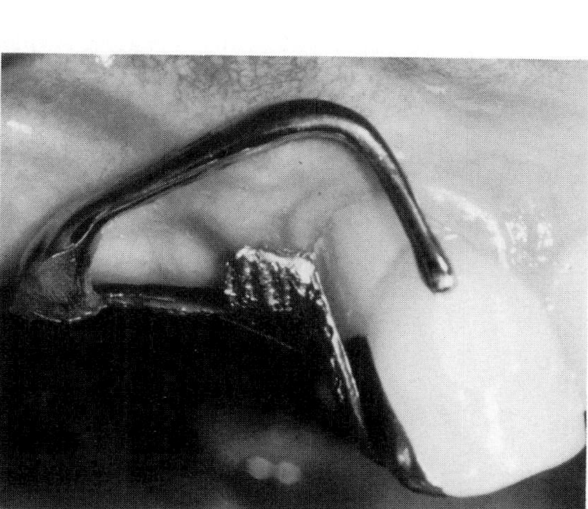

Figure 7–3 ■ The vertical portion of the I bar is positioned parallel to the long axis of the tooth. (Note the unattached tissue with blood vessels.)

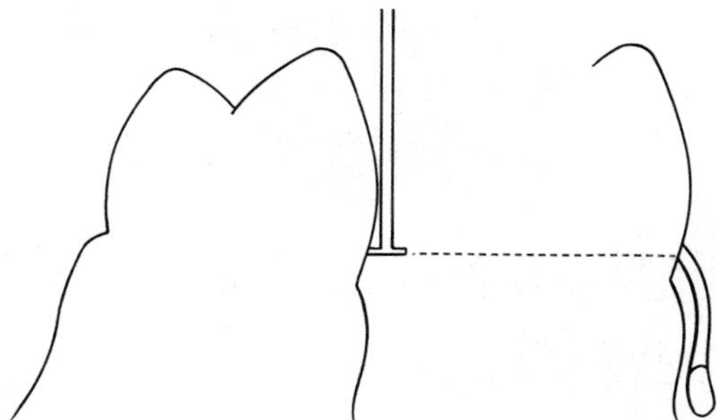

Figure 7–4 ■ The amount of tooth undercut engaged determines the amount of retention from the retainer. The undercut gauge is used to determine the amount of undercut.

the tooth to where it enters the denture base in order to prevent tissue hypertrophy (Fig. 7–6A and B).

Suprabulge Retainers

A suprabulge retainer is a direct retainer that begins at the occlusal portion of the tooth and extends onto the tooth, crossing the survey line and extending into a tooth undercut. An example of the suprabulge retainer is the circumferential retainer (Fig. 7–7). Factors causing concern with use of the circumferential retainer are greater area of tooth contact, interference with tooth-tissue contours (Fig. 7–8), and potential to torque abutment teeth in extension situations in which there is denture movement (Fig. 7–9).

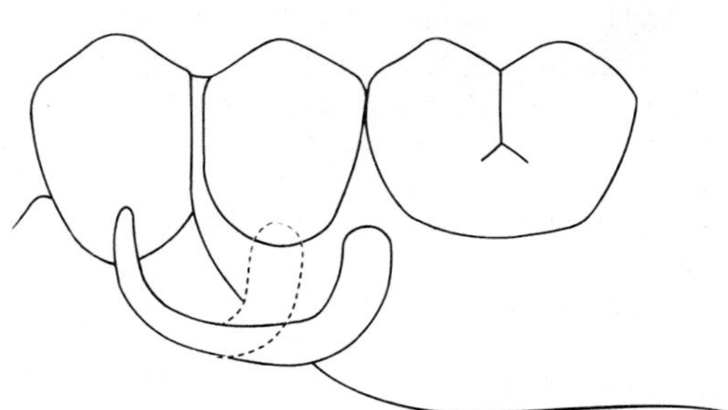

Figure 7–5 ■ The origin of the retainer is positioned or joins the partial casting between the denture teeth so as not to interfere with the placement of the prosthetic tooth.

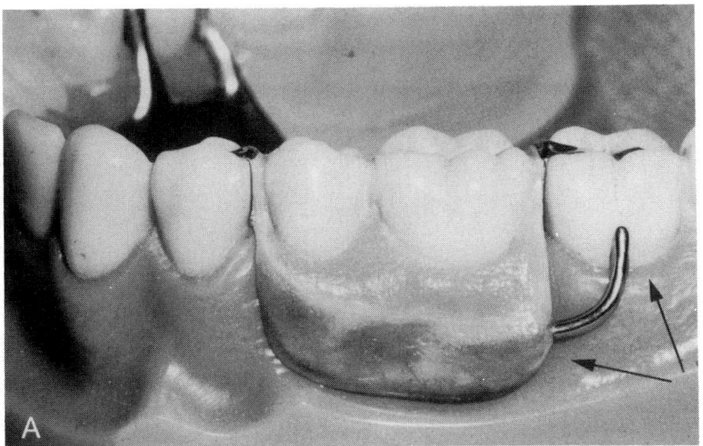

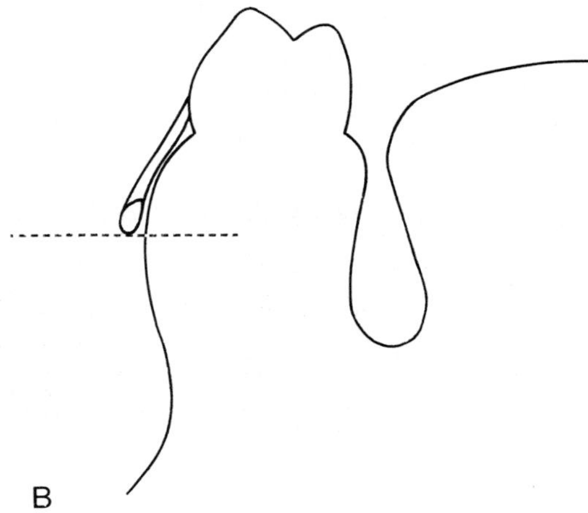

Figure 7–6 ■ *A*, Space is provided under the retainer where it crosses the tissue from tooth contact to junction with the plastic of the denture base. *B*, The space between retainer and tissue is approximately the thickness of 30-gauge wax. This space is necessary to prevent tissue hypertrophy.

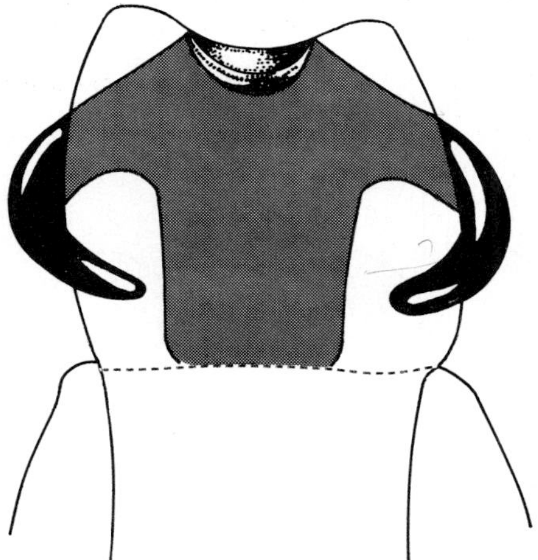

Figure 7–7 ■ The suprabulge or circumferential retainer originates at the occlusal surface of the tooth and extends around the tooth to terminate in a tooth undercut.

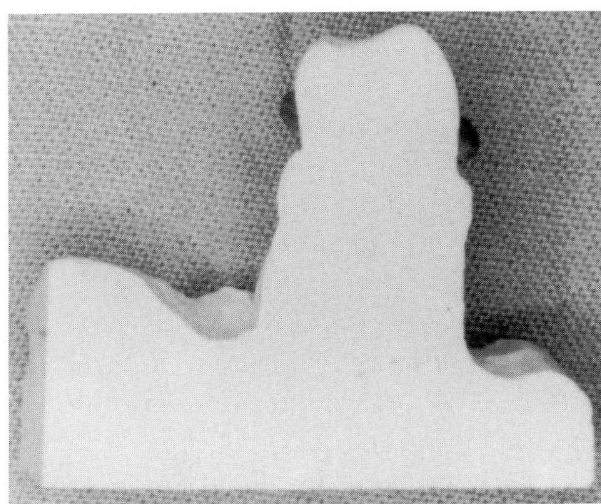

Figure 7–8 ■ The anterior-posterior view demonstrates circumferential retainer interference with the tooth-tissue profile.

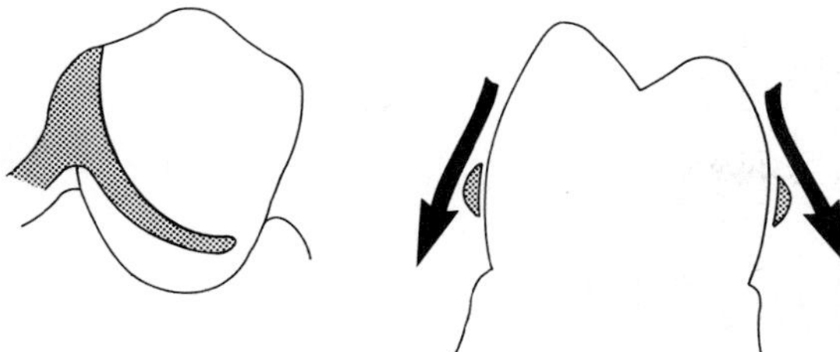

Figure 7–9 ■ Circumferential retainers can interfere with food flow and could grip and torque the tooth when there is movement of the prosthesis.

RETENTION AUGMENTED BY DENTURE BASES

The denture base augments retention of both maxillary and mandibular prostheses by the adhesive and cohesive phenomena between the base and the mucosa (Fig. 7–10). For the mandibular prosthesis, atmospheric pressure and weight can augment retention, but for the maxillary prosthesis, these factors require additional retention considerations.

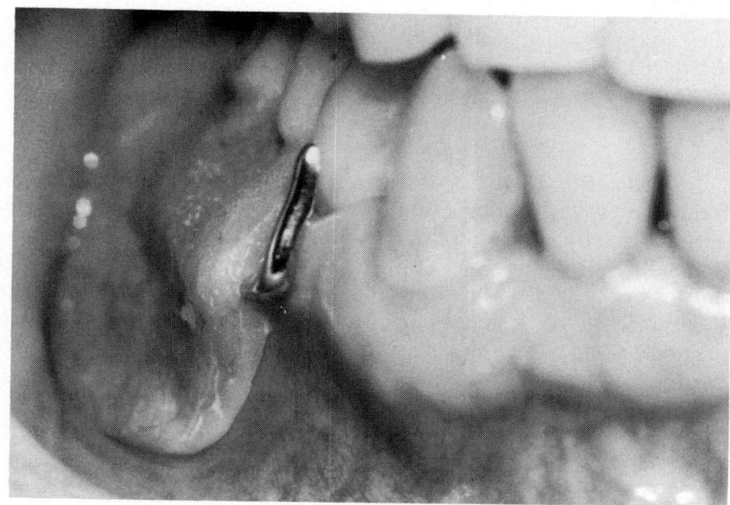

Figure 7–10 ■ Close adaptation of the denture base to the mucosa assists retention. (Note that the I-Bar retainer has a minimum of metal displayed for better esthetics.)

REFERENCES

Academy of Prosthodontics: Glossary of Prosthodontic Terms. St Louis, CV Mosby Co, 1968.

DeVan MM: The nature of partial denture foundation—suggestions for its preservation. J Prosthet Dent 2:210, 1952.

Fisher RL and Jaslow C: The efficiency of an indirect retainer. J Prosthet Dent 34:24, 1975.

Kratochvil FJ: Influence of occlusal rest position and clasp design on movement of abutment teeth. J Prosthet Dent 13:114–124, 1963.

Krol A: Clasp design for extension base removable partial dentures. J Prosthet Dent 29:408, 1973.

Steffel V: Planning removable partial dentures. J Prosthet Dent 12:524, 1962.

chapter 8

Types of partial dentures

Identification of the types of removable partial dentures should be done by use of a short, simple, easily understood, universal system that allows for precise communication with dental peers and with laboratory personnel.

There are two basic types of partial dentures, (1) *toothborne partial dentures* and (2) *extension partial dentures.*

Toothborne Partial Denture

The toothborne partial denture is self-explanatory in that the forces in function are borne primarily by the remaining natural teeth, which in turn transmit these forces to the periodontal ligament and to the bone structure for support (Fig. 8–1A and B). This type of partial denture is virtually synonymous with the fixed partial denture, if basic concepts are employed in the design plan. For the toothborne prosthesis, the rests can be placed in any position as long as they exert the forces in the long axis of the tooth. This requires positioning of the rest in the center of the tooth or on both sides of the tooth. The partial denture should always provide the greatest possible bracing, stability, and support for all remaining teeth in that arch.

Extension Partial Denture

The extension partial denture presents a unique situation in dental treatment, in that it relies upon two entirely different sources of support. In one instance, the support is derived through the tooth from the periodontal ligament and bone; the other source of support is the mucosa that covers the bone (Fig. 8–2A, B, and C). However, mucosa is not designed to act as a direct support tissue or to withstand the forces of occlusion. Its primary function is to cover the bone and the cervical area of the tooth while supplying necessary nourishment and acting as a protective mechanism to the tooth and surrounding structures.

After the removal of teeth, the mucosa forms coverage for that entire surface. When a denture base is placed over the mucosa and an occlusal force is applied, the mucosa is placed in a most unnatural situation. It is literally compressed between the hard surface of the denture base and the surface of the bone, and the blood supply is inhibited (Fig. 8–3A). If the nutrient supply to the bone and periosteum is compromised, change or resorption of the bone structure can result. The mucosa is not structured to withstand a pinching or compressive force and cannot function as it does under normal conditions.

A factor that dentists and patients must accept is that the extension partial denture, with its combination of tooth and mucosal support, causes an uneven or unequal balance of movement. This occurs because the mucosal support allows more movement of the prosthesis than does the tooth-supported portion of the prosthesis. This factor must be fully understood and analyzed in planning the partial denture design for functional movement. The amount of movement that will occur depends upon several circumstances: (1) the area of support; (2) the type and thickness of mucosa; (3) how well

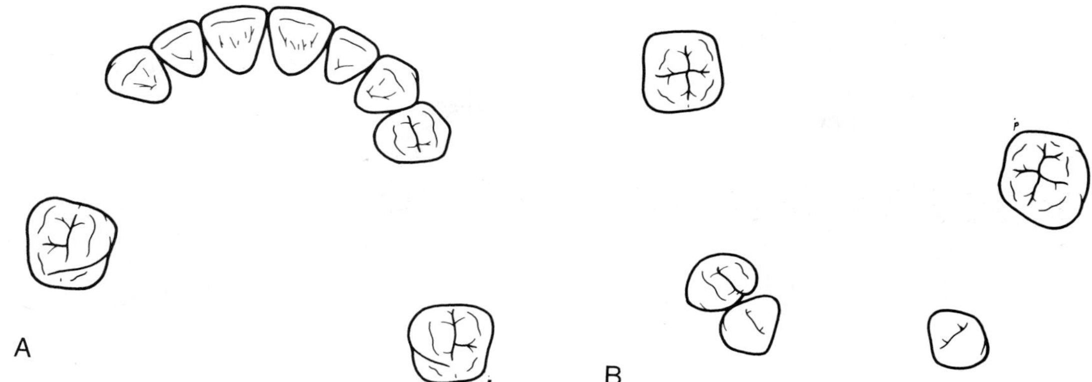

Figure 8–1 ■ *A*, Maxillary toothborne situation: Support will be provided by existing teeth. *B*, Mandibular toothborne situation: The prosthesis will restore function within the confines of the remaining teeth.

the edentulous area is used, that is, accuracy of impression and insertion adaptation; (4) refinement of the occlusal factors at completion and insertion of the prosthesis; (5) physiologic response of the individual patient, which, in turn, is dependent upon many biologic factors.

In planning the extension partial denture, the first point to consider is the location of the axis of rotation, which is determined by the position of the rests and, specifically, that part of the rest which is closest to the edentulous area (Fig. 8–3B and C). The most important and greatest movement to consider is the *movement that results during function* rather than the movement that occurs during removal.

All parts of the partial denture on the edentulous side of the axis of rotation move in an arc or circle in the direction of the edentulous bone

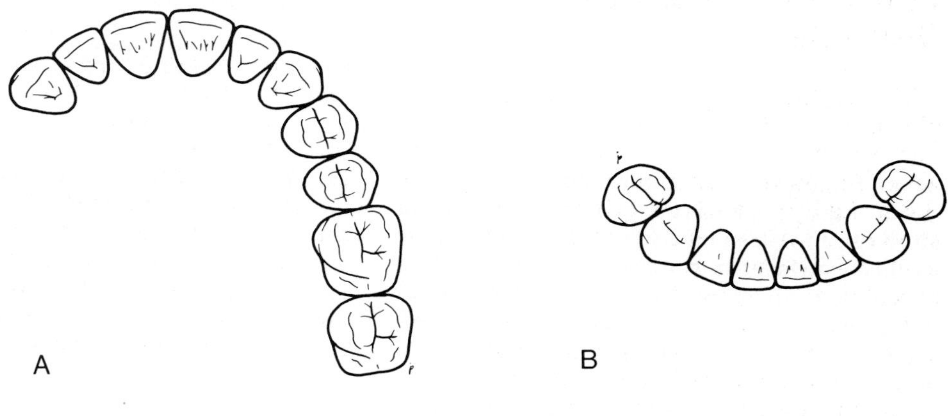

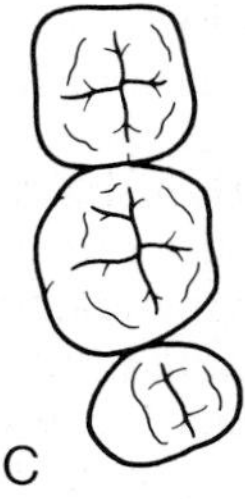

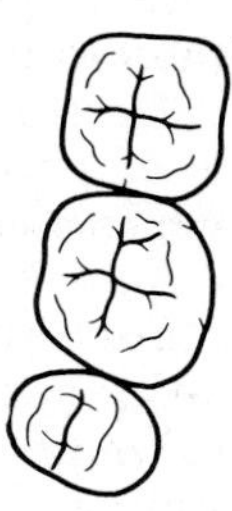

Figure 8–2 ■ *A*, Unilateral posterior extension: A combination of teeth and mucosa will provide support. *B*, Mandibular bilateral posterior extension: The partial denture will utilize a combination of teeth and edentulous area for support. *C*, Anterior extension partial denture situation.

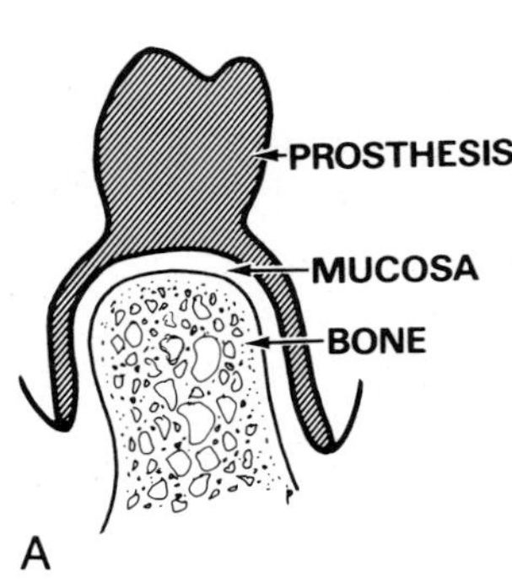

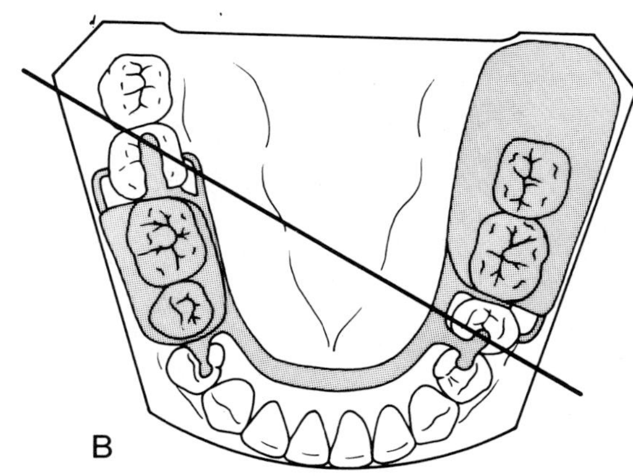

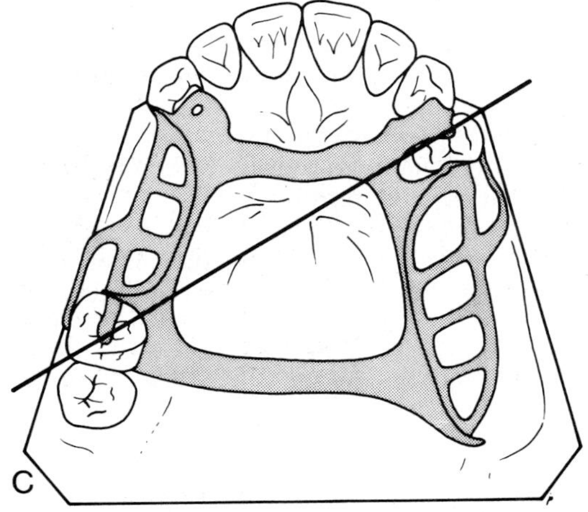

Figure 8–3 ■ *A*, Mandibular posterior extension partial denture: Mucosa provides denture support between bone and denture base. This is a most unnatural situation and tends to restrict blood supply to the mucosa. *B*, Mandibular unilateral extension partial denture: The rotation axis is located at the most posterior part of the rests adjacent to the edentulous area. *C*, Maxillary unilateral extension removable partial denture: Rotation axis.

when force is applied in the extension area. All parts of the prosthesis on the toothborne side of the axis of rotation tend to move away from the occlusal surfaces of the teeth (Fig. 8–4). Once this basic factor of movement around the axis of rotation is understood, it is possible to determine the direction of movement of all parts of the prosthesis in function or under occlusal load. If a position is taken looking down the axis of rotation and an imaginary series of circles is circumscribed extending outward from the center of the axis, the movement of all parts of the prosthesis can be visualized (Fig. 8–5).

Determination of this direction of movement is of paramount importance in placement of guide planes and retainers so that they do not torque, bind, or elevate the abutment teeth or other teeth in the arch. In some instances, these points of interference could actually become detrimental rotation points with incorrect designs.

Since the portion of the rest closest to the edentulous area becomes the axis of rotation, the rest preparation on the tooth at that point should be a perfect *half sphere* to provide an ideal rotation situation (Fig. 8–6). This rotation area should be about the size of a number 6 or 8 round bur and should be highly polished.

POSITIONING THE AXIS OF ROTATION TO PROVIDE THE BEST SUPPORT FOR THE EDENTULOUS AREA

A prime objective when planning treatment for a partially edentulous arch is to utilize all remaining tissues to their greatest potential. The edentulous area provides the best support when forces are directed at right angles to the surface of the mucosa and bone (Fig. 8–7A). Placement of the rest in relation to the edentu-

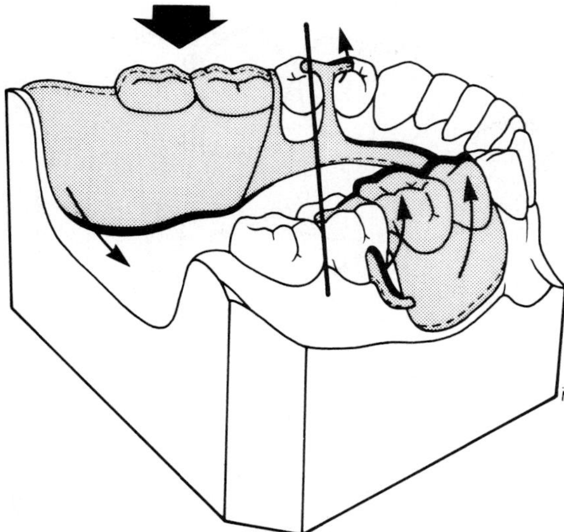

Figure 8–4 ■ Occlusal force applied —all parts of the prosthesis on the edentulous side of the rotation axis move toward the mucosa in an arc around the axis. All parts of the prosthesis on the toothborne side of the axis move in an arc away from the occlusal surface of the teeth.

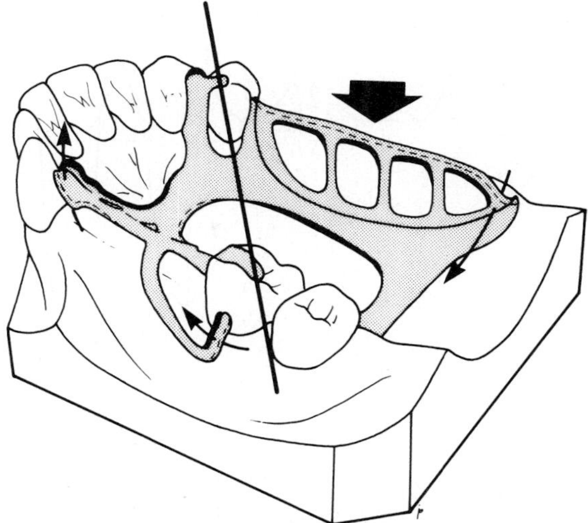

Figure 8–5 ■ A view looking directly down the rotation axis, diagramming the circles of movement.

lous area in an extension situation determines the rotation axis, which, in turn, determines the direction of movement of the prosthesis against the mucosa and bone.

Placement of the rest on the occlusal surface of the abutment tooth next to the edentulous area results in direct horizontal movement of the prosthesis at the gingival portion of the tooth (Fig. 8–7B). Little or no vertical support is obtained from the tissue next to the abutment tooth. This movement is at an angle to the supporting tissues and tends in movement to pinch or roll the mucosa between the bone and denture base.

As the rotation axis is moved anteriorly or away from the edentulous area (Fig. 8–7C), the arc of rotation becomes greater, and more of the denture base force is delivered in a vertical direction (Figs. 8–7C and D). Lowering of the rotation axis toward the gingiva improves the direction of force; consequently it is advisable to lower the rotation point whenever possible (Fig. 8–7E).

DIRECT EFFECT OF REST PLACEMENT ON ABUTMENT TEETH

Placement of a rest immediately adjacent to the edentulous area of an extension partial denture tends to pull or tip the tooth toward the edentulous area (Fig. 8–8); this has the effect of

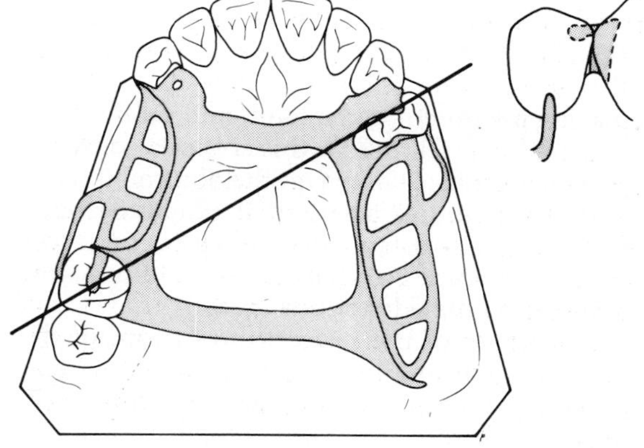

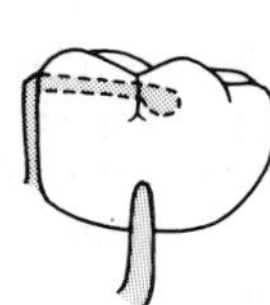

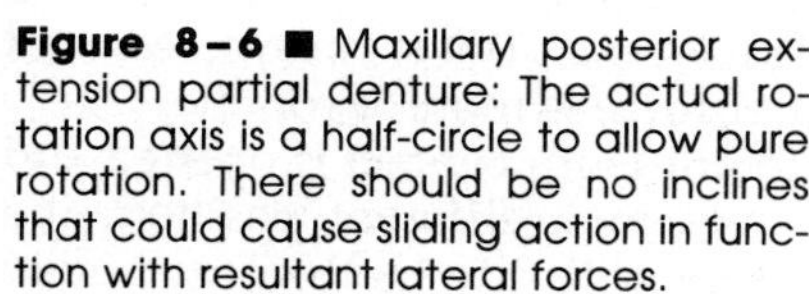

Figure 8–6 ■ Maxillary posterior extension partial denture: The actual rotation axis is a half-circle to allow pure rotation. There should be no inclines that could cause sliding action in function with resultant lateral forces.

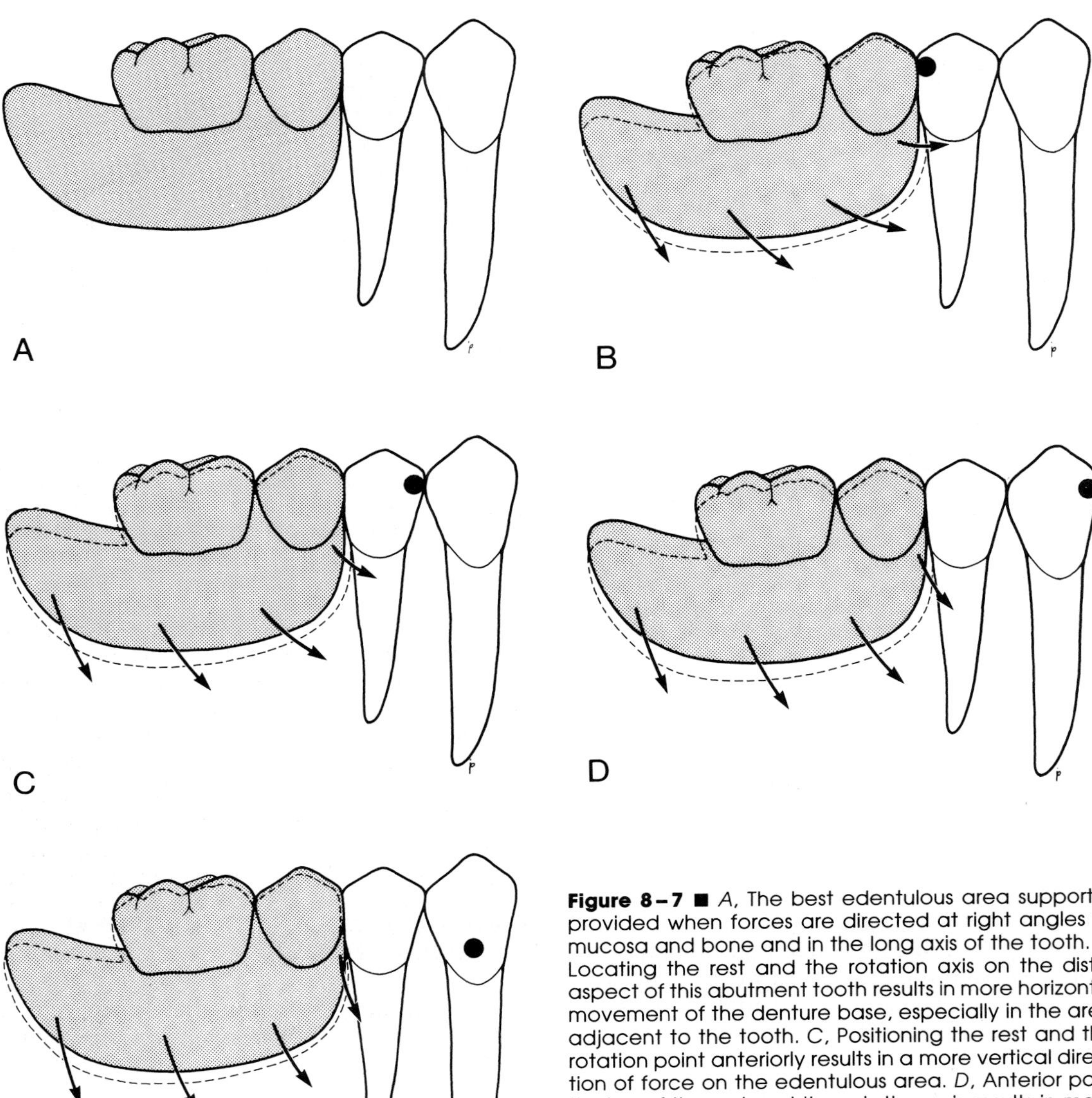

Figure 8–7 ■ *A*, The best edentulous area support is provided when forces are directed at right angles to mucosa and bone and in the long axis of the tooth. *B*, Locating the rest and the rotation axis on the distal aspect of this abutment tooth results in more horizontal movement of the denture base, especially in the area adjacent to the tooth. *C*, Positioning the rest and the rotation point anteriorly results in a more vertical direction of force on the edentulous area. *D*, Anterior positioning of the rest and the rotation axis results in more advantagous support from the denture base area. *E*, Lowering of the rest and the rotation axis results in the most ideal condition for denture base support.

placing a wrench on the tooth and producing a tipping force. Clinically, this is observed by the presence of space between the abutment tooth and the tooth adjacent to it. Radiologically, there is usually osteoblastic activity or bone loss at the tooth apex and at the crestal bone area adjacent to the edentulous area.

Placement of the rest on the surface of the tooth away from the edentulous area produces a tipping force in the opposite direction (Fig. 8–9). The identical amount of force from occlusal function is delivered to the tooth-rest area; however, the direction of force tends to move the abutment tooth toward remaining teeth, producing a tight interproximal contact and utilizing other teeth besides the single abutment tooth to help control the position of teeth and prosthesis. The wrench effect is reversed, and the direction of force is more favorable.

If the abutment tooth contact is opened and the tooth moves to a different position, the prosthesis moves with the tooth. This bodily

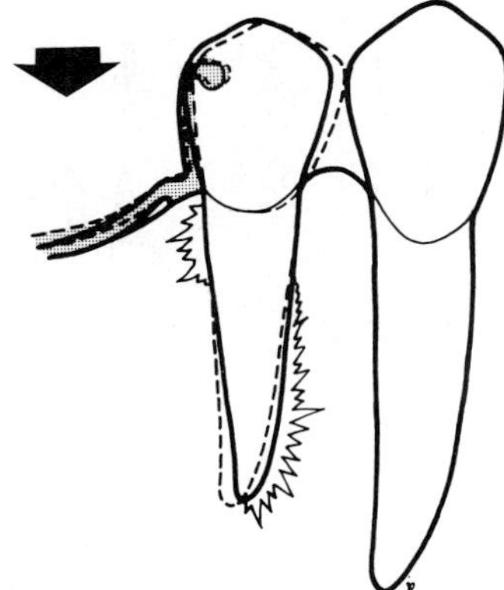

Figure 8–8 ■ Placement of the rest adjacent to the extension edentulous area may produce a tipping force during function, which opens the contact between teeth and moves the tooth, causing mobility and bone loss.

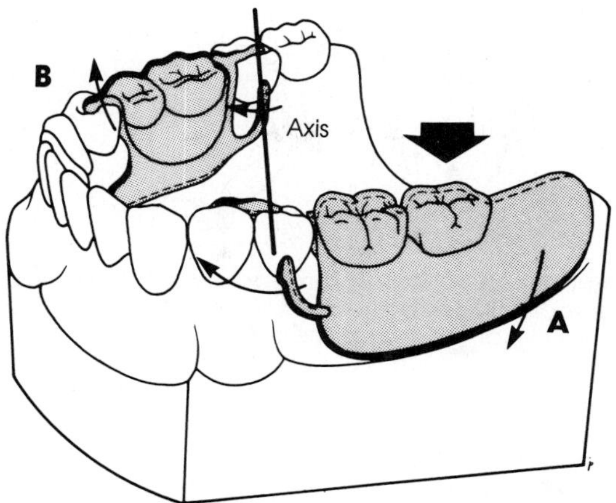

Figure 8–10 ■ The direction of retainer movement is determined by the location of the rotational axis. Note the direction of movement on both sides of the rotation axis at points A and B.

movement disrupts the occlusion developed at the time of insertion and produces occlusal interferences, which, in turn, cause excessive force to be placed on the remaining teeth and on the edentulous area (Fig. 8–8).

DESIGN AND POSITIONING OF THE RETAINER

Movement of retainers on an extension partial denture in function is determined by the rotation axis (Fig. 8–10). Directional movement of the retainers must be controlled so that contact is diminished or eliminated when the partial denture moves from a passive position to a functional movement position. The contact engagement of the retainer should occur only in a *removal* action. For example, given a mandibular posterior extension situation (Fig. 8–11), in which the rotation axis is on the mesial occlusal surface of the abutment tooth, the retentive tip of the I bar is placed at the point of greatest circumference of that premolar on the facial surface (Fig. 8–12) and moves downward and forward under occlusal load, disengaging from the tooth (Fig. 8–11). As the rest and the rotation axis are moved farther away from the extension area, the retainer tip disengages more rapidly during occlusal function (Figs. 8–13 and 8–14). It is not advisable to position the

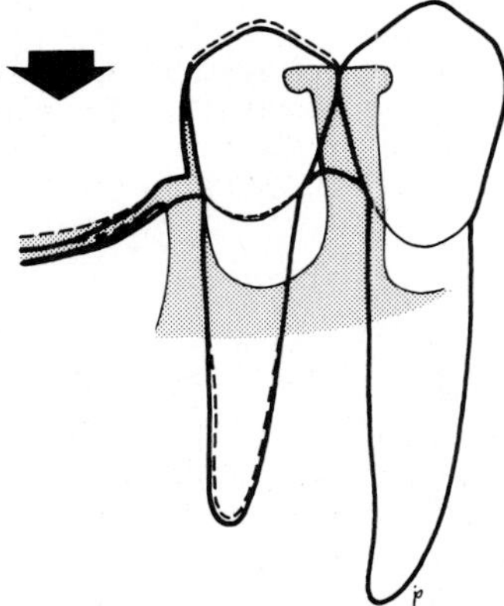

Figure 8–9 ■ Moving the rest away from the edentulous area produces a direction of force that tends to maintain contact with adjacent teeth, resulting in multiple tooth support and acceptable directions of force.

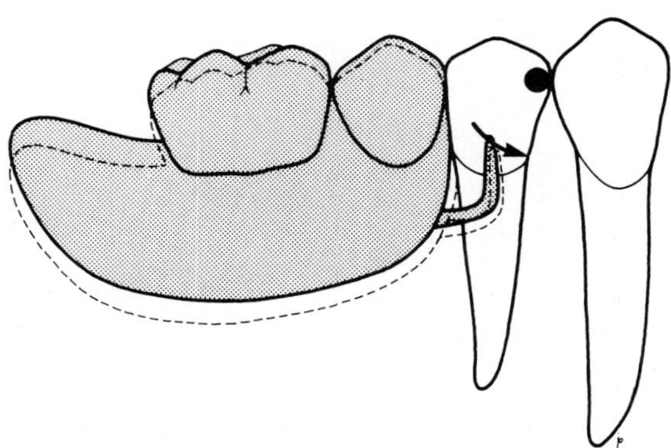

Figure 8–11 ■ Anterior positioning of the rest results in forward and downward movement of the retainer during occlusal force, preventing torque on the tooth.

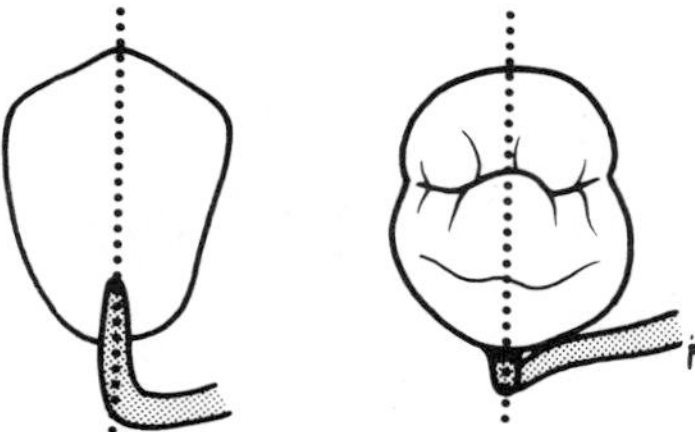

Figure 8–12 ■ Occlusal and facial view. The retainer contact is placed at the point of greatest mesial-distal curvature of the tooth. The retainer will then disengage under the force of functional biting.

retentive tip of the retainer distal to the center of the tooth or distal to the point of greatest circumference of the tooth, since any forward movement of the retainer may torque the tooth and harm the supporting structures (Fig. 8–15).

RETAINER POSITIONED FORWARD OF THE AXIS OF ROTATION

The retentive portion of a retainer should not engage an undercut *forward of the axis of rotation* in an extension situation, since that part of the prosthesis moves upward in function (Fig. 8–16) and will tend to torque the tooth. The periodontal ligament acts as a sling and exerts a pull on the bone when loaded occlusally. A lifting action on the tooth is abnormal and may cause periodontal problems (Fig. 8–17).

If a retainer is placed anterior to the rotation point, it is placed at the height of contour without engaging the undercut area and lifts free of contact during function. The retainer may be placed on the canine for two reasons: (1) Contact with the tooth provides some retention because of parallelism and friction between the lingual rest and the retainer (such as the retention of a full gold crown provided by parallel preparation). (2) If there is a possibility of posterior abutment tooth loss, a replacement tooth could be added to the prosthesis as an immediate procedure at the time of the loss. The retainer could then be altered and recontoured to engage an undercut area and to provide the necessary retention.

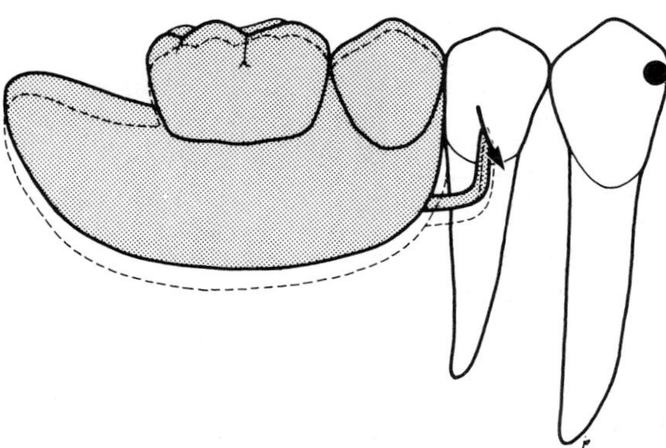

Figure 8–13 ■ Moving the rotation axis forward provides quicker retainer disengagement and diminished possibility of tooth torque caused by the retainer.

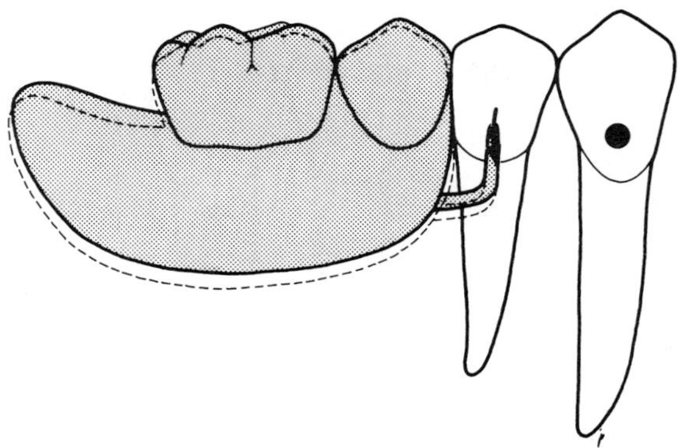

Figure 8–14 ■ Lowering the rotation axis produces the most ideal retainer movement. Note that the retainer contact is positioned in the center of the tooth.

Attention must be given to position and placement of the retainers on the opposite side of the arch from the extension side. When the prosthesis moves in function, that movement is reproduced throughout the partial denture. Retainers on all teeth in all parts of the mouth move according to the basic laws of physics and must be designed to prevent tooth engagement, except against removal activity; Figure 8–3B illustrates this point. The lingual retainer on the molar engages a tooth undercut, and in biting function moves downward and forward, disen-

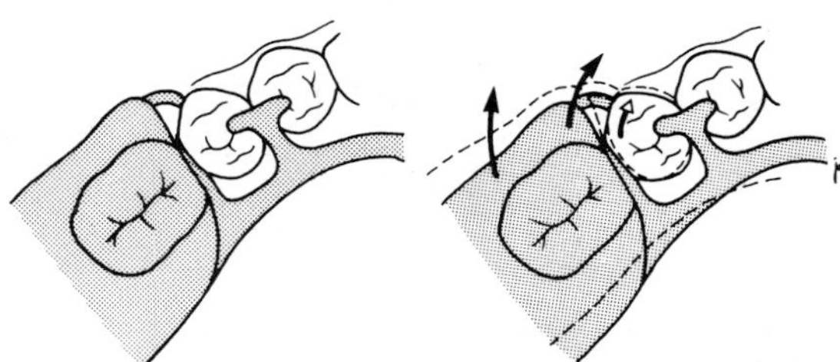

Figure 8–15 ■ Occlusal view. The retainer *must not* be placed behind the greatest curvature of the tooth in an *extension* situation because it could torque the tooth as the retainer moves forward in function.

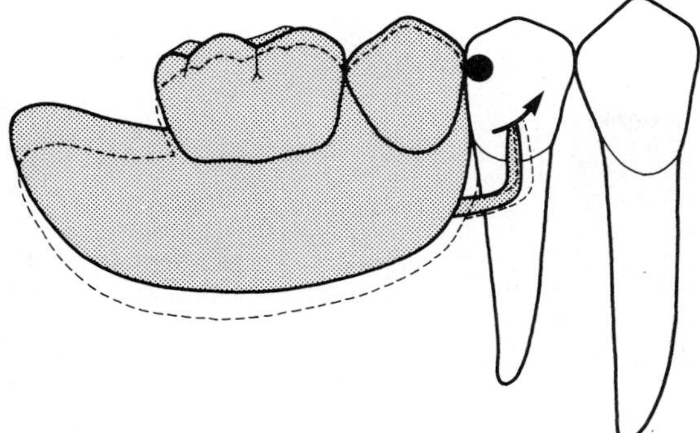

Figure 8–16 ■ If the rotation axis or the rest is placed between the retainer and the extension denture base, the retainer moves upward, engaging and torquing the tooth when the patient applies occlusal force.

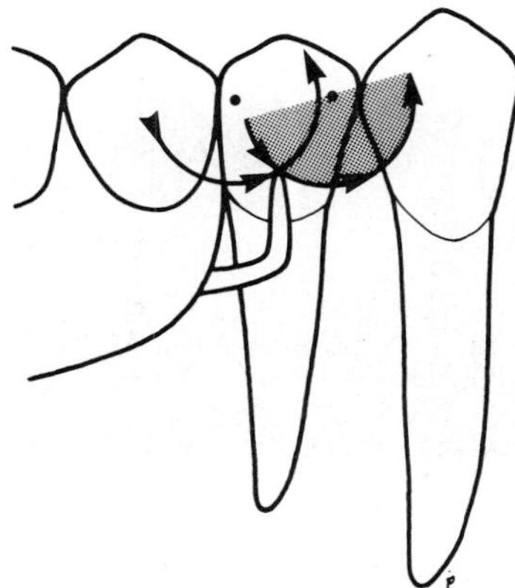

Figure 8–18 ■ Rest placement at a mesial or distal location controls the rotation axis, which has a profound influence on the direction of movement of the retainer contact area.

gaging tooth contact. During a removal motion it engages and provides retention.

A review of the physics and the geometry of an extension removable partial denture in function demonstrates the influence that rest placement has on the direction of movement of the retentive portion of the retainer. Moving the rest position from a distal to a mesial location on one tooth can change the direction of movement of the retainer 180 degrees (Fig. 8–18). Retainer position must always be coordinated with rest position so that the retainer disengages from tooth contact during closure movement of the mandible.

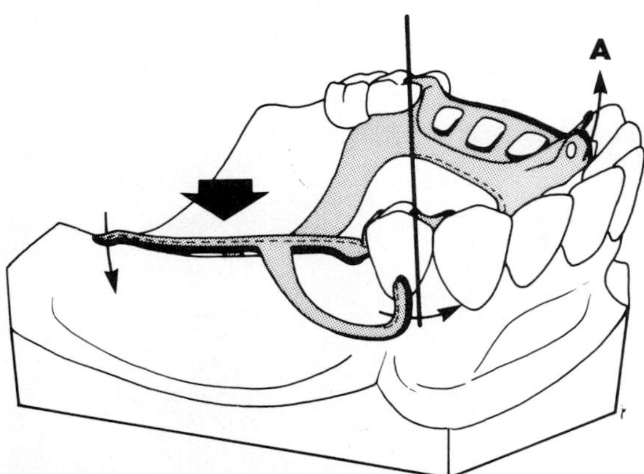

Figure 8–17 ■ All parts of the prosthesis forward of the axis of rotation lift off the teeth when the edentulous area is loaded. If a retainer is placed on the canine (point A), it *should not* engage the undercut, or it will tend to lift the canine, with resulting periodontal involvement.

DIAGONAL PLACEMENT OF THE AXIS OF ROTATION

In some instances, design of the partial denture casting results in one end of the rotation axis occurring low on a tooth next to the gum, as in the case of a lingual cervical rest on a canine, with the other end of the axis high on the occlusal surface of a tooth such as the second premolar (Fig. 8–19). This high-low axis position develops unusual directional movement of all parts of the prosthesis when in function. Most diagrammatic analysis is done in two planes; however, function in three planes must be considered.

When the position of the rotation axis is anterior on one side of the arch and posterior on the opposite side (Fig. 8–10), the direction of movement of all parts of the prosthesis is more difficult to analyze. In many instances, final assessment must be made intraorally at the time of the casting try-in.

A special effort must be made to prevent any portion of the casting that might be contacting an inclined tooth surface from becoming a rotation point; not only does this affect the movement direction of the retainer and other parts of the partial denture, but it also tends to move the tooth out of position and allows the prosthesis to move against the tissue, causing recession and damage.

Movement of Guiding Surfaces in Function

Other portions of the extension prosthesis are affected by functional movements and by the

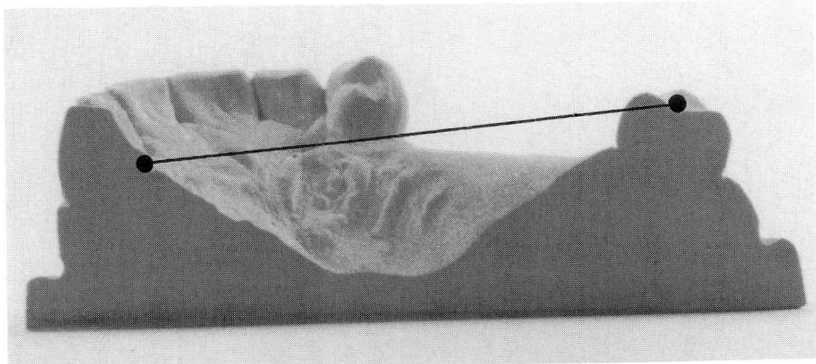

Figure 8–19 ■ A high-low rotation axis develops angular movements of the prosthesis in function. Close assessment of possible torquing action is indicated at the time of casting try-in.

axis of rotation. Of particular concern are the guiding surfaces of the casting, which contact the surface of the teeth next to the edentulous area (Fig. 8–20), and the connectors, which extend from the major connectors to the rests (Fig. 8–21).

The rationale for complete contact of the metal casting at the crestal gingival tissues has been presented. However, it must be noted that when the partial prosthesis moves in function, these guiding surfaces may bind or become sliding rotation points (Fig. 8–22A and B). To prevent this binding of prosthesis on teeth, it is necessary to *physiologically adjust* the casting in the mouth. Each tooth has its own individual movement that is normal; teeth have different root configurations that influence their movement and function. This individual movement can be buccal, mesial, distal, lingual, or a slight turning of the tooth or a combination of these movements.

It is not possible on an inanimate stone cast to engineer or design a partial denture casting that allows for all individual teeth idiosyncrasies and different functional movements; thus, the need for adjustment of the casting in function in the mouth.

Physiologic Adjustment Procedure

When the casting is returned from the laboratory, it is carefully inspected as to design and is compared with the design submitted on the diagnostic cast. Fit of casting to all surfaces of the cast is verified (Fig. 8–23). All internal surfaces are inspected for sharp points, small bubbles, or voids.

Place the casting in the patient's mouth and check for complete seating of all rests. Check adaptation of all other parts of the casting for proper adaptation to teeth and mucosa (Fig. 8–24).

When the casting is properly seated, a disclosing medium is applied to all surfaces that contact tooth structure. One excellent disclosure medium is gold rouge painted on the metal

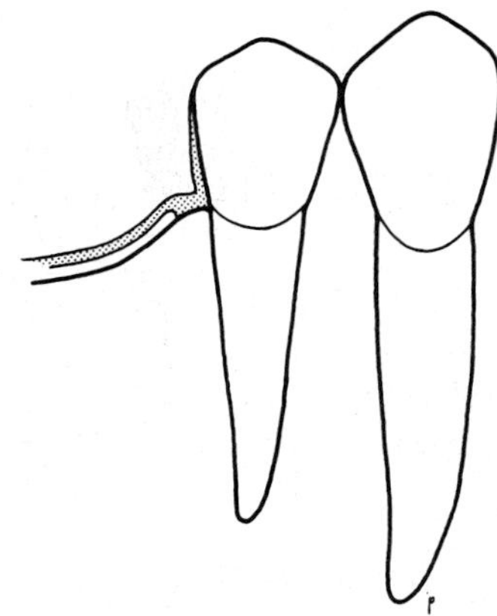

Figure 8–20 ■ The guiding surfaces of the casting are designed to contact the surface of the tooth and the crestal mucosa.

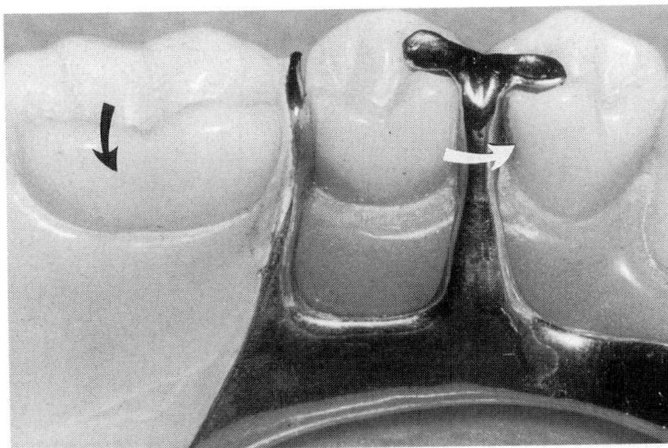

Figure 8–21 ■ Lingual view, mandibular posterior extension prosthesis. The lingual strut between the premolars and the distal guiding surface could bind or torque the teeth as the prosthesis moves in function.

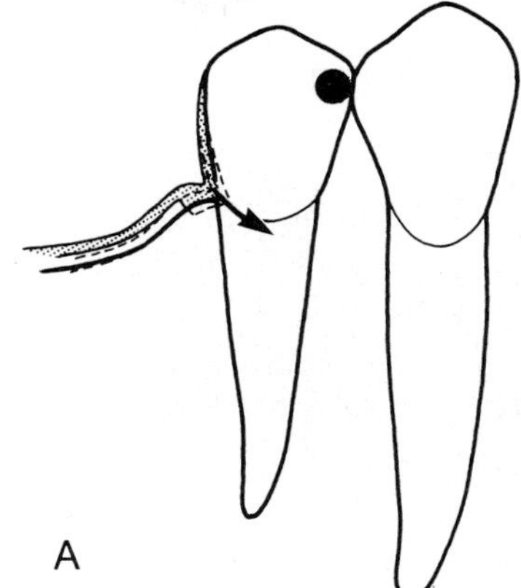

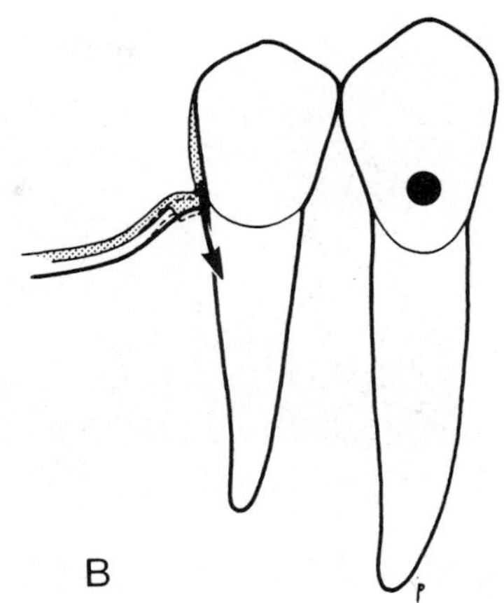

Figure 8–22 ■ *A*, In function, the distal guiding surface could engage the tooth surface, producing a torquing action. *B*, Lowering of the rotation axis greatly reduces the potential for binding of the distal guiding surface.

surface using chloroform to dissolve the rouge (Fig. 8–25). The chloroform quickly evaporates, leaving a thin coat of dry rouge that marks readily to show tooth contacts (Fig. 8–26). The casting is placed in the mouth and moved as in biting function, with heavy pressure applied (Fig. 8–27). This pressure produces some of the tooth movement that occurs during function as well as casting contact against the teeth (Fig. 8–28). Binding contact areas on guiding surfaces next to edentulous areas are readily identified and relieved with grinding stones or carbide burs (Figs. 8–29 and 8–30).

It is especially important to investigate contact areas between teeth, where the casting extends to the rests on occlusal surfaces (Figs. 8–21 and 8–31). Contact in these areas during function may create a wedging action, which forces the teeth apart. Adjustment is continued until the casting moves easily in function, with the rest at the axis of rotation rolling smoothly in its rest seat without lifting.

This physiologic adjustment establishes a safety factor for abutment teeth: If there is excessive movement of the prosthesis due to bone resorption or poor edentulous area support, the forces transmitted to the abutment teeth remain in the long axis of the teeth.

LINGUAL DESIGN CONSIDERATIONS FOR THE EXTENSION PARTIAL DENTURE

The effects of partial denture movement on teeth have been discussed as they relate to tooth

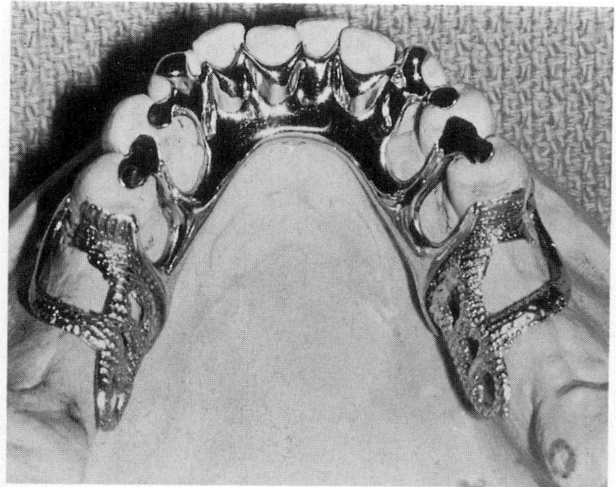

Figure 8–23 ■ The casting is carefully inspected for proper adaptation to teeth and to tissue areas. The casting is compared to the design on the diagnostic cast. The undersurface is checked for sharp points or voids.

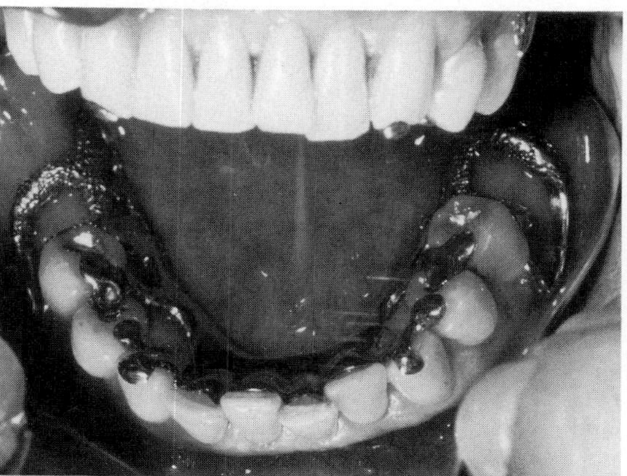

Figure 8–24 ■ The casting is placed in the mouth and checked for proper adaption and fit to teeth and mucosa. (See also Color Plate 1, p XVII.)

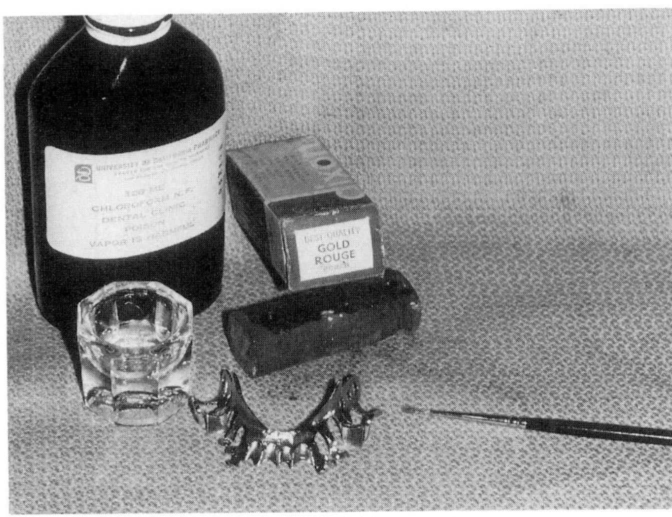

Figure 8–25 ■ Disclosing medium is used to demonstrate areas of binding. (See also Color Plate 1, p XVII.)

contact on facial, mesial, and distal points. The effects of such movement on the lingual aspect need to be considered.

All forces and denture movements affecting the abutment teeth that have been described could also occur on the lingual surface of the teeth. To prevent potential torquing of teeth, the casting does not contact the lingual surface of the posterior teeth. An exception is the placement of lingual struts; they cross the tooth soft tissue junction at right angles to the occlusal plane or long axis of the tooth for maximum self-cleansing and drop to the junction of the unattached mucosa, where they turn to follow the crest of the unattached mucosa (Fig. 8–31). With this design, the potential for teeth becoming torqued from the lingual aspect is minimized, and tooth-tissue junctions are kept as open as possible.

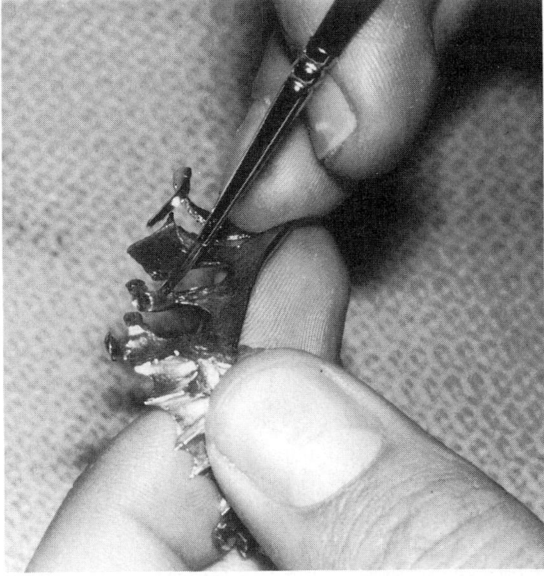

Figure 8–26 ■ Gold rouge dissolved in chloroform is painted on the casting surfaces that contact the teeth. Dry with air to produce a good disclosing surface. (See also Color Plate 1, p XVII.)

EVALUATION OF OTHER RETAINER DESIGNS

Other types of extracoronal retainers are the circumferential retainers as described by

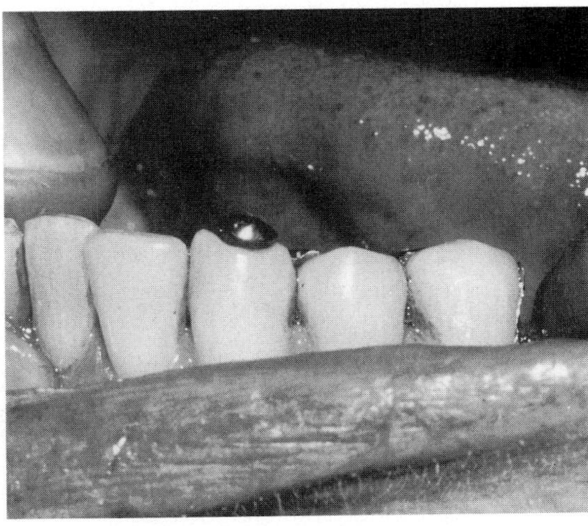

Figure 8–27 ■ Movement with heavy pressure, simulating functional movement, is produced in the mouth. (See also Color Plate 2, p XVIII.)

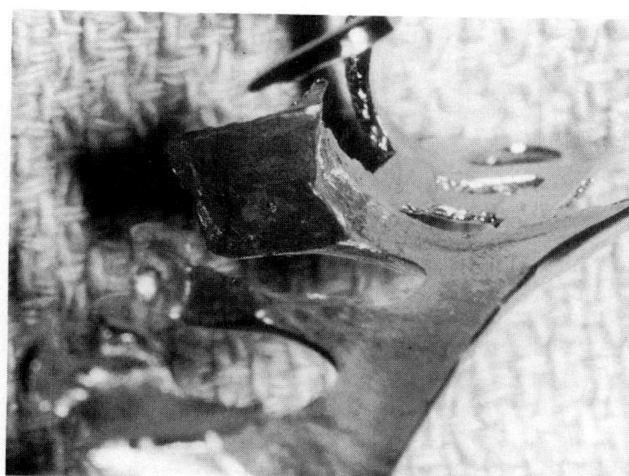

Figure 8–28 ■ Areas of contact or binding are identified as light areas where the disclosing medium is rubbed off. Struts placed between teeth must be carefully checked. (See also Color Plate 2, p XVIII.)

DeVan. They may be suprabulge (Fig. 8–32) (attached to the casting at the occlusal surface of tooth) or infrabulge (Fig. 8–37) (attached to the casting from a soft tissue or apical direction). The important point to be considered regarding retainer movement is that all the elements are part of a single casting, and therefore the prosthesis moves as a unit (Fig. 8–32). The basic

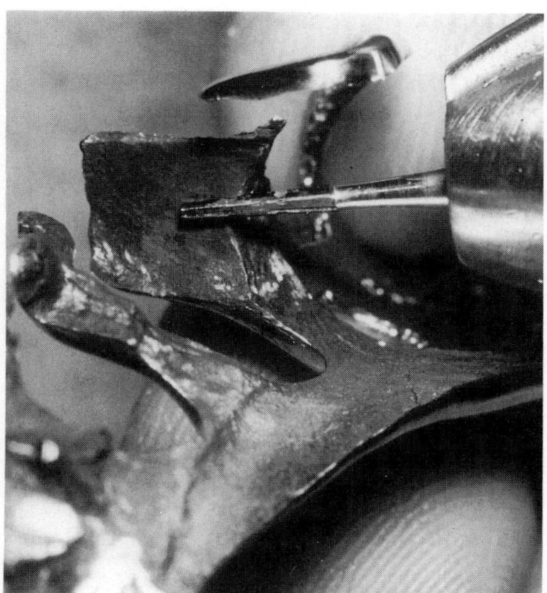

Figure 8–29 ■ Areas of heavy contact are relieved with a high speed carbide bur or stone. The procedure is repeated until the casting rotates smoothly without lifting in the rest areas that form the rotational axis. (See also Color Plate 2, p XVIII.)

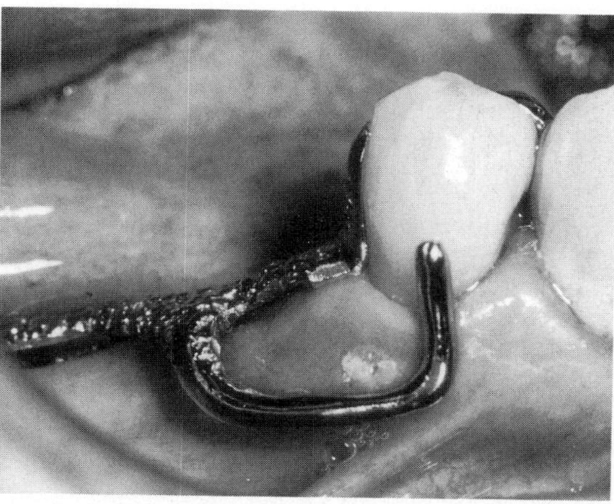

Figure 8–30 ■ Adjustment results in a well-adapted casting that allows functional prosthetic movement, keeping forces in the long axis of the abutment teeth without producing torquing forces. (See also Color Plate 2, p XVIII.)

factor in the direction of movement is the relationship of the retainers to the axis of rotation. An analysis of all retainer systems is presented to help in the understanding of forces affecting abutment teeth.

Suprabulge Circumferential Retainer

The circumferential retainer is commonly used to provide retention for the prosthesis (Fig. 8–32). The retentive part is the terminal end of the casting, which usually engages a tooth undercut. Analysis of the effect of function or movement employing a distal rotating axis illustrates the forces exerted on the tooth (Fig. 8–33).

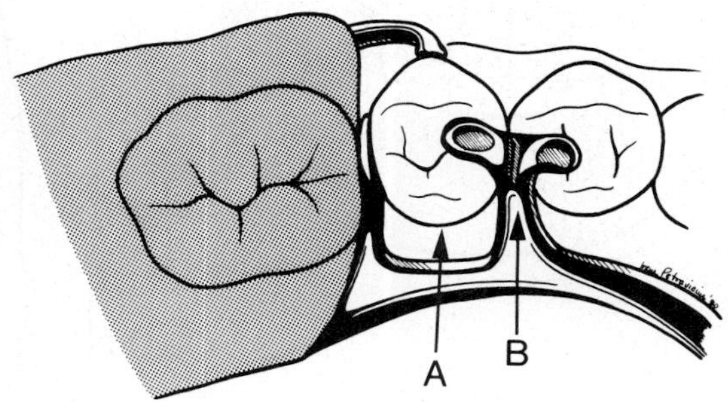

Figure 8–31 ■ The casting is designed so as not to engage the lingual tooth surface at point A. The lingual strut, B, is placed parallel to the long axis of the tooth until it reaches unattached mucosa before continuing anteriorly or posteriorly as the lingual bar.

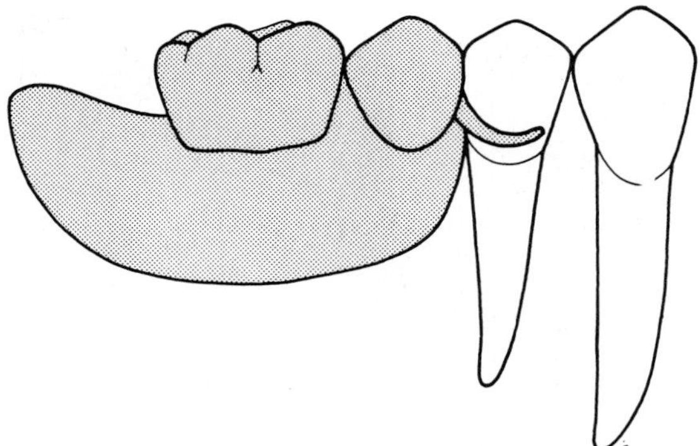

Figure 8–32 ■ Evaluation of the suprabulge circumferential retainer. The completed prosthesis is cast as a single unit and moves a unit. A basic concept in prosthetic design is the prevention of movement of the abutment tooth by the prosthesis.

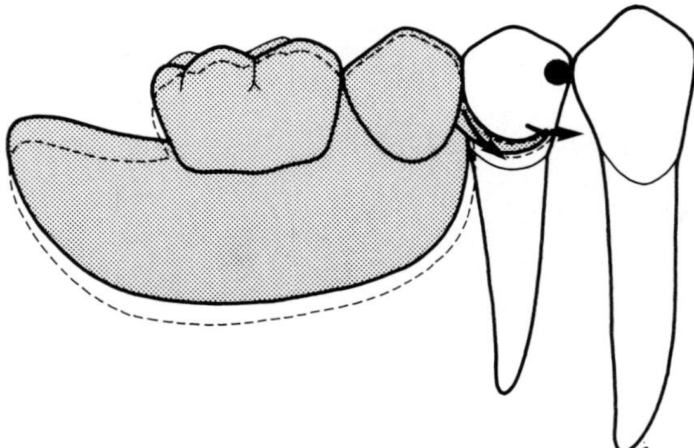

Figure 8–34 ■ Anterior rest and rotation axis. The distal portion of the retainer moving forward may engage and torque the tooth.

Moving the rotation axis to the mesial aspect of the tooth changes the direction of movement of the retainer (Fig. 8–34). However, the potential for torque is present because the distal portion of the retainer curves around the tooth, as seen when observed from an occlusal view. Any contact of the casting with the tooth at this point tends to rotate the tooth.

Moving the axis of rotation farther forward (Fig. 8–35) again changes the direction of retainer movement. However, anytime a retainer crosses the survey line of the tooth and makes contact above and below the survey line, it has a *grip* on the tooth, and as the retainer moves, so moves the tooth. (Fig. 8–36).

Infrabulge Circumferential Retainers

The infrabulge circumferential retainer (Fig. 8–37) manifests the same physical geometric movements as those demonstrated by the suprabulge circumferential retainer. The direction of retainer movement is controlled by the position of the axis of rotation. If the retainer crosses the survey line on the tooth or wraps around the distal curvature of the tooth, it has the potential to torque the abutment tooth in function (Figs. 8–38 through 8–41). Again, the amount of movement of the extension base depends upon the proper utilization of the residual ridge, proper occlusion, and the physiologic stability of the edentulous ridge.

Recommended Retainer Design and Position

A full understanding of factors involved in movement of the extension partial denture in-

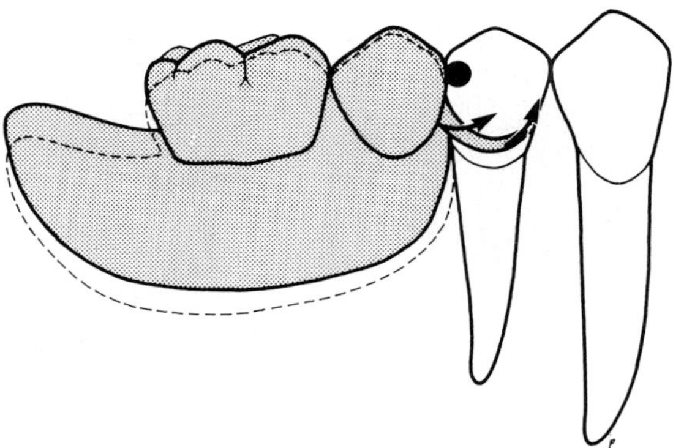

Figure 8–33 ■ Mandibular extension prosthesis with a distal rest and a circumferential retainer. If the retainer terminal engages the tooth undercut and excessive movement occurs, the tooth may be torqued.

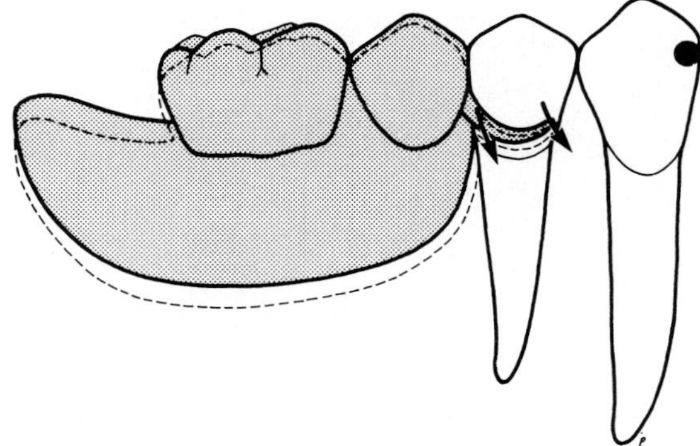

Figure 8–35 ■ The rest and the rotation point are moved anteriorly. At the point where the retainer crosses the survey line it could torque the tooth or actually become the rotation point during function.

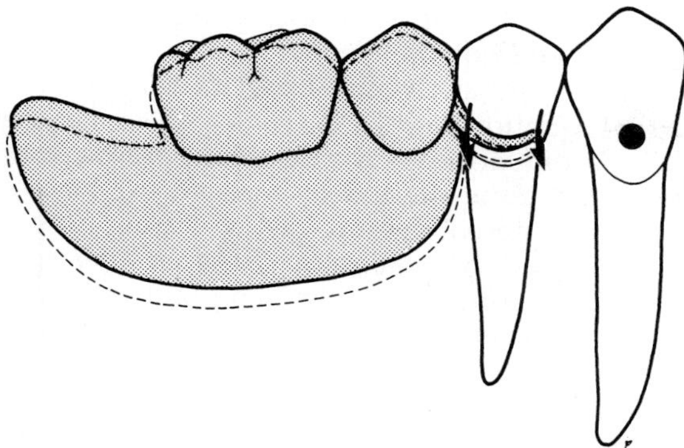

Figure 8–36 ■ Lowering the rotation point and the anterior rest will *not* prevent pressure by the circumferential retainer on the tooth.

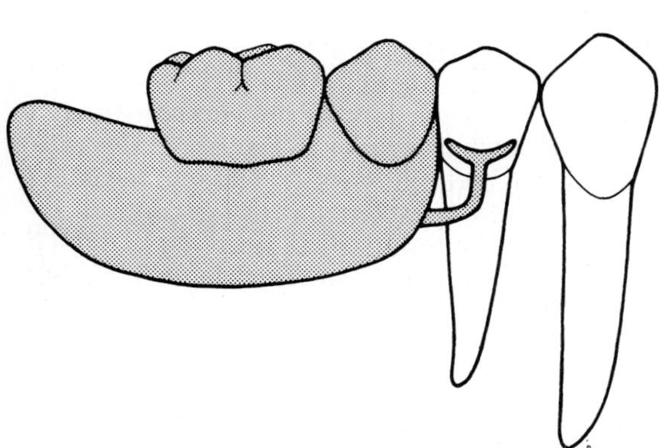

Figure 8–37 ■ The infrabulge T-shaped retainer.

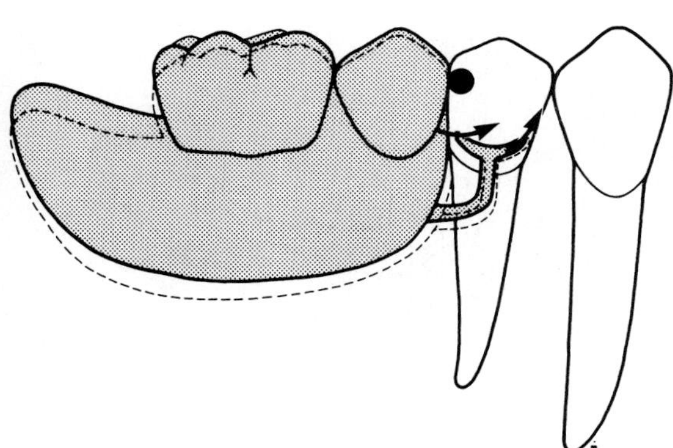

Figure 8–38 ■ Use of the distal rest or rotation axis in conjunction with the infrabulge T retainer tends to pull the tooth posteriorly and to torque it as the distal wing of the retainer moves forward.

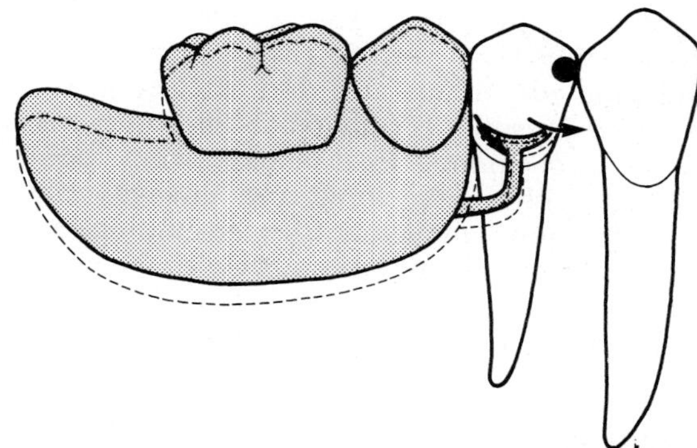

Figure 8–39 ■ Placing the rotation rest anteriorly *will not* remove the potential torquing action of the distal arm of the T retainer.

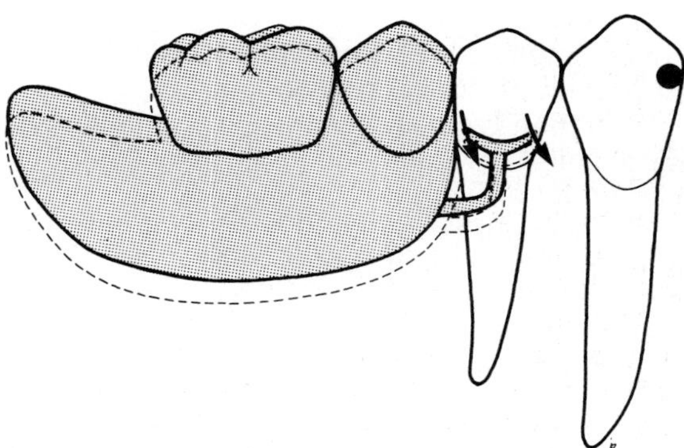

Figure 8–40 ■ Moving the rotation axis further forward does not eliminate the possibility of torque; the factors of excessive tooth area contact and engagement of distal tooth contour remain.

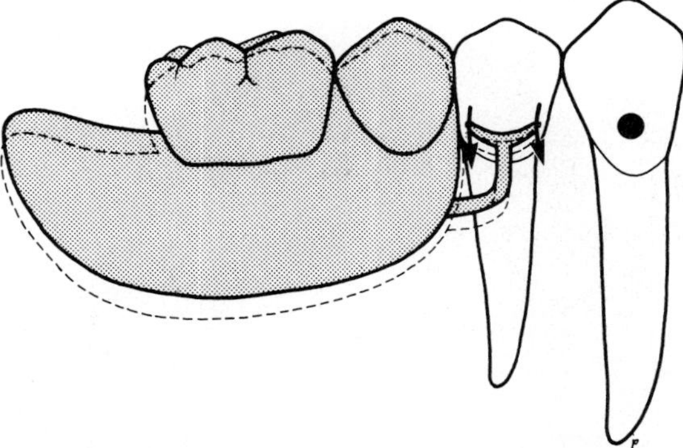

Figure 8–41 ■ Moving the rotation axis forward and down improves the direction of movement of the denture base and the retainer. *However*, if the T-bar retainer crosses the survey line of the tooth, it will exert *torquing* action on the tooth when the partial prosthesis is in function.

dicates that the most stable results can be obtained when (1) the rotation axis is placed away from the edentulous area and as close to the bone as possible; (2) the I-bar infrabulge retainer is positioned to disengage from tooth contact with biting force and engage only against removal movement; (3) the guiding surfaces keep basic position contact with the tooth but do not engage the tooth in function (Figs. 8–11, 8–13, and 8–14).

PHOTOELASTIC ANALYSIS OF PRESSURE ON TOOTH AND BONE SUPPORTING REMOVABLE PARTIAL DENTURES

The philosophic basis and clinical procedures for removable partial denture design presented in this chapter were successful, according to the evaluation of clinical results.

With the advent of photoelastic techniques, it is possible to evaluate the procedures from the standpoint of laboratory research.

Three major premises of treatment with removable partial dentures are that

1. The force of greatest concern is the occlusal biting force.

2. The force on the abutment teeth should be exerted and controlled primarily through the rest.

3. The direction of delivered force should be along the long axis of the tooth for the best advantage of the periodontal ligament, and the potential for tilting or torquing the abutment tooth should be minimized.

Photoelastic analysis can provide the following information:

1. A comparison of the directions of force on teeth and bone exerted by a distal extension removable partial denture casting during function *before and after the casting has been adjusted.*

2. A recording of the direction and position of force on teeth and bone when the partial denture is *in simulated function.*

The distal extension removable partial denture tested (Fig. 8–42) was designed with an anterior rest on the abutment tooth. All other aspects of its design followed the principles recommended and described in this text. The casting was tested before and after physiologic adjustment.

A photoelastic replica of the mandible was fabricated (Fig. 8–42). This model was made with individual simulations of (A) the entire tooth, (B) the periodontal ligament, and (C) the bone portion of the mandible (Fig. 8–43).

A removable partial denture was constructed on this model according to the principles outlined in the text (Fig. 8–42). The metal casting was relieved to prevent soft tissue contact, except over the edentulous denture base, which contained a uniform 2-mm thick layer of rubber base impression material placed on the edentulous ridge to simulate the resilience of mucosa (Fig. 8–44).

The photoelastic plastic model was mounted on a table in the center of a straining frame that

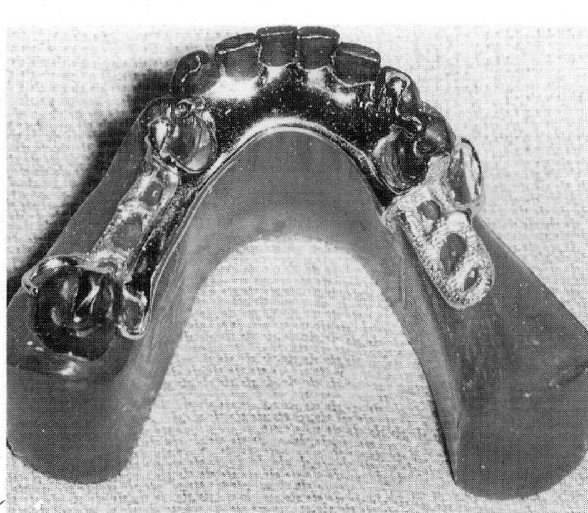

Figure 8–42 ■ The partial denture design to be tested in place on the photoelastic model.

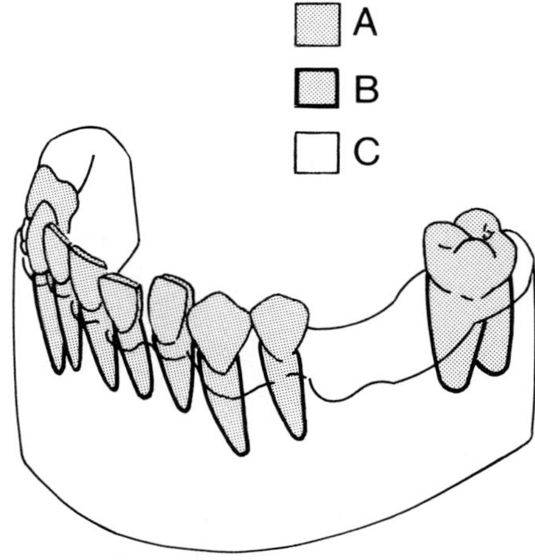

Figure 8–43 ■ The photoelastic model is constructed with three different hardnesses of photoelastic plastic for the three different areas: *A*, the entire tooth; *B*, the periodontal ligament; *C*, bone.

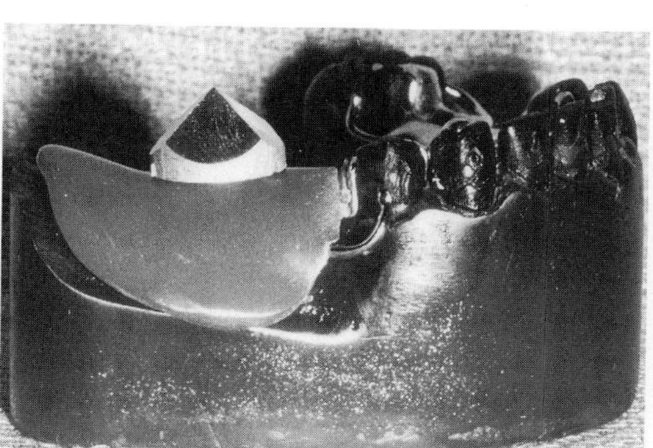

Figure 8–44 ■ The tissue side of the denture base has a 2 mm thickness of rubber base material to simulate mucosa. The metal pyramid on the occlusal surface permits a load to be delivered in various directions.

could rotate 360 degrees (Fig. 8–45). A fixed light source was placed in the center of the model. The model was rotated around the light source for viewing and photographing of all teeth and supporting structures while the denture was under a controlled load.

A metal cone with the four sides machined to 45-degree angles was prepared and attached to the occlusal surface of the denture base so that

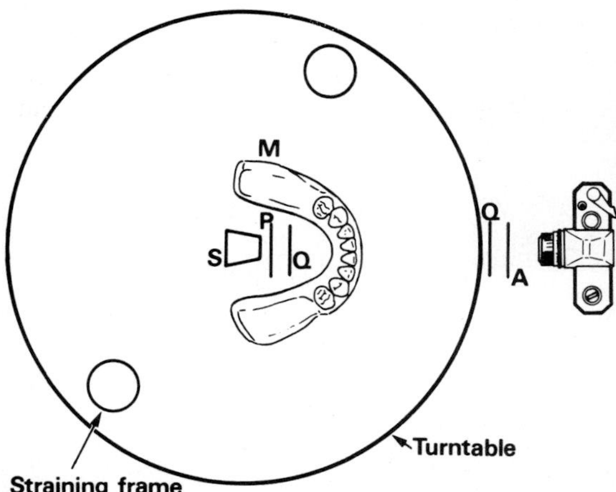

S FIBER OPTIC LIGHT SOURCE
P POLARIZATION
Q QUARTER WAVE PLATE - CIRCULAR POLARIZED LIGHT
A ANALYZER - POLARIZER
M MODEL - BIREFRINGENT PLASTIC

Figure 8– 45 ■ The arrangement of the model on a turntable with the placement of light, lens, and camera. S = Fiberoptic light source; P = polarization; Q = quarter wave plate—circular polarized light; A = analyzer—polarizer; M = model—bifringent plastic.

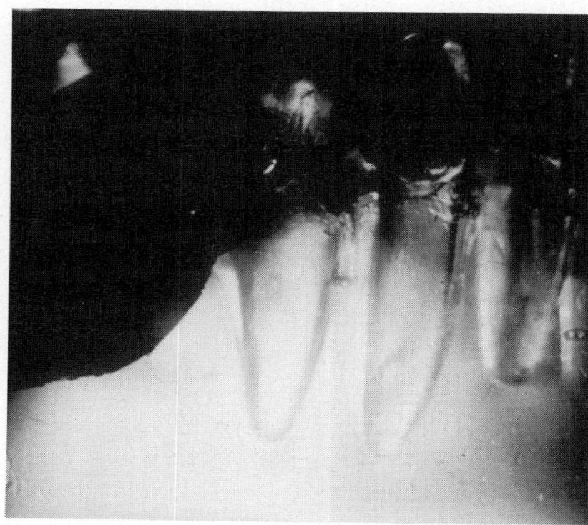

Figure 8–46 ■ A control picture of the photoelastic model with no pressure applied. (See also Color Plate 2, p XVIII.)

loads could be delivered in different directions to simulate occlusal, buccal, lingual, mesial, and distal forces. Opposite the light source and at the same level were cameras to record results.

A load was delivered to the distal extension portion of the removable partial denture. The results showed the difference in force area and location before and after the casting was adjusted.

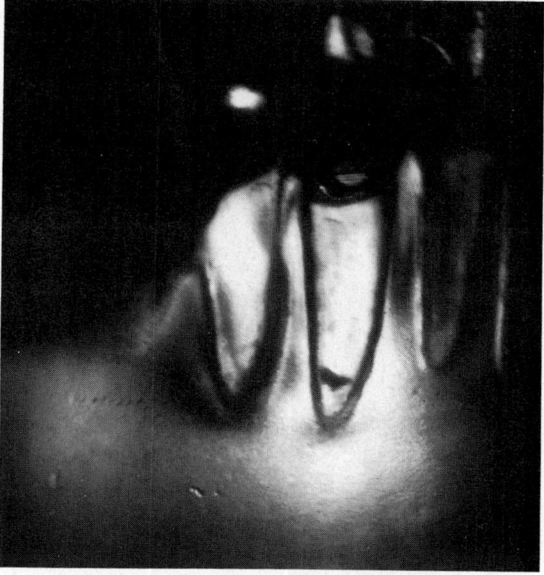

Figure 8–47 ■ The unadjusted casting in place, with a vertical load of 25 lb applied. Note the lateral force areas. (See also Color Plate 3, p XIX.)

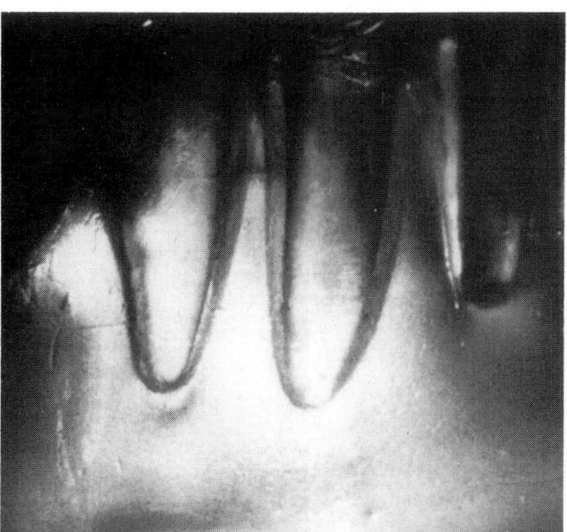

Figure 8–48 ■ The casting is physiologically adjusted—a 25-lb vertical load is applied. Note that lateral force areas have disappeared, and the forces are concentrated around the apex and in the long axis of the tooth. (See also Color Plate 3, p XIX.)

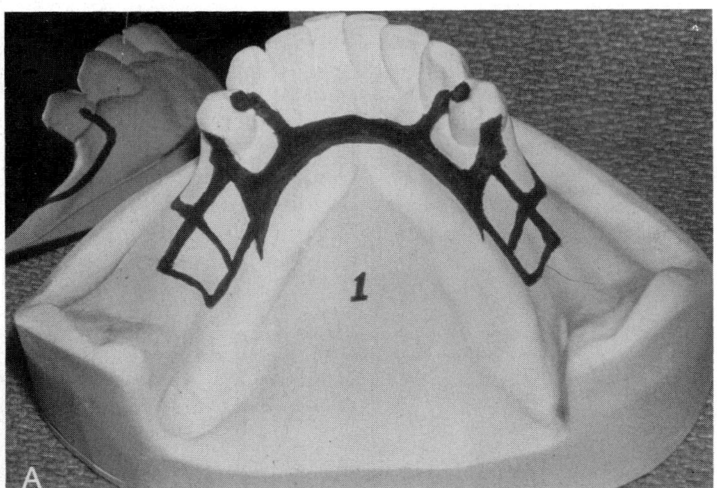

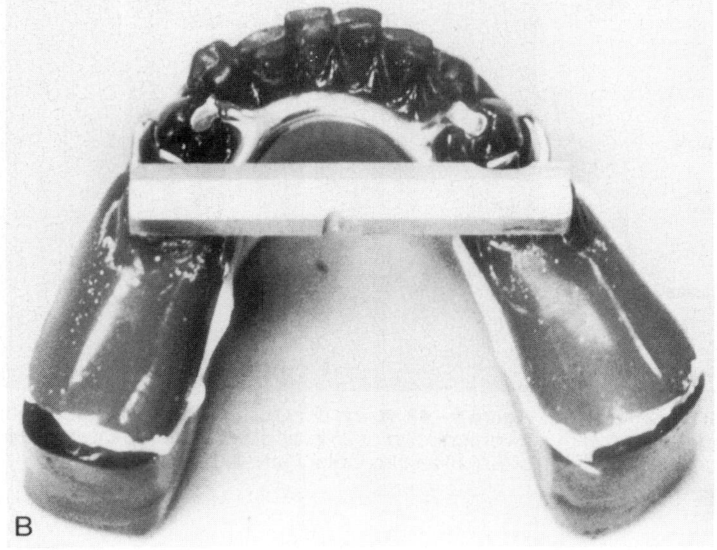

Figure 8–49 ■ *A*, Test design 1: Mesial rests, cast buccal I bars, and distal guide planes. *B*, Bilateral distal extension prosthesis with simulated mucosa under denture base and loading bar.

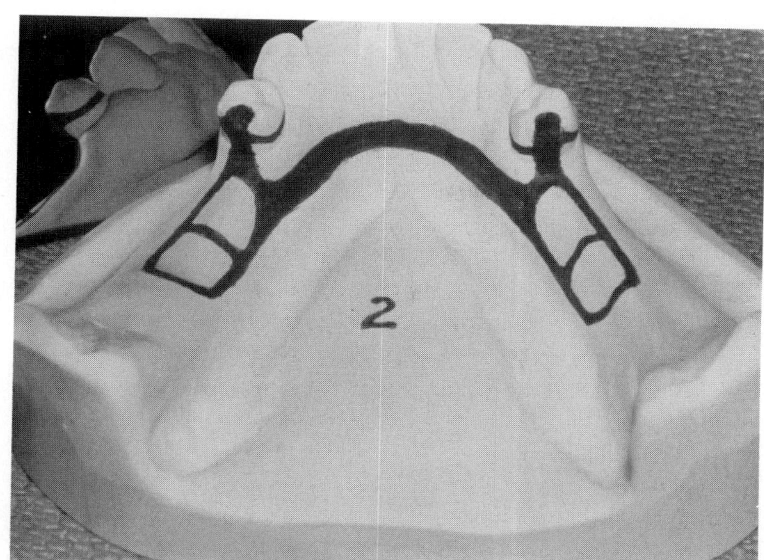

Figure 8–50 ■ Test design 2: Distal rests and cast circumferential retainers.

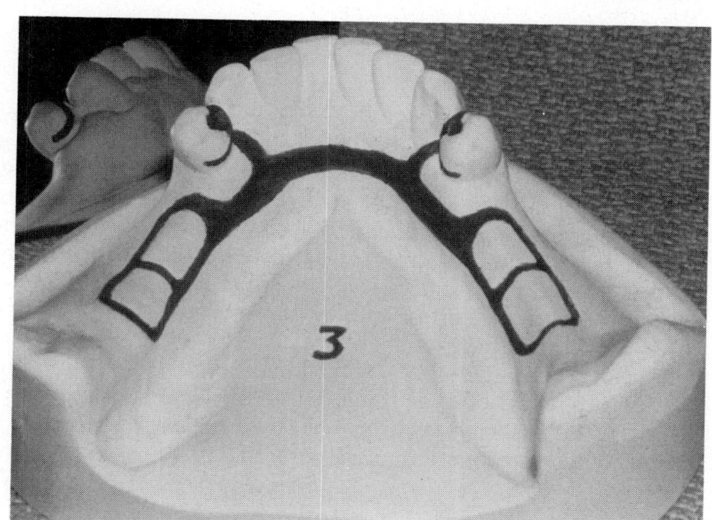

Figure 8–51 ■ Test design 3: Mesial rests and cast circumferential retainers.

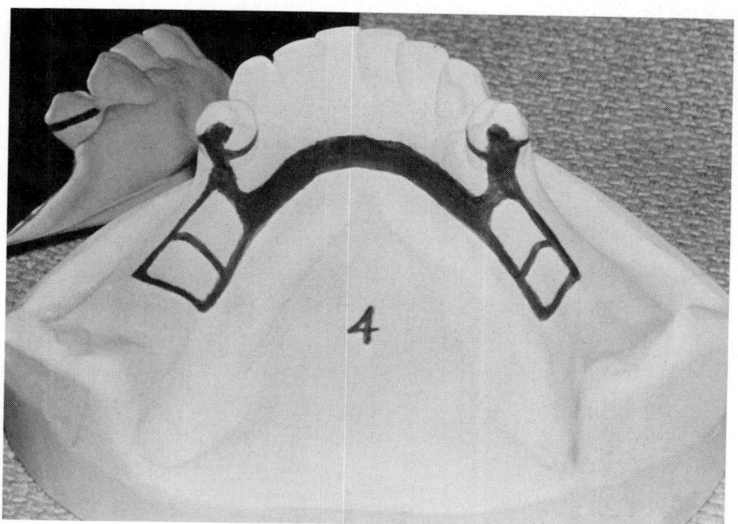

Figure 8–52 ■ Test design 4: Distal rests, 18-ga wrought wire facial retainers and cast lingual reciprocation.

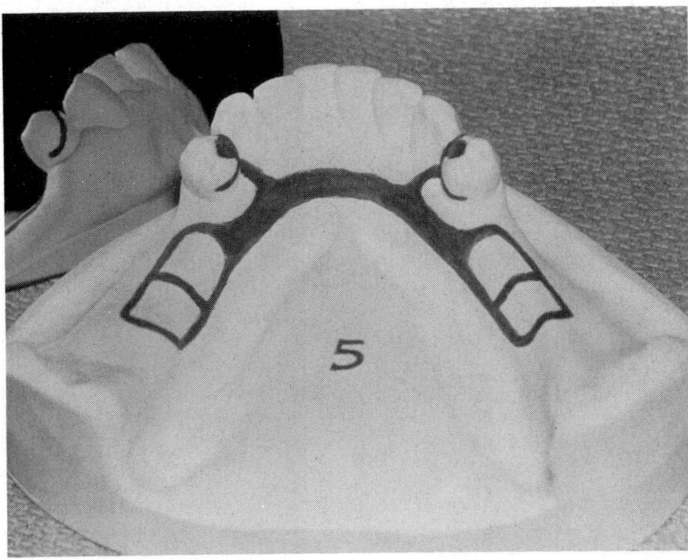

Figure 8–53 ■ Test design 5: Mesial rests, 18-ga wrought wire facial retainers and cast lingual reciprocation.

Vertical occlusal loading to the distal extension base with the casting *unadjusted* produced extensive pressure areas concentrated in the bone along the mesial apical surface of the root and the distal crestal bone. This can be seen by comparing the experimental and the control photographs (Figs. 8–46 and 8–47), in which the posterior tipping or tilting action of the abutment tooth and the extensive *lateral forces* on the periodontal ligament, periodontal membrane, root, and bone are demonstrated.

When the casting was adjusted to allow for physiologic movement in function, the force pattern was concentrated equally around the apex of the abutment tooth (Fig. 8–48). The line of force within the root of the tooth was straight and unbroken and in the center of the tooth. The periodontal membrane presented an even, unbroken appearance on both mesial and distal surfaces, which indicated even, downward pressure on the tooth. The force to the abutment tooth is delivered on the long axis, providing the most advantageous support. This demonstrates that *physiologic adjustment* of the metal contacts against the teeth on the distal extension removable partial denture castings *is*

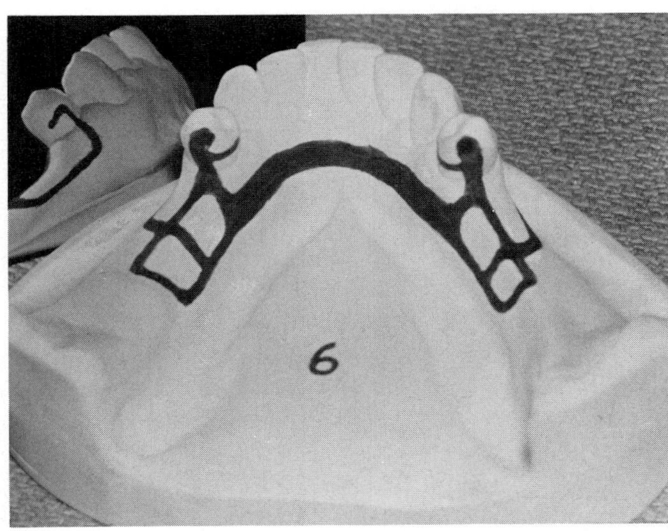

Figure 8–54 ■ Test design 6: Distal rests and cast facial one-half T-bar retainers.

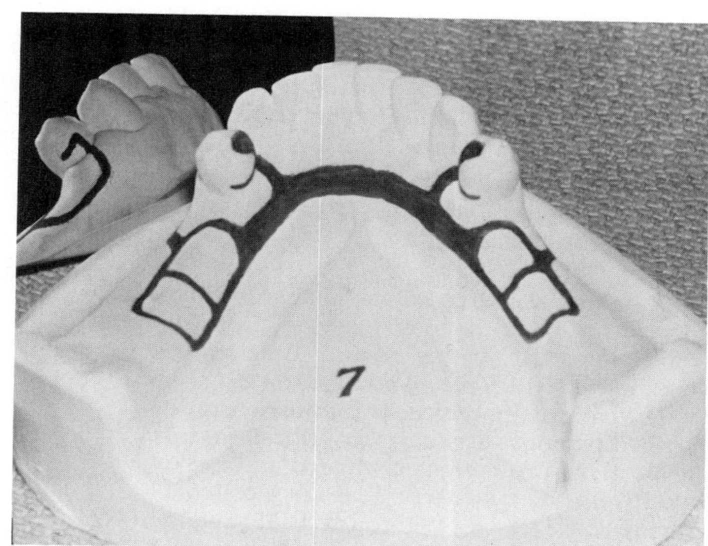

Figure 8–55 ■ Test design 7: Mesial rests and cast facial one-half T-bar retainers.

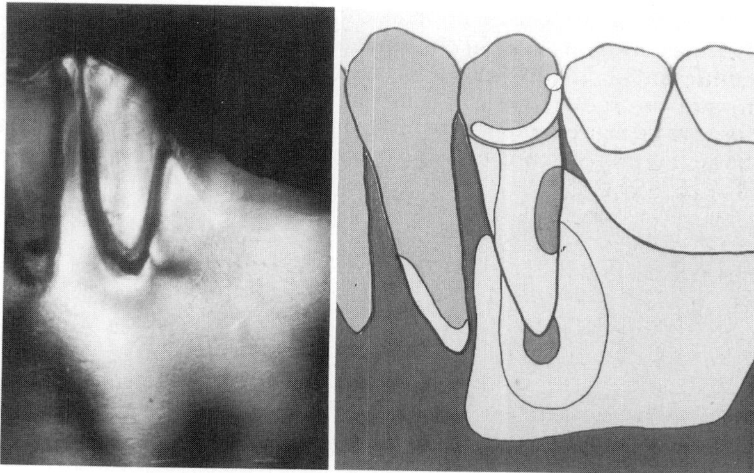

Figure 8–56 ■ *Excessive lateral forces* produced by distal rests in conjunction with mesial retention, which tend to move the clinical crown distally. Left side: Photoelastic result. Right side: Diagrammatic representation of forces. (See also Color Plate 3, p XIX.)

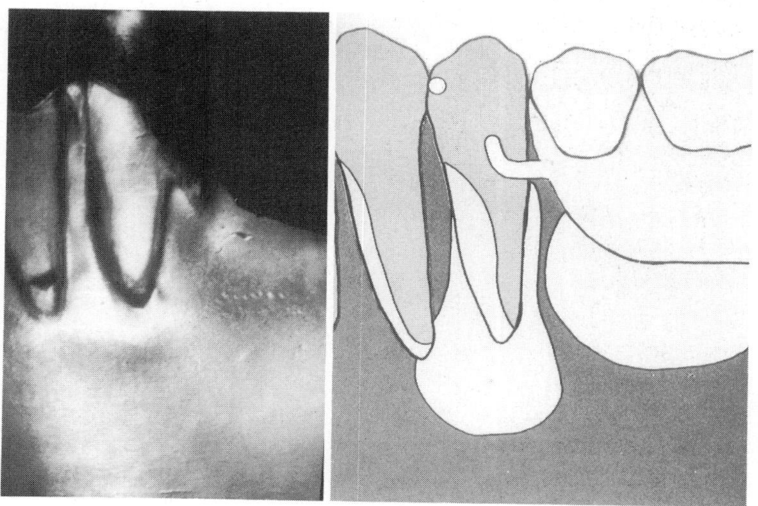

Figure 8–57 ■ The *best results* were produced by placing the rests of the extension partial denture in an anterior position in conjunction with I-bar retainers. The forces are in a more vertical direction. Left side: Photoelastic result. Right side: Diagrammatic representation of forces. (See also Color Plate 3, p XIX.)

necessary in order to minimize tipping and torquing movement on the abutment teeth.

EVALUATION OF VARIOUS PARTIAL DENTURE DESIGNS

The photoelastic technique enables evaluation of several of the most commonly used removable partial denture designs to determine the directions of force on abutment teeth.

The basic method used for the previously described photoelastic study was utilized for this evaluation. The designs compared and evaluated were seven of those that are most commonly used (Figs. 8–49 through 8–55) and included a combination of rests or rotation points and different types of retainers.

The conclusions were as follows:

1. A distal rest or a rotation axis located next to the edentulous area in conjunction with circumferential retainers tends to move and torque the tooth severely, causing horizontal force to be exerted on periodontal ligament and bone (Fig. 8–56A and B).

2. *Mesial* rests or rotation points located away from the edentulous area in conjunction with *properly positioned* I-*bar retainers* orient forces in a more favorable vertical direction (Fig. 8–57A and B).

REFERENCES

DeVan MM: Preserving natural teeth through the use of clasps. J Prosthet Dent 5:208, 1955.

Kratochvil FJ: The influence of occlusal rest position and clasp design on movement of abutment teeth. J Prosthet Dent 13:114, 1963.

Kratochvil FJ and Caputo AA: Photoelastic analysis of pressure on teeth and bone supporting removable partial dentures. J Prosthet Dent 32:52, 1975.

Kratochvil FJ and Vig RG: Principles of Removable Partial Dentures. UCLA Health Sciences Bookstore, 1979.

Lythe R: Soft tissue displacement beneath removable partial and complete dentures. J Prosthet Dent 12:34, 1962.

Thompson W, Kratochvil FJ, and Caputo AA: Evaluation of photoelastic patterns produced by various designs of bilateral distal-extension removable partial dentures. J Prosthet Dent 38:3, 1977.

Wright K, Mech EM, and Yettram A: Reactive force distributions for teeth when loaded singly and when used as fixed partial denture abutments. J Prosthet Dent 42:411, 1979.

chapter 9

Partial denture design principles and design sequence

Design Principles

The basic philosophy of treatment is to plan the best partial denture design for a given arch and to prepare the mouth for the ideal prosthesis. The patient who has missing tissues requires preparation and assistance, as described under basic principles. Periodontal disease and unusual configurations of soft tissue and tooth positions can jeopardize long-term success. It is best to resist compromising basic design principles whenever possible by performing proper mouth preparation.

Design Sequence

It is necessary to have an organized, orderly, definite design sequence when designing the removable partial denture casting. To this end, the support and rigid parts that control the partial denture *are placed first,* since their design and position control placement and design of other parts of the denture. The design sequence is accomplished in this order:

1. Rests
2. Major connectors
3. Minor connectors
4. Denture base connectors
5. Retainers

The rationale and principles for use and design of these five parts of the casting have been described and discussed in previous chapters. The design in detail is now formulated into the actual treatment plan on the diagnostic casts, which are a three-dimensional replica of the oral condition of the patient to be treated. The design is precise, detailed, and serves as an organized treatment plan for mouth preparation and for communication with other doctors for specific treatment and with the prosthetic laboratories. It also serves as a patient record for future reference.

MAXILLARY DESIGN SEQUENCE

Occlusal Rests (Fig. 9–1)

The extension, exact position, and width of each rest is precisely and clearly outlined on each tooth that will receive a rest. The molar rest on the toothborne side extends at least to the center of the tooth to ensure that occlusal forces are exerted in the long axis of the tooth. Further extension of the rest across the tooth is determined by the need to restore occlusal plane and occlusion. *Diagnostic casts mounted in centric relation are necessary for analysis* of rest design and position.

The premolar rest on the extension side is placed on the mesial side of the tooth because of the rotational factors described and discussed in Chapter 8. A rounded, ball-and-socket type of rest is used to allow pure rotational movement of the extension prosthesis during function.

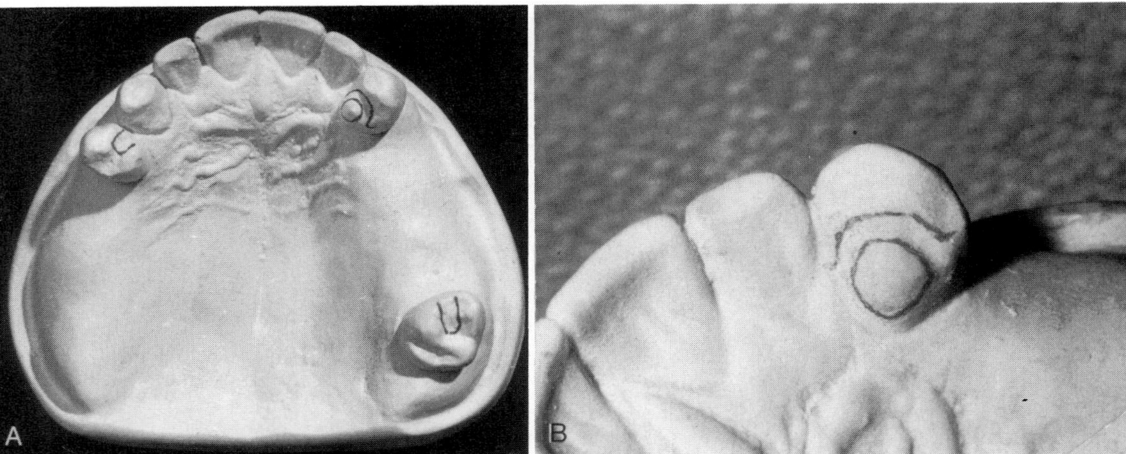

Figure 9–1 ■ *A*, Maxillary design sequence: Step 1. Place the occlusal rests in exact position. Note that the right side is toothborne, with rests in the center of the tooth; the left side is an extension situation, with an anterior or mesial rest. *B*, Anterior rest is open in the center to visualize complete seating of the rest and for easy cleaning.

The canine rest is positioned where the most positive rest seat can be prepared, compatible with occlusion and anterior guidance. Location of this rest is determined by the mounted diagnostic casts. The rest is open in the central portion (Fig. 9–1B) for visualization of proper seating in the rest preparation and for ease of cleaning, in that the bristles of the denture cleaning brush can protrude through the opening and keep the rest seat area clear of debris.

Major Connectors (Fig. 9–2)

The design joins all rests and edentulous areas with a rigid connection to ensure control of position. The anterior portion of the circularly designed major connector is placed in the valley of the ridge to reduce marginal bulk and tongue interference. Posteriorly, the extension does not continue beyond the vibrating line of the palate. The design carries the metal well into the edentulous hamular notch area. The finish line on the right or toothborne side is positioned to allow easy placement of the prosthetic teeth plus sufficient space for plastic material to secure the prosthetic teeth to the metal casting.

On the edentulous or left side, the metal is designed to be more towards the middle of the palate to provide maximum exposure of the edentulous ridge for the greatest area coverage by the denture base for support.

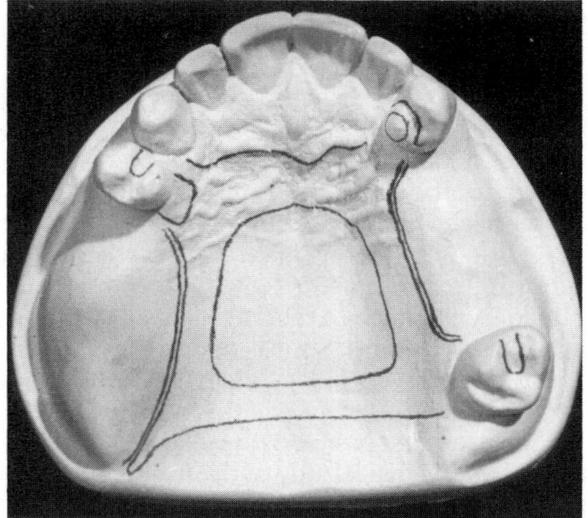

Figure 9–2 ■ Maxillary design sequence: Step 2. The maxillary major connector is of circular design for increased strength and rigidity.

Minor Connectors (Proximal Plates) (Fig. 9–3)

The minor connectors are designed to place metal coverage over the mucosa at the tooth-tissue junction. The metal should extend onto the tissue for at least 2 mm (Fig. 9–4). The facial extension covers and protects any tissue depressions, and the facial portion extends over the curvature of the ridge. In some instances, such as on the molar, the minor connector provides the connection between the rest and the major connector. The portion of the minor connector contacting the tooth at the tooth-tissue junction provides lateral or horizontal bracing at a tooth contact closest to the bone, which is most desirable.

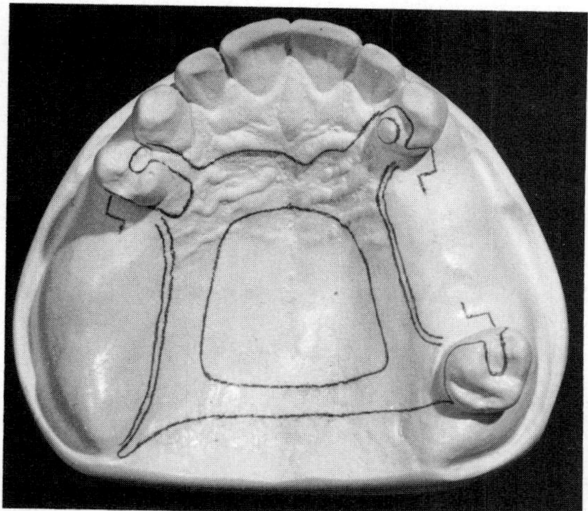

Figure 9–3 ■ Maxillary design sequence: Step 3. Minor connectors cover the side of the tooth and extend onto the mucosa for a minimum of 2 mm.

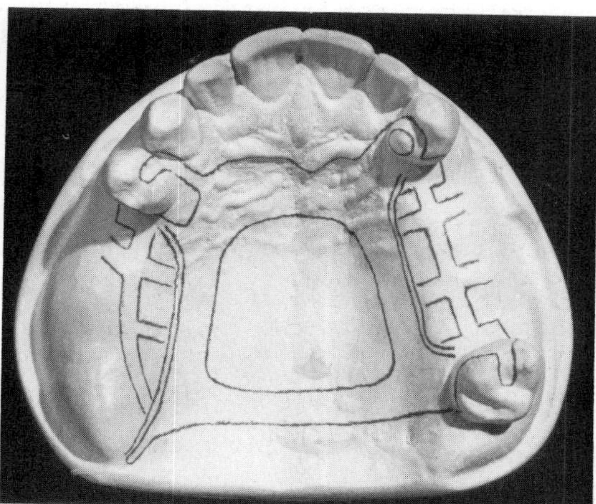

Figure 9–5 ■ Maxillary design sequence: Step 4. Denture base connectors are positioned on the crest of the ridge or to the lingual side so as not to interfere with the placement of denture teeth.

Note that the casting is designed well away from the tooth-tissue junction on the lingual side (Fig. 9–4).

Denture Base Connectors (Fig. 9–5)

The positions of the denture base connectors, which provide retention for the plastic and the teeth that compose the denture base, are determined by the requirements for the placement of prosthetic teeth. Connectors that interfere with tooth placement cause esthetic and retention difficulties. To eliminate these problems, the connectors are placed on the crest and the lingual side of the ridge away from the facial surface.

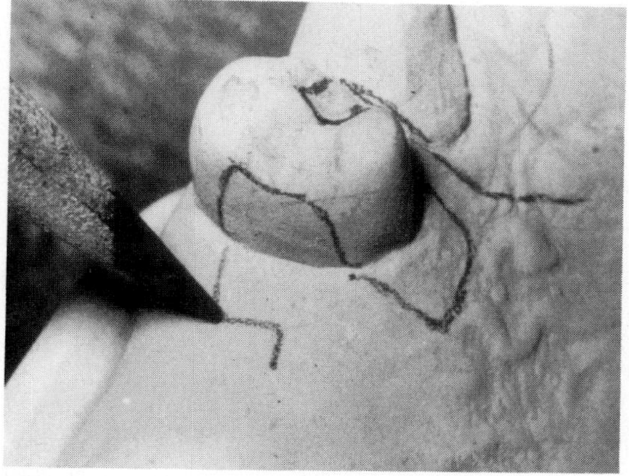

Figure 9–4 ■ All parts of the prosthesis that contact the tooth and the tooth-mucosa junction are designed in metal.

Note: The location of the posterior portion of the connector on the edentulous side is well to the lingual side and away from the crest of the tuberosity in order to minimize intraarch interference where there is restricted space. The double finish lines on the cast indicate a finish line on the ridge side and the tongue side of the casting that will form a positive union of the plastic and the metal.

Retainers (Fig. 9–6)

Location of the retention portion of the retainer is determined by the abutment tooth contour, at the retention areas and movement of the prosthesis in function. The retention portion is positioned first and designed to cross the tooth-tissue junction at right angles and to continue in the direction of the long axis of the tooth. It is continued, if possible, onto unattached mucosa, where it turns in a horizontal direction.

The retainer is joined to the denture base connector at the crest of the ridge (Fig. 9–7).

When viewed from the facial aspect (Fig. 9–8), the tapered design of the retainer can be visualized with the bulkier portion at the junction with the denture base connector and located at the interproximal area of the denture teeth. Junction at this location causes the least interference with placement of the prosthetic teeth and enhances esthetics.

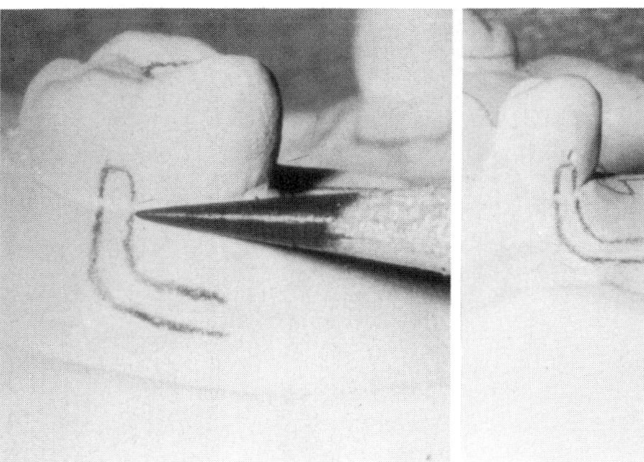

Figure 9–6 ■ *A*, Maxillary design sequence: Step 5. The retention portion of the retainers is positioned for the proper undercut position. *B*, The retainer is designed to join the denture base retention where there is the least interference with prosthetic tooth placement.

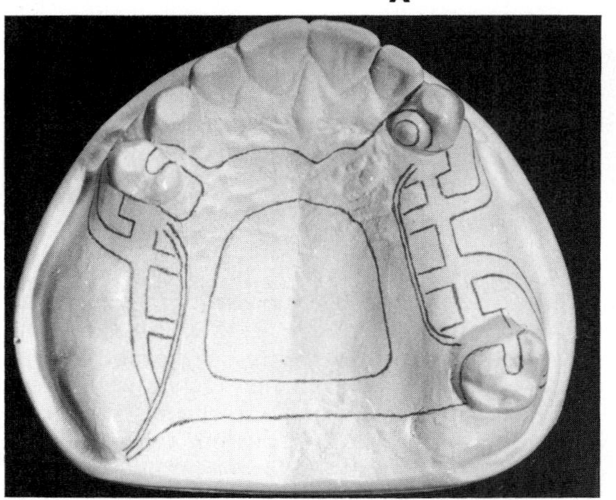

Figure 9–7 ■ The retainers are joined to the denture base connectors at the interproximal area between the denture teeth.

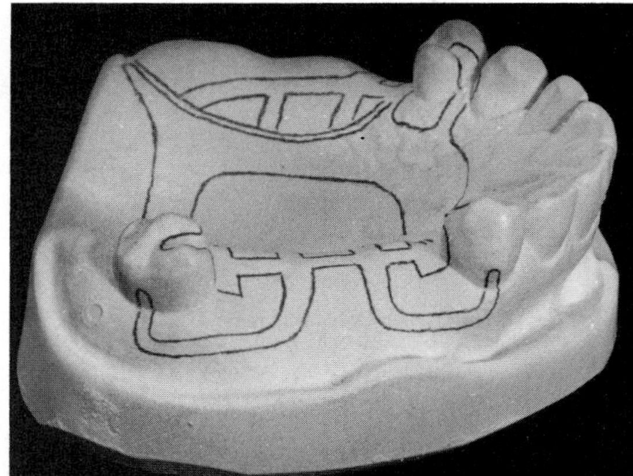

Figure 9–8 ■ The side view illustrates the retainer crossing the tooth-tissue junction in a vertical direction at right angles to unattached gingiva before the horizontal direction begins.

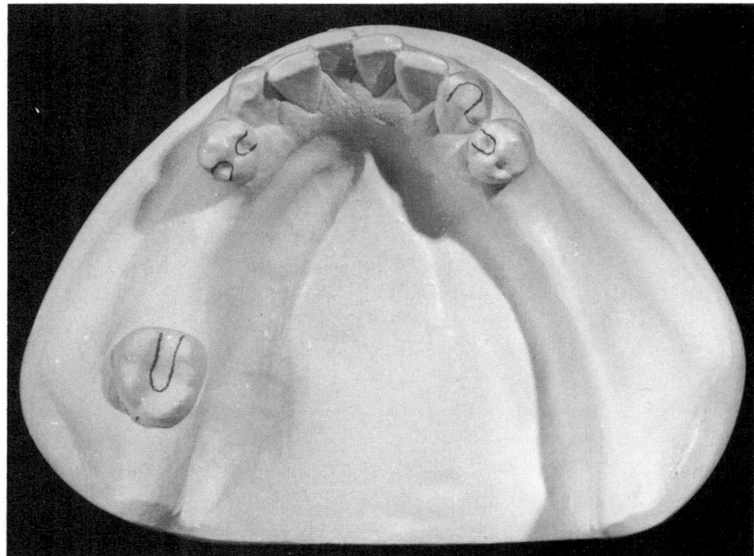

Figure 9–9 ■ Mandibular design sequence: Step 1. Occlusal rests are selected for support, restoration of occlusion, and axis of rotation in extension situations.

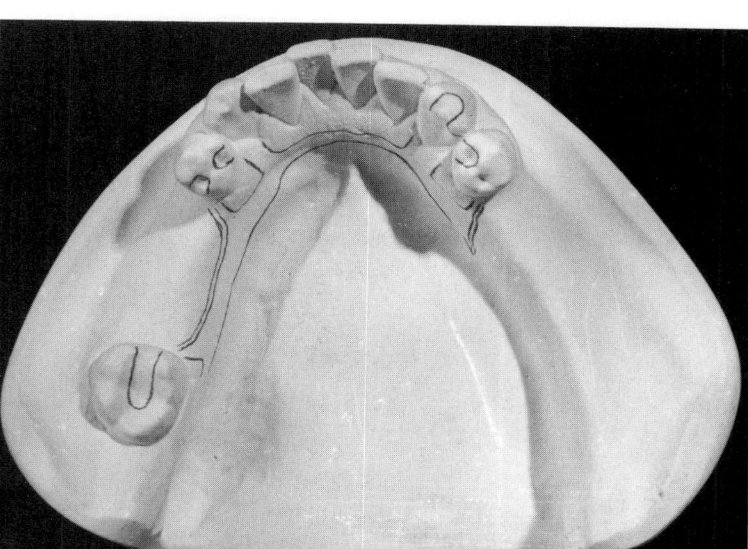

Figure 9–10 ■ Mandibular design sequence: Step 2. The lingual bar or complete lingual coverage is positioned to provide a rigid design compatible with existing anatomy.

MANDIBULAR DESIGN SEQUENCE

Occlusal Rests (Fig. 9–9)

The rests provide the support and control points between tooth and prosthesis, so they are positioned *first*. Where an incisal rest is required, as, for instance, on the right canine, it is designed to cover and restore the entire functional area. The mesial and distal rests on the left premolar may be joined together for greatly increased strength, since this is a nonocclusal area.

Major Connectors (Fig. 9–10)

Rigidity for the mandibular major connector is more difficult to provide, since it is not possible to employ the circular design in this arch. Greater bulk is necessry to produce the rigid connection between the rests and the edentulous area. When the lingual bar is the design of choice, it should be positioned on unattached mucosa wherever possible and well away from the tooth-tissue junction. The bar can be extended into the lingual area as far as functional anatomic structures permit in order to gain the required bulk for rigidity.

Where casting crosses the tooth-tissue junction, it should be at right angles to the junction to minimize food impaction and should continue to unattached gingivae before the horizontal portion begins. The space between the crest of the mucosa and the lingual bar should be as open as possible (Fig. 9–11).

Minor Connectors (Fig. 9–12)

The minor connectors are positioned to cover the side of the tooth and to extend onto the mucosa at the tooth-tissue junction for a minimum of 2 mm. The design should provide metal

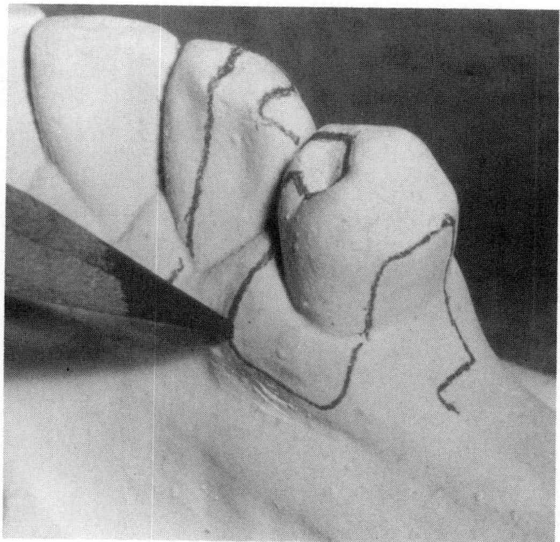

Figure 9–11 ■ The lingual bar is positioned on unattached gingiva as far as possible from the tooth-tissue junction.

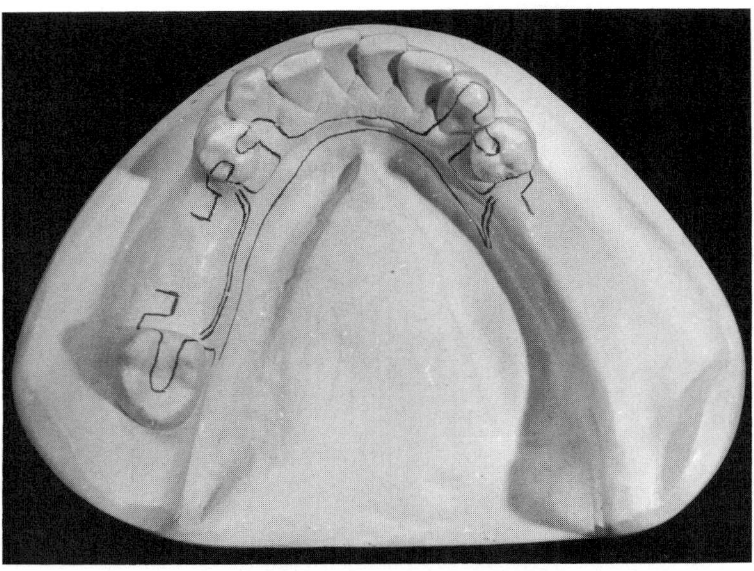

Figure 9–12 ■ Mandibular design sequence: Step 3. Minor connectors cover the tooth-tissue junction and contact the tooth at the mucosa as close to the bone as possible for the most favorable leverage to brace against lateral movement.

contact at all points where the prosthesis contacts the tooth or the tooth-tissue junction.

Denture Base Connectors (Fig. 9–13)

Denture base connectors are positioned on the crest of the ridge and toward the lingual side to reduce interference with denture tooth placement. On the edentulous or right side, an area of critical concern is the junction with the major connector (Fig. 9–14). This is an *area of frequent fracture or flexure* and must be designed with additional bulk and a fan-shaped union *for maximum strength.* Note the position of the finish line in this area; it is placed well to the distal side of the tooth and curved into the edentulous portion, where there is extensive bone and tissue loss. Placement of the bulky plastic-metal junction in this area restores the contour of lost tissues without infringing on tongue space. The superior border of the lingual bar is located as far from the tooth-tissue junction as possible.

On the toothborne side of the arch (Fig. 9–

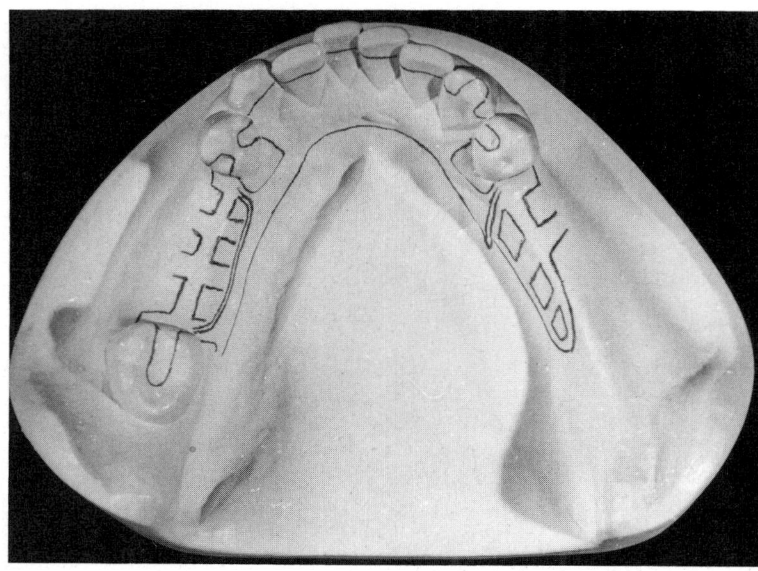

Figure 9–13 ■ Mandibular design sequence: Step 4. Denture base connectors are located on the crest of the ridge and on the lingual side to provide attachment of the denture base.

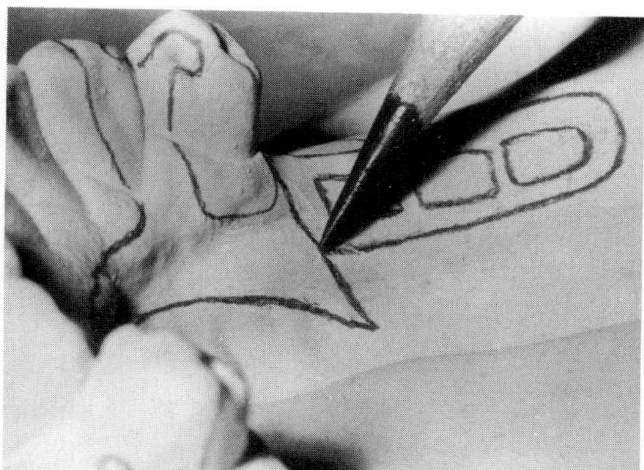

Figure 9–14 ■ A *strong* union at the junction of the denture base connector and the major connector is essential to prevent flexure or breakage. Note the posterior sweep of the finish line well into the edentulous area.

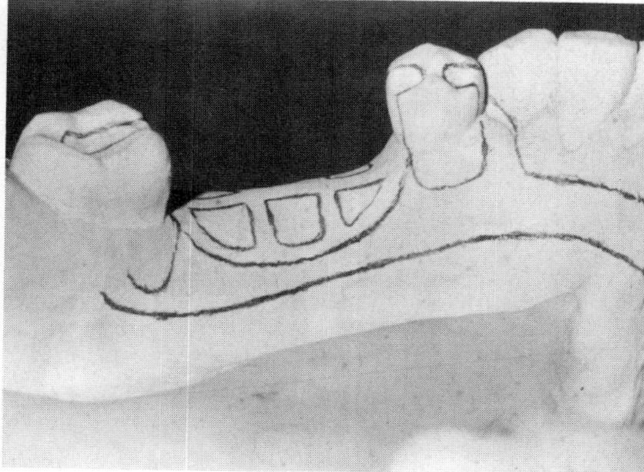

Figure 9–15 ■ The major connector forms the inferior border of the denture base and a finish line on the toothborne side of the arch.

15), the major connector forms the inferior border of the prosthesis to provide maximum strength with minimum bulk and provides a junction point for the denture base connector as well as a lingual finish line area.

Retainers (Fig. 9–16)

The retainers are designed and positioned to provide retention as required and to allow the proper placement of the denture teeth for good esthetics.

In the mandibular arch, the contour of the tissues on the facial surface can present extensive undercuts that require shorter vertical extension of the retainer before the horizontal portion is located (Fig. 9–17). A high attachment of the buccal frenum may require consideration for location of the arm of the retainer (Fig. 9–18).

A systematic approach with a step-by-step sequence develops a quick, practical design, which organizes planning treatment and provides for detailed communication with the laboratory.

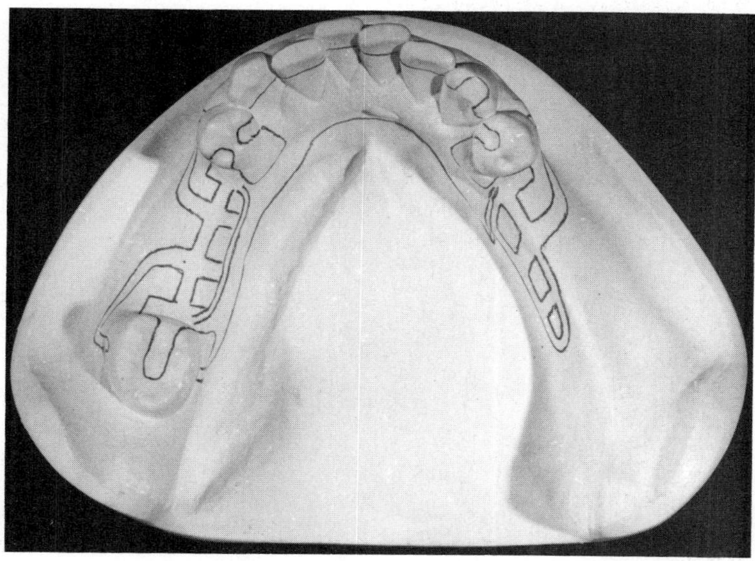

Figure 9–16 ■ Mandibular design sequence: Step 5. The retainers are positioned for proper retention and are attached to the denture base connectors.

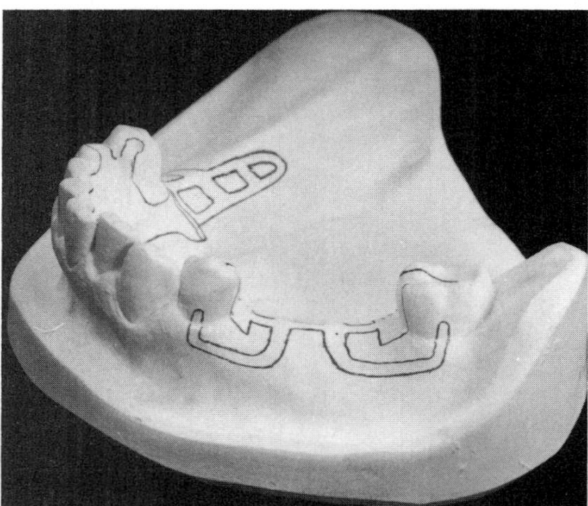

Figure 9–17 ■ The alveolar contour or tissue undercuts may influence the length of the vertical portion of the retainer.

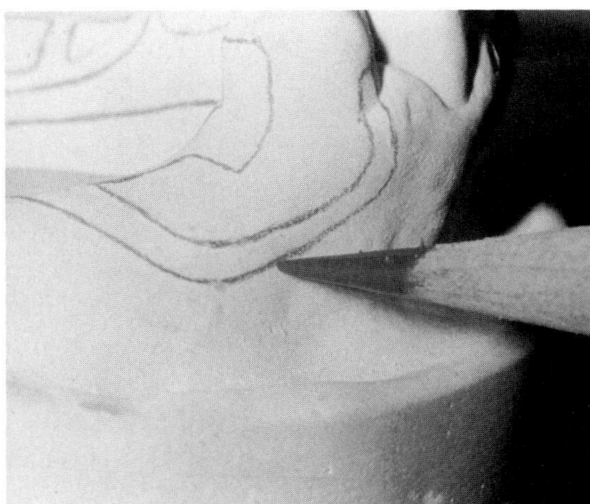

Figure 9–18 ■ The position and attachment of the buccal frenum and tissue topography require special consideration in the placement of infrabulge retainers.

REFERENCES

Berg T: I-Bar: myth and countermyth. Dent Clin North Am 23:45–75, 1979.

Girardat RL: History and development of partial denture design. J Am Dent Assoc 28:1399, 1941.

Kratochvil FJ: Influence of occlusal rest position and clasp design on movement of abutment teeth. J Prosthet Dent 13:114–124, 1963.

Kratochvil FJ and Vig RG: UCLA Removable partial denture syllabus. Los Angeles, UCLA, 1968.

Krol AJ: Removable partial denture design: an outline syllabus. San Francisco, Bookstore, University of the Pacific School of Dentistry, 1976.

Miller EL: Systems for classifying partially edentulous arches. J Prosthet Dent 24:25, 1970.

Potter RB et al: Removable partial denture design: a review and a challenge. J Prosthet Dent 17:43–68, 1967.

Schmitz AH: Partial denture planning and design. J Am Dent Assoc 35:562, 1947.

Steffel VL: Current concepts in removable partial denture service. J Prosthet Dent 20:387, 1968.

chapter 10

The most advantageous treatment position (MAP)

The removable prosthesis provides position control and stabilization of the remaining teeth and unites the entire arch. Stability depends upon basic principles of design and construction determined by the patient's remaining oral structures and physical condition.

A basic premise of treatment is to design the proper prosthesis for a given situation. The prosthesis design should not be compromised by existing pathologic conditions or by malposition of the teeth. The basic principle is to prepare the mouth to receive the necessary and proper prosthesis. Sound design principles are the major factor in prosthesis construction. When a draftsman prepares a blueprint, he first establishes a base line, and all other lines are drawn in relation to that one position or line. This is the basic concept of establishing a treatment position. The basic position selected for the cast, which is a reproduction of the patient's arch, establishes this base line for all planning, design, and fabrication. The primary objective is to establish a position of the cast that places teeth and associated tissues in the *most advantageous position* (MAP) for treatment with the partial denture. The MAP is determined by the following factors.

Guiding surfaces ■ These determine how the prosthesis moves into position.

1. Guiding surfaces may be the mesial or the distal portions or both surfaces of the teeth next to edentulous areas (Fig. 10–1).
2. Other guiding surfaces can be the surfaces of teeth contacted by the rigid part of the prosthesis (Fig. 10–2).

Retention areas ■ The ideal retention area is close to the tooth-tissue junction. Retention areas influence selection of the MAP, since a given cast position may demonstrate

1. Correct retention areas.
2. Lack of retention areas.
3. Excessive retention areas.

SURVEY INSTRUMENT

The surveyor is used to evaluate and measure the relationship to the basic cast position of all structures and parts of the prosthesis.

The survey instrument is a basic paralleling device that demonstrates the parallelism or lack of parallelism of all surfaces to a base line or a fixed cast position. It consists of the following elements:

1. A survey instrument with a vertical arm extended at right angles to the base (Fig. 10–3). A small analyzing rod is attached to the arm, which visually demonstrates the relationship of any part of the cast to a selected path of insertion (Fig. 10–4).
2. The cast platform or table that is adjustable and holds the cast in a definite position (Fig. 10–3).

Procedure to Establish the Most Advantageous Position

Place the diagnostic cast on the survey table.

1. Establish a basic position with an "eye

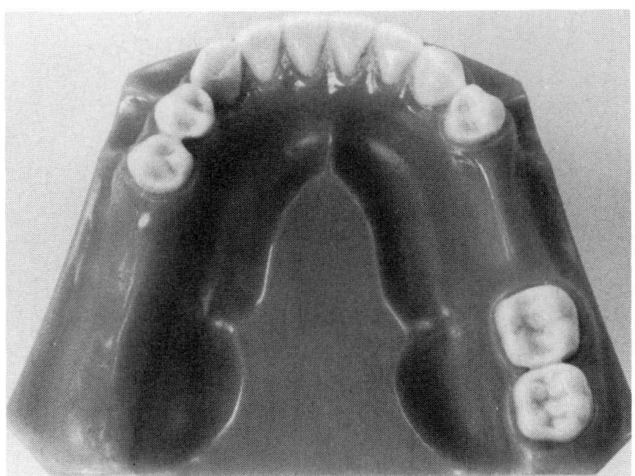

Figure 10–1 ■ The primary guiding surfaces that determine the insertion for the partial denture are the tooth surfaces adjacent to the edentulous areas.

survey," by placing the survey table with cast in place on a bench and standing directly over the center of the cast (Fig. 10–5).

2. Adjust the cast via the adjustable survey table, until guiding surfaces and retention area undercuts are equal or as parallel as possible.

Place the survey table with the cast in place onto the base of the survey instrument (Fig. 10–3).

1. With the analyzing rod in place, check the parallelism of the guiding surfaces (Fig. 10–6A and B).

2. Check the retention areas for necessary undercuts to provide retention, or demonstrate lack of undercuts (Fig. 10–7).

3. Check for tissue undercuts (Fig. 10–8).

Make adjustments of the cast position to estab-

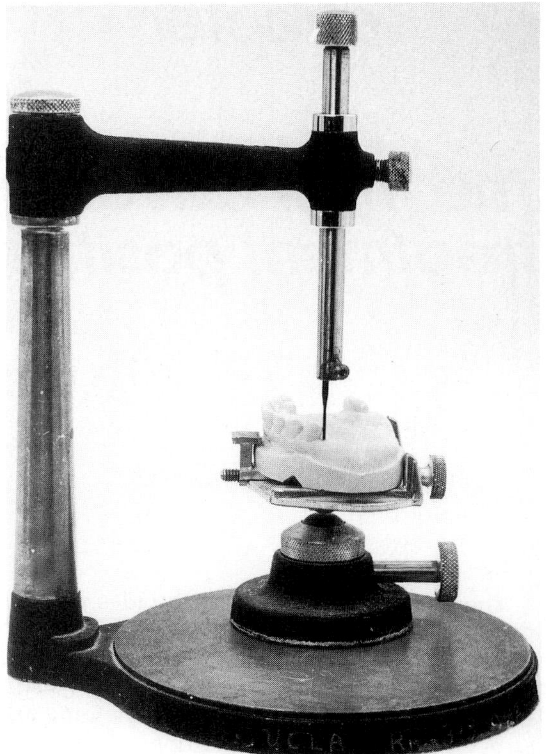

Figure 10–3 ■ The dental surveyor is a basic instrument for comparing the parallelism of one surface to other surfaces at a given position.

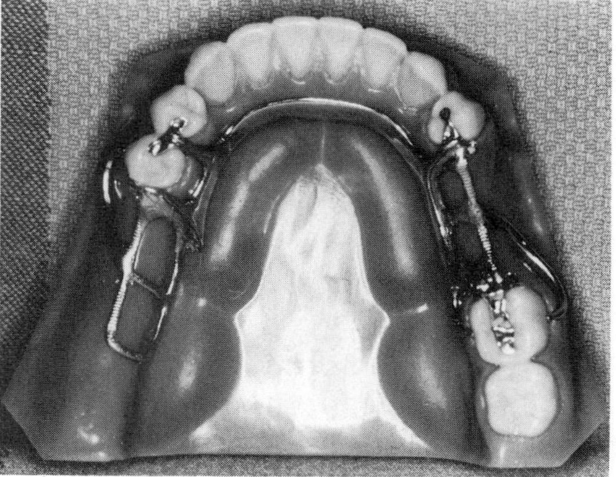

Figure 10–2 ■ Additional guiding surfaces are areas where the partial casting contacts the interproximal surfaces of teeth, such as between the two premolars.

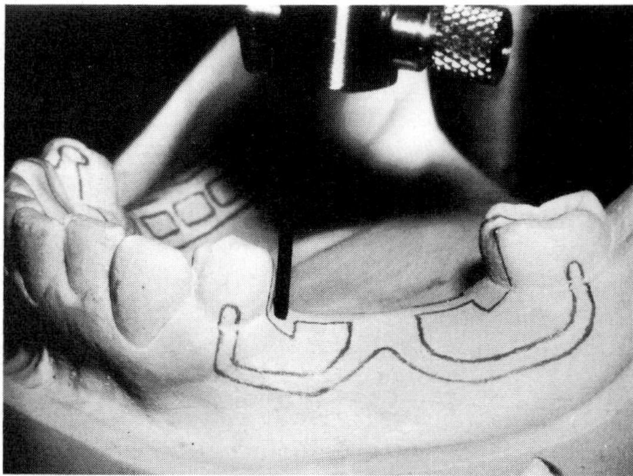

Figure 10–4 ■ The analyzing rod attached to the vertical arm of the instrument demonstrates the parallelism of one tooth surface to other tooth surfaces at a given cast position.

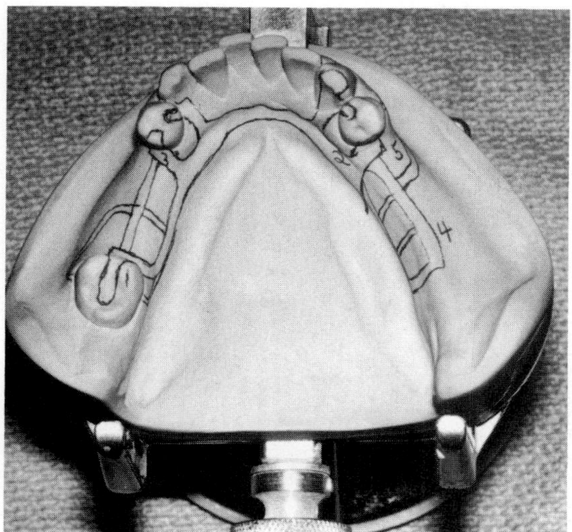

Figure 10–5 ■ Make an *"eye survey"* to place the cast in the *most advantageous position.* Stand directly over the cast and make the guiding surfaces as parallel as possible by adjusting the position of the cast.

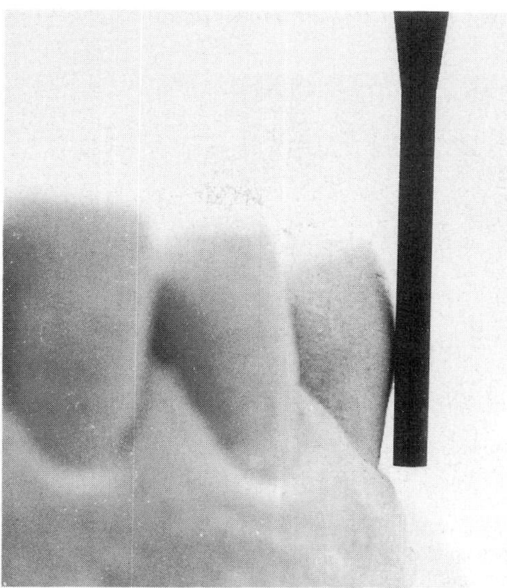

Figure 10–7 ■ Areas of teeth that will be used for retention are evaluated for position and amount of undercut.

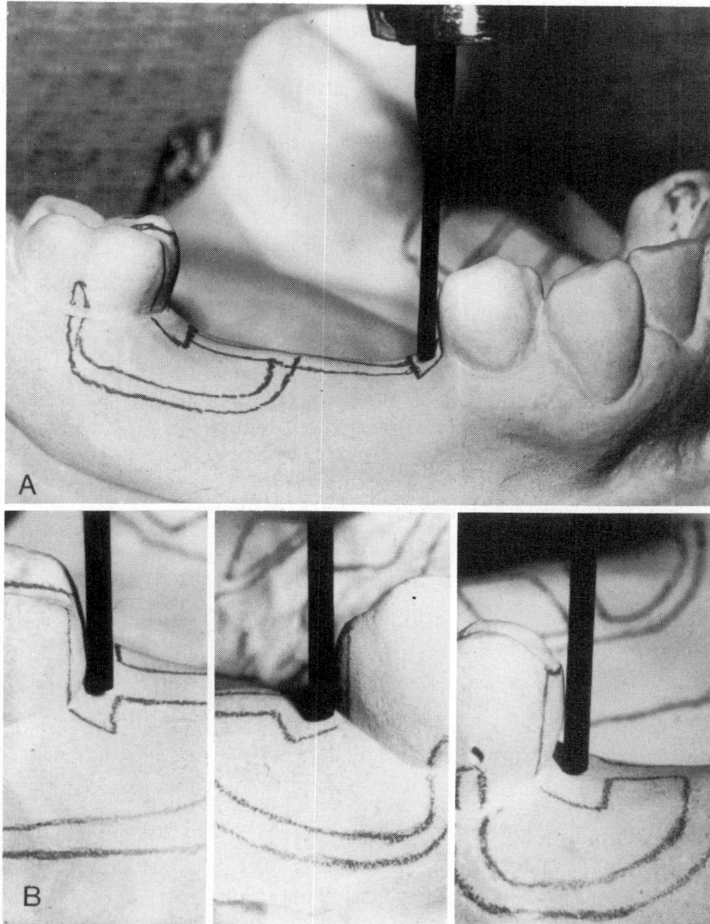

Figure 10–6 ■ *A,* Check the guiding surfaces of all teeth to be contacted by the denture for parallelism to the diagnostic rod. *B,* All guiding surface areas on each abutment tooth are checked for *space* at the *tooth-tissue junction,* as illustrated on the premolar in the picture on the right.

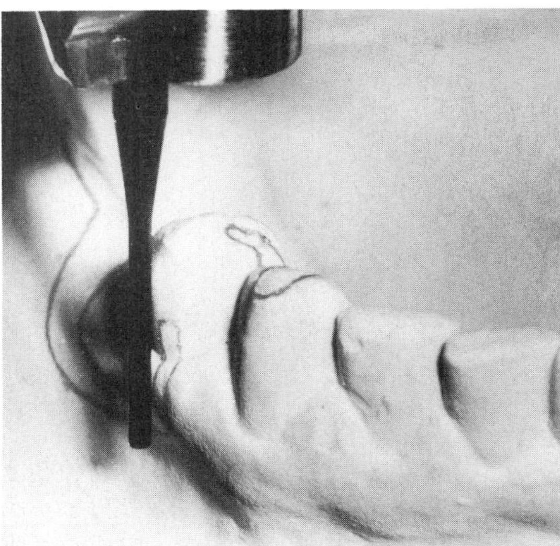

Figure 10-8 ■ Tissue undercut areas are evaluated for placement of the infrabulge retainer.

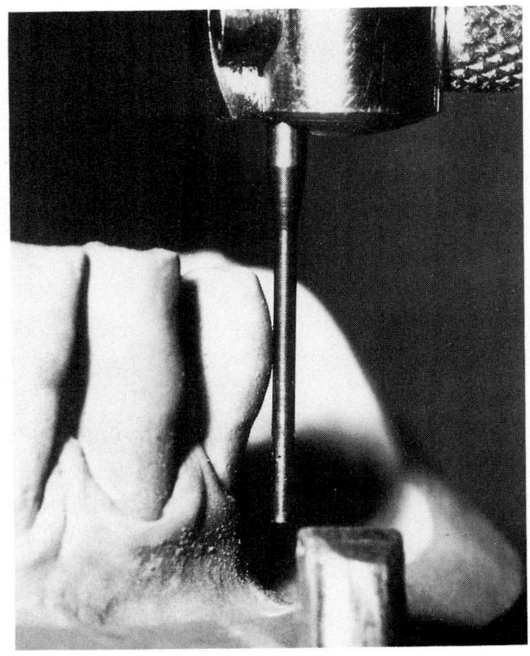

Figure 10-10 ■ Retention areas that will place the retainer too high on the tooth or too far away from the mucosa require tooth preparation on the facial side to move the retainer inward with lower contact.

lish the best possible position. Keep the occlusal plane as close to a *horizontal position* as possible.

1. Do not permit one tooth that is out of normal alignment to dictate a grossly tipped cast position (Fig. 10-9).
2. Position the cast to the advantage of the other teeth in the arch and adjust or restore the malaligned tooth to conform to the teeth in normal position.
3. Retention areas can be altered and recontoured to remove excess undercut areas or to provide proper contours for retention (Fig. 10-10).

Eliminate spaces and voids

The ideal situation is to position the cast so that all parts of the prosthesis will contact teeth and soft tissues with no space remaining (Fig. 10-11A and B) to avoid a *soft tissue reaction.*

Soft tissue reacts to a space or void in either of two ways: It may hypertrophy into the space, creating deep pockets, or it may recede, especially if irritated by food impaction (see Chapter 4). Maneuver the cast into different positions to locate the position that will present the least or smallest voids or areas of undercut.

Procedure for Recording the Most Advantageous Position of the Cast

Tripoding is the method used to record the determined cast position for reproduction at a

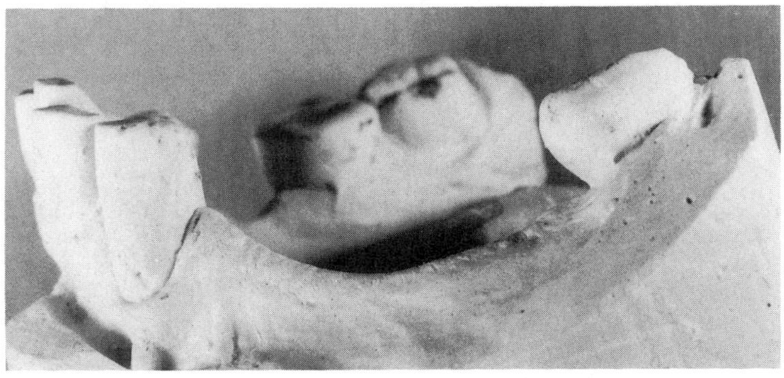

Figure 10-9 ■ Do not let one tooth in an abnormal, tipped position influence the path of intersection. Establish the best position with the other abutment teeth, then alter the malpositioned tooth with a restoration for parallel contour.

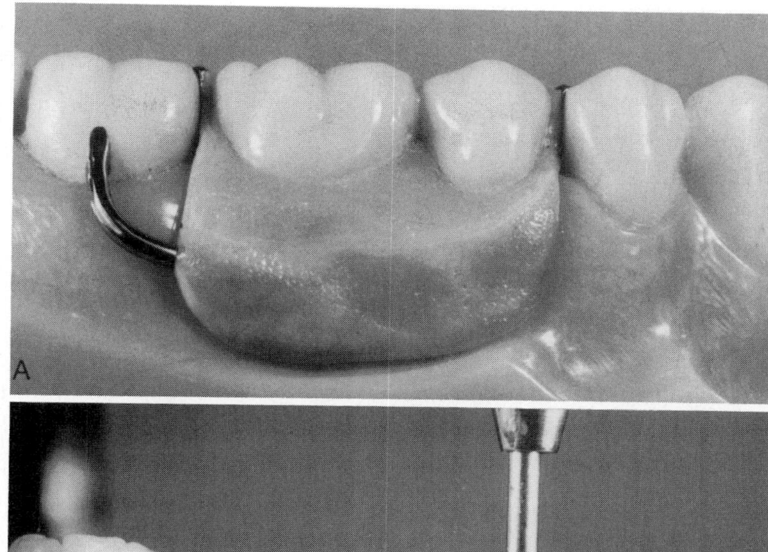

Figure 10–11 ■ *A*, The ideal path of insertion allows seating of the prosthesis with complete elimination of all spaces and voids. *B*, To achieve parallel guiding surfaces requires planning, measurement, and tooth preparation.

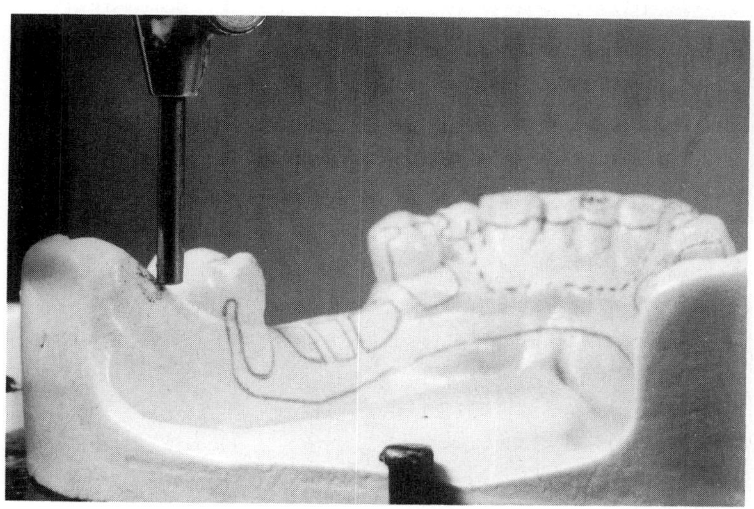

Figure 10–12 ■ *With the cast fixed in the MAP on the surveyor table, the vertical arm of the surveyor is fixed in a position that allows the tip of the diagnostic rod to touch the cast in three widely separated areas.* This allows removal and replacement of the cast in the identical MAP.

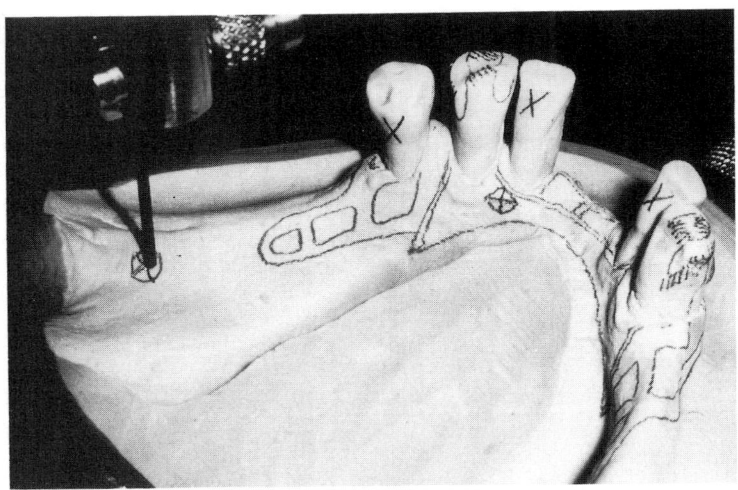

Figure 10–13 ■ The tripod marks are circled in red for easy identification at a later date for the laboratory procedures.

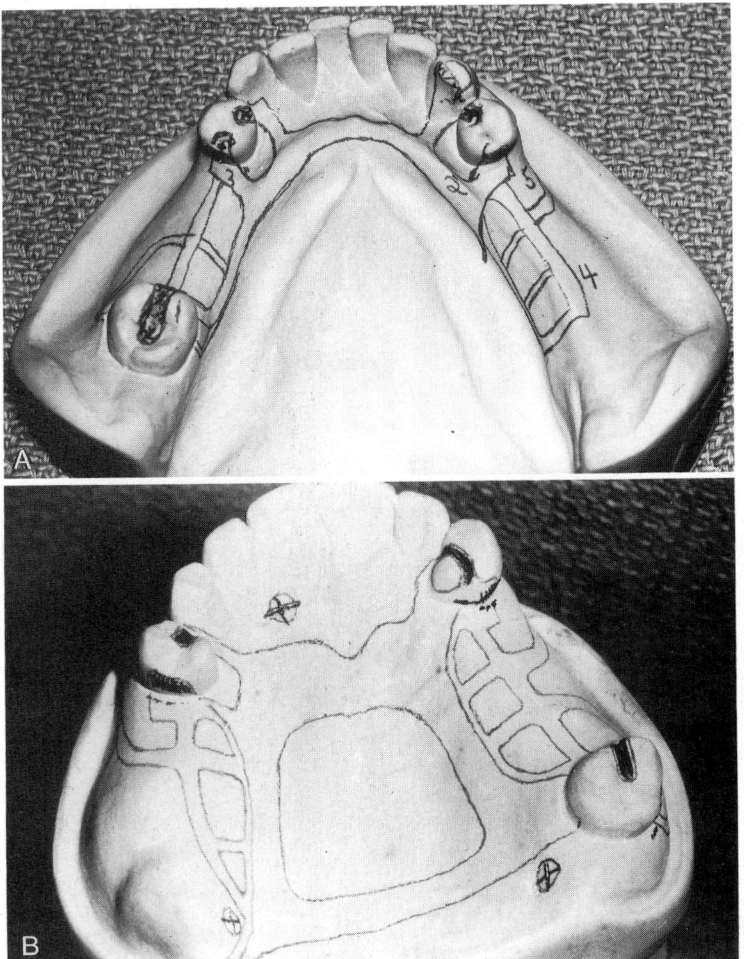

Figure 10–14 ■ *A*, A completed mandibular diagnostic cast is shown, with the detailed design marked in red and the areas requiring mouth preparation for guiding surfaces and rests marked in blue, as determined by the MAP. It is ready to be "tripoded." *B*, A completed maxillary diagnostic cast is shown.

later date in the laboratory, during fabrication procedures.

1. Place the survey table with the cast in the desired position on the base of the survey instrument.

2. Position the surveyor arm with the analyzing rod in place so that the tip touches the cast at three points as far removed from each other as possible (Fig. 10–12).

3. *Fix the surveyor arm* with the set screw, and mark three points on the cast with a carbon pencil. Circle the mark with red pencil for easy location at a later time (Fig. 10–13).

The reason for tripoding is to be able to remove the cast from the survey table and then return the cast to the identical position at a later date by reversing the above procedures. Exact repositioning is necessary at the laboratory, when the master cast is sent for fabrication of the metal casting.

Analysis of the Guiding Surfaces

With the analyzing rod in place, all portions of the teeth that will be guiding surfaces are inspected.

1. Areas on the teeth that produce undercut or open spaces are marked with a blue pencil as a guide for tooth alteration during mouth preparation (Fig. 10–14A and B).

2. It may be advantageous to make preparations on the cast before performing this procedure in the mouth in order to evaluate final contours or to demonstrate the need for restorations. *The ideal method is to estimate all spaces by preparing parallel guiding surfaces.*

Evaluation of Retention Areas

The rigid metal casting fitting against the guiding surfaces of the teeth stabilizes them in a controlled position in relationship to the retainers, whose purpose is to engage tooth undercuts and to hold the prosthesis in place (Fig. 10–15).

A measuring instrument can be placed on the surveyor to accurately determine the position and placement of the retainer for the required retention. The undercut gauges are manufactured so as to measure a set amount of distance.

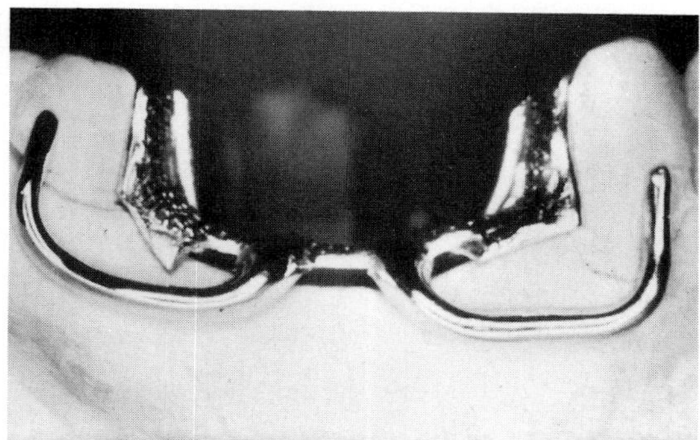

Figure 10–15 ■ Parallel guiding surfaces provide excellent bracing between remaining teeth for stabilization.

The amount of retention required is 0.010 in or 0.25 mm (Fig. 10–16).

Place the undercut gauge with its shank touching the tooth surface. Move the surveyor arm until the tip of the gauge touches the tooth surface. *Both shank and tip must touch the tooth simultaneously.* The point of contact with the tip of the gauge is a 0.010-in undercut (Fig. 10–17). If there is contact of the retainer against the tooth to the gingival side of this point, retention will be increased. If retainer contact is superior or occlusal to this point, retention will be less.

EXCESSIVE RETENTION AREAS

It is desirable to keep the retention contact as close to the gingival portion of the tooth as pos-

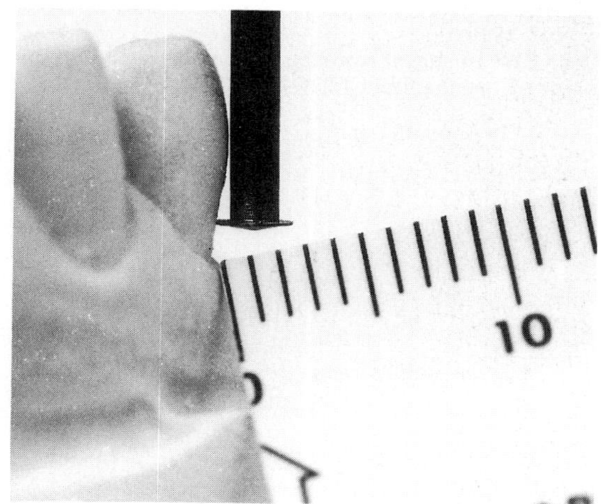

Figure 10–16 ■ The exact *location, amount,* and *position* of required retention is determined with a measuring device—the undercut guage. Any contact of the retained tooth *below* the undercut gauge *increases* retention. The ideal amount of retention is 0.010 inch.

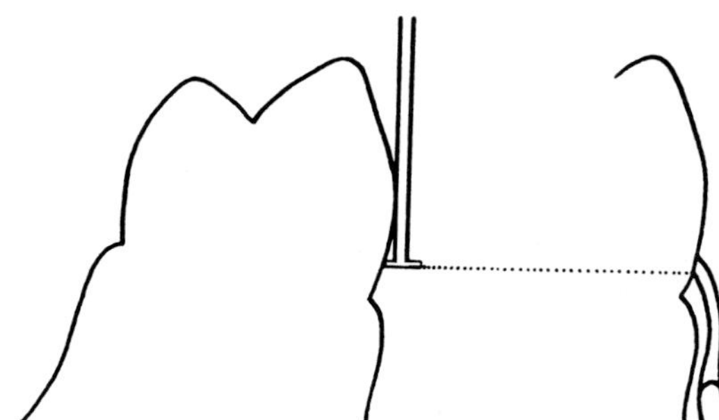

Figure 10-17 ■ The undercut gauge locates the exact position for placement of the retainer contact.

sible. In some instances, tooth contour or position creates excessive space at retention areas. This can result in esthetic problems, since the retainer is positioned close to the occlusal surface of the tooth. Recontour the tooth or the restorations to remove excessive contacts if necessary. A vertical groove can be placed, through which the I bar can slide to reposition the retention area closer to the cervix of the tooth or to move the arm of the retainer closer to the gingival tissue, if necessary (Fig. 10-18).

All areas of alteration are marked in blue on the cast for easy identification during mouth preparation.

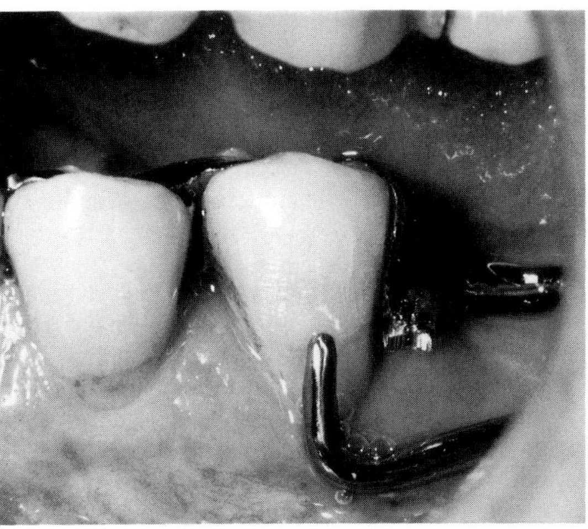

Figure 10-18 ■ In situations in which there is excessive facial contour of the tooth, a groove is placed in the tooth above the tip of the retainer, which allows the retainer to be positioned lower on the tooth and closer to the mucosa.

REFERENCES

Applegate OC: Use of the paralleling surveyor in modern partial denture construction. J Am Dent Assoc 27:1937-1407, 1940.

Donn BW: Treatment planning for removable partial dentures. J Prosthet Dent 1:247-255, 1961.

Frechette AR: Partial denture planning with special reference to stress distribution. J Prosthet Dent 1:700-707, 1951.

Glann GW and Appleby RC: Mouth preparation for removable partial dentures. J Prosthet Dent 10:698-706, 1960.

Henderson D and Seward TE: Design and force distribution with removable partial dentures: a progress report. J Prosthet Dent 17:350-364, 1967.

Schorr L and Clayman LH: Reshaping abutment teeth for reception of partial denture clasps. J Prosthet Dent 4:625-633, 1954.

Zoeller GN: Block form stability in removable partial dentures. J Prosthet Dent 22:633-637, 1969.

Zoeller GN and Kelly WJ Jr: Block form stability removable partial prosthodontics. J Prosthet Dent 25:515-519, 1971.

chapter 11

Diagnosis and treatment planning

Attitudes and Objectives of Doctor and Patient

Diagnosis and treatment planning consideration have been deliberately positioned at this part of the book so that the principles of partial denture design can be considered when treatment is being planned. The rationale is to have available the objectives and principles of the treatment before treatment planning is considered. At this time, diagnosis and treatment planning can be coordinated, utilizing the philosophies outlined in the previous chapters.

GENERAL PATIENT EVALUATION

Appraisal of a patient begins when he or she walks through the door of the office. General gait, appearance, coordination, and demeanor are especially pertinent in patients who will be treated with a removable prosthesis. Good physical coordination is essential, since the patient must be instructed and conditioned for the treatment and for use of the removable prosthesis.

The patients must realize that they are central in the coordination of the entire treatment effort and that their ability to cooperate is a major factor in successful treatment.

FIRST APPOINTMENT ENCOUNTER

The patient is approached and evaluated as an individual at the first meeting. This meeting takes place at an equal physical level, with both patient and doctor either standing or sitting (Fig. 11–1). Patients can feel threatened and dominated by the doctor standing over or above them. It is desirable to first establish the relationship on a professional but equal basis.

Physiologic Factors

Evaluate the patient's attitude, facial expressions, and muscle tone, especially of the face, cheeks, and neck. Observe basic facial forms and expressions, noting peculiar habits. Continue to observe coordination, as this is a good evaluation of the ability to control and use a prosthesis.

Psychologic Factors (DeVan's Evaluation)

1. The patient must have the will to adjust to and use dentures.
2. Patient may have the need for dentures but not the will to adjust to dentures.
3. There may be the need and the will but not the physical ability to use a prosthesis.
4. The dentures must be accepted as part of the body.
5. The doctor must take the patient's need and turn it into a want.

Patient-Doctor Relationship

The first impression is most important from the patients' point of view. They are evaluating you in much the same manner that you are

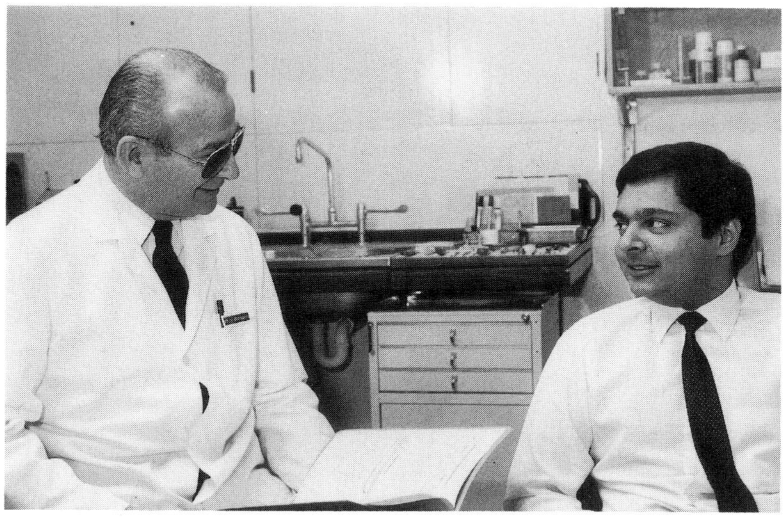

Figure 11–1 ■ In the first meeting with the patient, the doctor is at an equal physical level to enhance patient-doctor rapport and to create a more comfortable atmosphere.

evaluating them. Do not stand over patients at the first meeting; sit down beside them at an eye-to-eye level. Standing over patients gives them an uncomfortable feeling and indicates that some type of immediate treatment is about to begin, for which they may not be prepared (Fig. 11–2). All patients are interested in what is going to happen to them. Explain what you are going to do, even in the basic examination. Explain all other procedures *briefly,* in lay terms.

Evaluate whether you will have to exert yourself to like the individual or whether future visits will be a pleasure and you will enjoy them. Patient-doctor feelings can influence your attitude and, possibly, the success of the treatment.

Remember—patients have a treatment and complaint history to tell; *let them tell it completely.* Listen to the history in detail, since it may influence the success of your treatment.

MAINTENANCE OF PATIENT HEALTH—PHYSIOLOGIC AND PSYCHOLOGIC

Many patients presenting for treatment are in the partially edentulous categories and will require removable partial dentures. It is most rea-

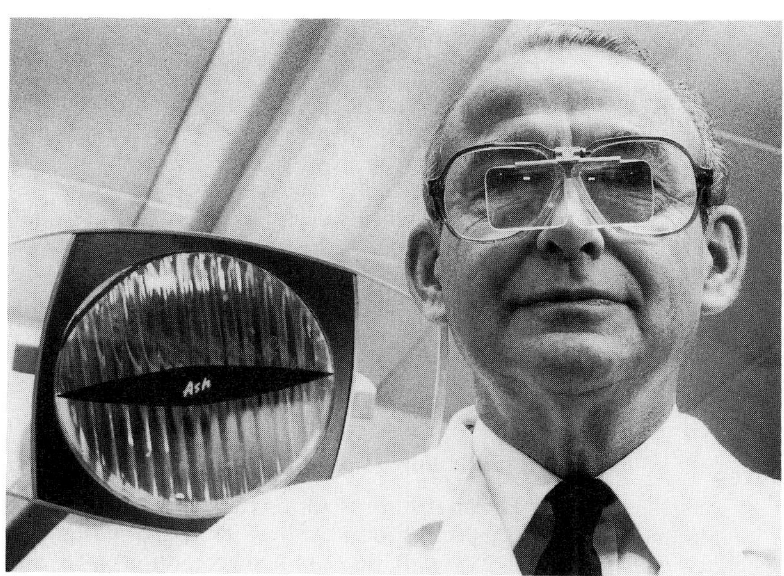

Figure 11–2 ■ A first association or meeting should *not* present an intimidating or superior situation.

sonable to plan this treatment with a primary objective being to preserve and maintain the tissues of the mouth, in conjunction with the treatment of the pathologic condition that may be present. If the removable partial denture treatment procedures receive the same consideration in appraisal and planning as do the other areas of oral treatment, they can achieve equal success.

Do not promise or imply that you can restore to the patient his or her original capabilites, as is often possible in an individual tooth restoration. Do not give the patient the impression that you or anyone else can accomplish this feat, but do give assurance that you will do your best to maintain the remaining oral structures and to control further degeneration. You may be able to make significant improvements in esthetics, but do not stress the ability to restore the masticating ability that was present prior to the loss of natural structures.

Diagnosis

There are three areas of consideration in diagnosis:

I. Physiologic
II. Structural
III. Psychologic

When planning any type of restoration, you must start at the foundation, and then work upward. You cannot start in the middle and work toward both sides. You must know what structures are available for support and what forces will be encountered to challenge that support. In other words, there must be a systematic approach; your thoughts and methods must be organized or you will soon become lost. Every doctor develops his or her own method to best plan procedures, which is as it should be—as long as the method is systematic!

I. **Physiologic considerations.** Evaluate basic coordination and physiologic functions of each patient. What is this patient's potential to support a prosthesis?
   A. The mandible and its power sources are basic considerations. All the force that can be applied by the individual is supplied by the muscles.
      1. Physiologic forces are supplied by the
         a. Muscles of mastication
         b. Tongue
         c. Cheeks
         All apply force to the alveolus and prosthesis, which, in turn, transmit it to the teeth. Some force is applied directly to the teeth. Evaluate the condition, coordination, and appearance (basically healthy or unhealthy) of all these structures.
      2. Why is it necessary to replace lost tissue with a removable partial denture?
         a. To maintain, stimulate, and support the remaining teeth and supporting tissues in their proper positions in order to prevent further displacement or collapse of the oral situation.
         b. To aid mastication. In many cases the patient can masticate to his own satisfaction with remaining natural teeth. Replacement of occlusal surfaces may not be the most important reason for treatment with a partial denture.
         c. To improve or restore esthetics.
         d. To stabilize and support the temporomandibular joint.
   B. Saliva. This is always an important factor; it is the lubricant of the entire mechanism. (Many patients with constant soreness or irritation have very little saliva.)
   C. General health.
      1. Known diseases. These are diseases of which both you and the patient are aware, which are being kept under control as well as possible.
      2. Undetected or subclinical diseases. These are diseases that are unknown to both you and the patient, such as cardiac, urologic, and gastrointestinal diseases. Patients with undetected diseases often have unaccountable difficulties with constantly irritated oral areas. Many of these patients cannot be made completely comfortable. In many cases you will be able to advise the patient of possible physical problems and direct them toward proper treatment.
      3. Degree of success in treatment. It may be well to take a lesson from practitioners in the medical field. They are often satisfied when they can obtain a partial restoration of function. The disabled patient must accept his disability and must learn

to pace himself accordingly. The diabetic patient cannot eat what he did before the onset of the disease; the cardiac patient cannot play football; the orthopedic patient cannot do knee bends; and the partial denture patient cannot masticate with the force and vigor of previous times. Inability to meet the unrealistic expectations of the patient is one of the most common causes of denture failure.

D. Age. A 50 year old person does not usually enter the Olympic sprints. By the same token, do not try to make a 60 year old patient's masticatory system function like that of a 20 year old. As the patient grows older, he or she cannot expect this type of function; it simply is not possible because the older patient has less coordination, adaptability, and tissue response. These factors must be explained to him or her *before* treatment.

II. **Structural considerations.** Make an evaluation of supporting structures as to size, condition, and amount of force they can produce. What are the physical capabilities?

A. Muscles.

1. Evaluate their *size* and the amount of force they can generate. These two factors, which are usually related to age, determine the patient's ability to function. Muscles of large size can usually produce more force.
2. The muscle *attachments* may be a source of difficulty during the placement of the metal or acrylic resin portions of the denture (Fig. 11–3).
3. The presence of pathologic conditions indicated by fatigue, tenderness, or soreness is investigated, and specific treatment is considered. Patient history and palpation of structures are prime diagnostic tools.

B. Tongue. Observe the size and the position of the tongue (anterior or posterior). Estimate the amount of force a patient can produce with his tongue and his ability to coordinate tongue movements with your directions. Hold the tongue with gauze and examine lateral and inferior surfaces for disease or abnormalities (Fig. 11–4).

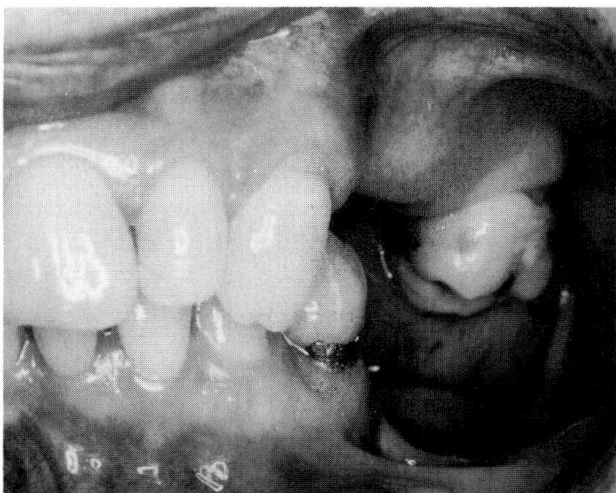

Figure 11–3 ■ The position or origin of muscle attachments and frenum influences the placement of denture base and retainers.

C. Bone structure.

1. Roentgenographic examination. This examination shows the amount and density of bone present, abnormalities (tori, spines, and so forth), disease, bone and tooth root contour, and unerupted teeth. Examination of the condition of the bone, especially around the most posterior teeth that will serve as abutments, gives a good index or guide for estimating how the bone is reacting to unusual forces and pressures and of how it will perform as a support for a prosthesis. Examine the cortical plate for continuity, thickness, or absence. Absence of cortical bone in a

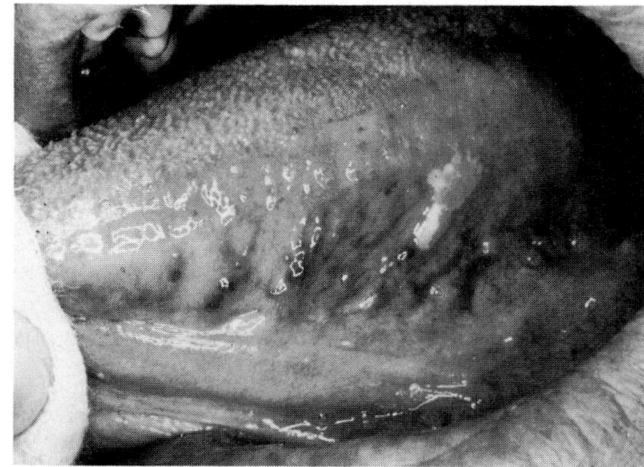

Figure 11–4 ■ The tongue is grasped with gauze and fully extended for examination and detection of pathology.

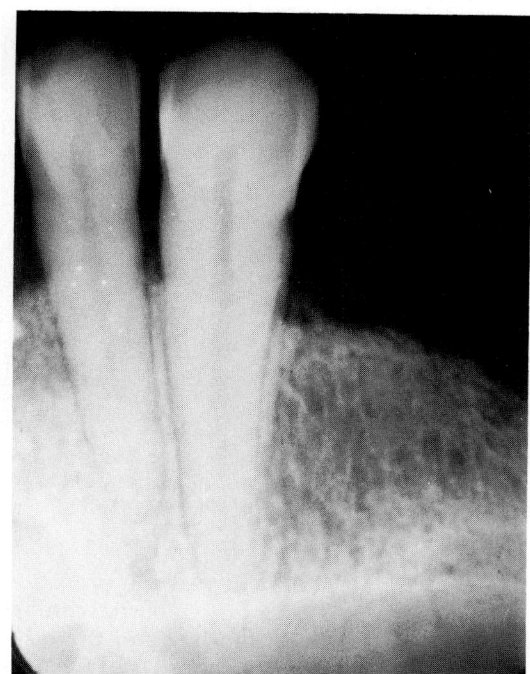

Figure 11–5 ■ The presence and continuity of cortical bone around remaining teeth is a good index of potential for support of the abutment tooth.

specific area that is bordered by a denture usually indicates excessive pressures either around roots or under the prosthesis as well as osteoclastic activity (Fig. 11–5).

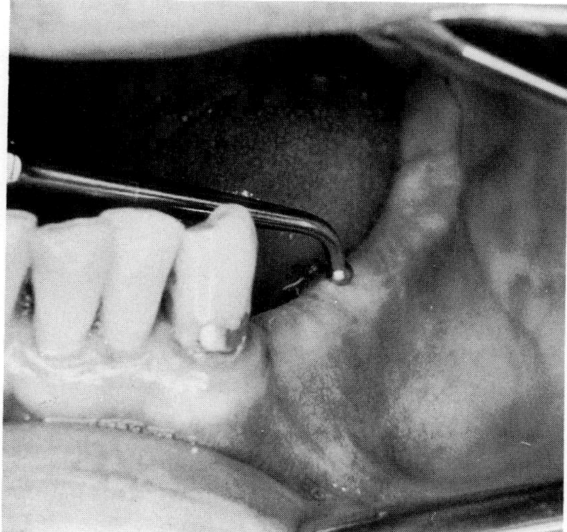

Figure 11–6 ■ Examination of the edentulous ridge is done to determine mucosa thicknesss, topograpy, and quality of tissue.

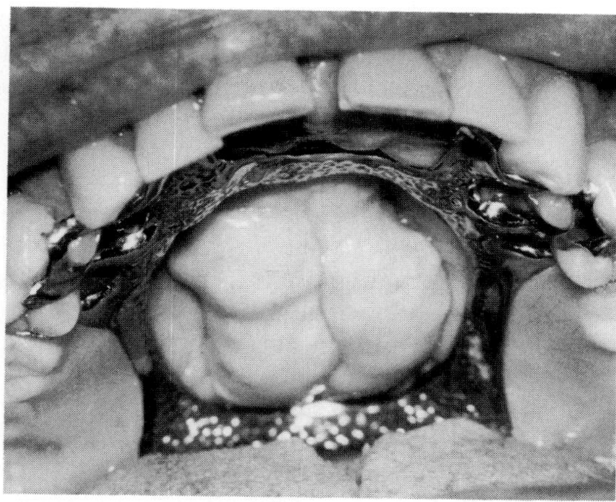

Figure 11–7 ■ Maxillary tori are evaluated for position and structure that could interfere with placement of the metal casting.

2. Clinical examination. This examination shows which areas are available for denture support (the size, shape, and contour of the edentulous support area) (Fig. 11–6). It demonstrates interfering structures, such as maxillary and mandibular tori and bony undercuts (Figs. 11–7 and 11–8).

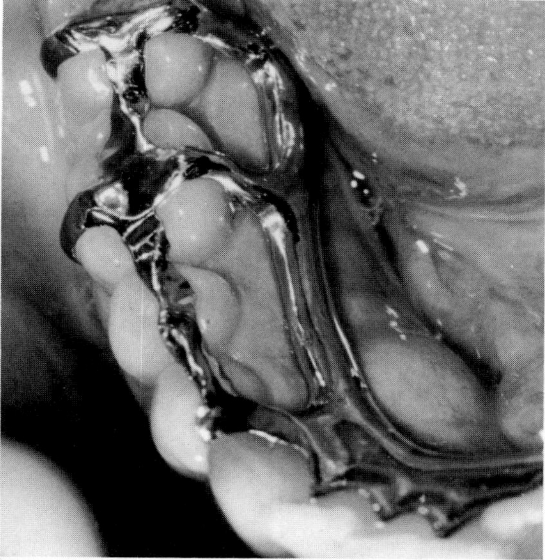

Figure 11–8 ■ Mandibular tori often interfere with placement and strength of the lingual major connector. In this situation, the continuous rest and circle design added to the casting strength and require minimum bulk of the lingual connector.

D. Periodontal ligament.
1. Roentgenographic examination. This examination demonstrates *thickness* and *continuity* of the periodontal ligament. It is one of the best indicators of what is going on at the time of diagnosis: Forces and pressures are indicated by the response of the periodontal ligament. Remember that a normal-appearing ligament indicates a tooth that is responding well to the current oral situation (Fig. 11–5).
2. Clinical examination. Check tooth mobility, depth of periodontal attachment, and appearance of the tissue around the tooth. Record the information.

E. Mucosa.
1. Observe the position of attached gingivae to ensure adequate attachment and proper position (Fig. 11–9).
2. Make a general appraisal of the mucosa of the entire oral cavity.
3. Evaluate the appearance, color, contour, area, and size of the usable portions of tissue for support. Evaluate muscle attachments, throat form, and hamular notch position as well.
4. Observe whether tissue areas are firm or flabby, and especially note and determine the causes of irritation and pathologic conditions.
5. *Palpate* the lips and cheeks between the thumb and forefinger. Look for hard areas that could indicate retention cysts or tumors and for tender or trigger areas. Repeat the procedure for the floor of the mouth, with one finger under the jaw and the other on the floor of the mouth. Observe the size and position of the sublingual glands.

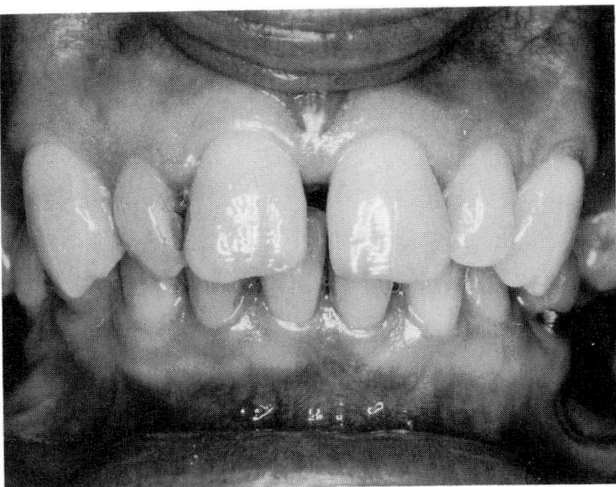

Figure 11–10 ■ A primary evaluation of the vertical dimension of occlusion by the use of phonetics may indicate the need to restore that dimension.

F. Teeth.
1. Observe the basic conformation of each arch and the relation of the arches to each other, and evaluate the overall conditions and approximation. Evaluate the *vertical dimension of occlusion* (VDO). Use of speech and phonetic assessment is most valuable for basic evaluation (Fig. 11–10).
2. Check the harmoniousness of centric relation with centric occlusion. Correction of disharmony must be a first priority.

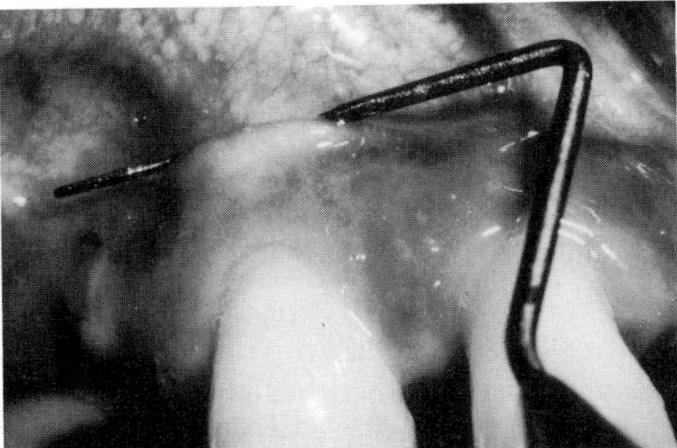

Figure 11–9 ■ The position and amount of attached gingivae will affect retainer placement, and a mucosa graft may be required.

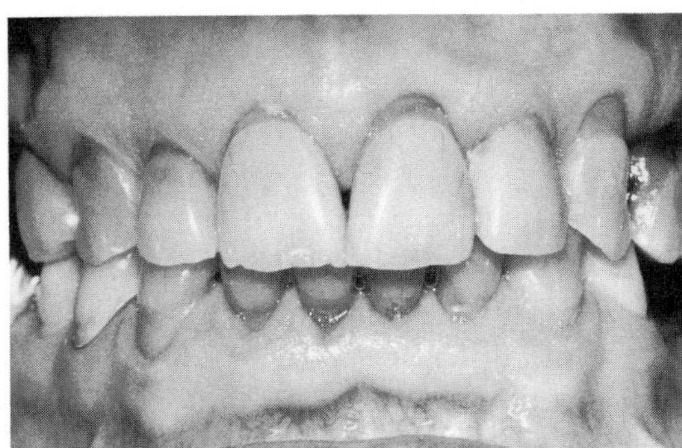

Figure 11–11 ■ The plane of occlusion at the correct vertical dimension of occlusion is assessed.

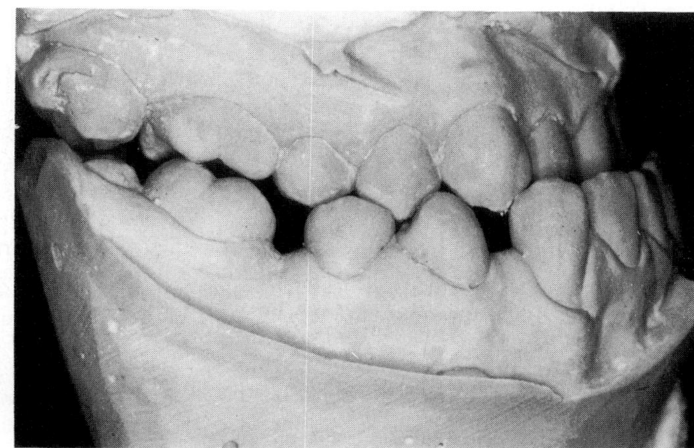

Figure 11-12 ■ Abnormal maxillomandibular relationships may require surgical intervention to improve esthetics and function.

3. Evaluate the position of the occlusal plane (Fig. 11-11).
4. Observe the size, length, and inclination of each tooth and crown. Evaluate form, shape, occlusal surface, and any pathologic condition, erosion, or abrasion.
5. Consider the size, shape, and condition of each root, where visible.
6. Record and evaluate caries and disease around teeth and existing restorations.

G. Temporomandibular joint. *Do not neglect the temporomandibular joint in diagnosis:* Feel it—listen to it—look at it.

1. Digital examination. Place a finger over the joint and have the patient go through all movements. Feel for "jumps" or irregular movements.
2. Auditory examination. Listen while the patient goes through all movements. Many patients with or without clinical complaints have an audible click or noise such as crepitus, indicating ligament or disk problems—a forewarning of difficulties in some situations.
3. Visual examination. Look at the head of the mandible as it moves the skin; "jerks" and "jumps" can be seen if they are present, indicating abnormalities.

H. General tooth arch considerations.

1. Interocclusal clearance in relation to the vertical dimension of occlusion. Evaluate this relationship by the use of phonetics. Loss of posterior tooth support often results in a great increase in interocclusal space.
2. Maxillomandibular relations. In cases of extreme skeletal Class II and Class III malocclusions, surgical correction may be considered (Fig. 11-12).
3. Diagnostic (study) casts. These must be available and mounted in centric relation for intelligent diagnosis and planning of treatment to be accomplished. Impressions for diagnostic casts are made at the first appointment (Fig. 11-13). *Diagnostic casts, properly mounted on the articulator*
   a. Demonstrate problem areas from the interarch standpoint.

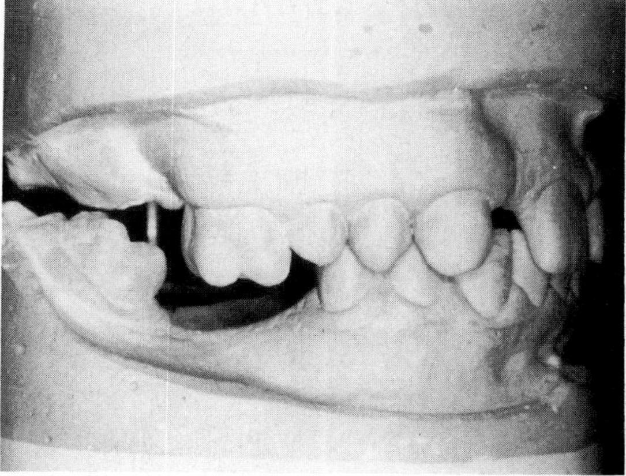

Figure 11-13 ■ Diagnostic casts mounted in centric relationship at the correct vertical dimension of occlusion are essential for intelligent diagnosis and treatment planning.

(1) Lack of space.
(2) Unequal space.
(3) Basic arch discrepancies in relation to each other.

b. Demonstrate usable areas for tissue support.
c. Demonstrate tooth and tissue undercuts.
d. Show problems associated with the *plane of occlusion,* show interference in movement, and also demonstrate the need for correction of the occlusal plane.
e. Show particular problems of rotated teeth.
f. Demonstrate the necessity for tooth alteration, surgery, and rest preparation.
g. Aid in planning the basic path of insertion.
h. Aid in planning the basic denture design.

III. **Psychologic considerations**

A. Can you meet the patient's expectations?
B. Can you expect cooperation in all treatment aspects?
C. Does the patient have a positive or a negative attitude?
D. Basic patient classification (Dr. House).
1. Philosophical.
2. Indifferent.
3. Exacting.
4. Hysterical.

Treatment Planning

Treatment planning must be considered together with diagnosis.

PATIENT ATTITUDE

Should this patient be treated with a removable partial denture? In some cases, the results of the evaluation from the initial diagnostic survey may indicate an apparent need for partial dentures. However, when careful consideration is given to patient attitude and mouth care, it is conceivable that more damage than good may result.

Example: The need for dentures has been explained to a patient, and the necessity for improvement of oral care to preserve the remaining teeth has been emphasized. When the patient returns for periodontal or operative procedures, there is no improvement in oral care.

In such a situation, it may be better to delay the partial denture treatment, because the basic prerequisite for a partial denture patient is above average oral cleanliness.

MAXILLOMANDIBULAR RELATIONS

Improvement may not be possible under existing conditions because of abnormal relation of maxilla to mandible or of remaining teeth to each other. Extensive surgical or orthodontic treatment or both may be indicated prior to prosthetic treatment (Figs. 11–12, 11–14, and 11–15).

1. In some instances of mandibular retrusion, there may be no remaining mandibular molars. However, when the mouth is closed in centric relation, mandibular second bicuspids may extend to the distal surface of the maxillary molars. In cases of this type, a partial denture serves no useful purpose.

2. Remaining mandibular teeth may all be located lingual to the maxillary teeth (Fig. 11–16).

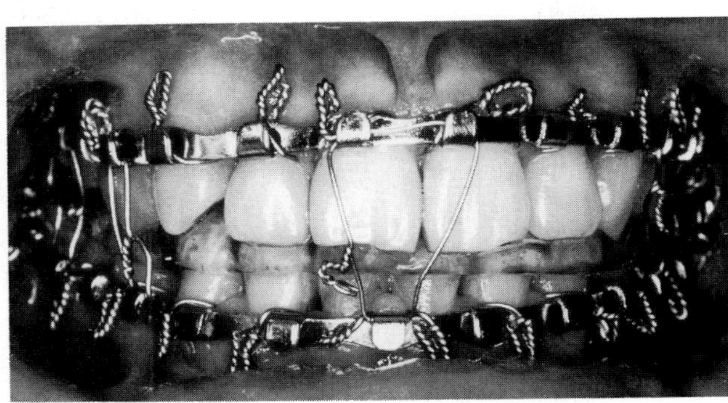

Figure 11–14 ■ Surgical repositioning of maxilla or mandible or both requires careful preplanning *prior* to the surgery in order to predict restorative results and improvement in occlusion.

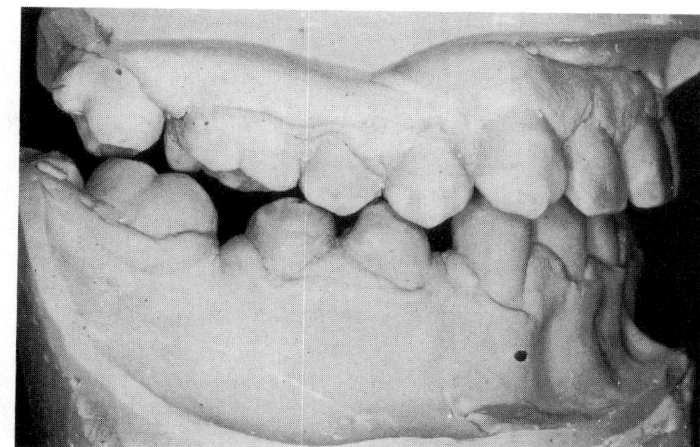

Figure 11–15 ■ Following surgical repositioning, extensive restorative procedures are usually necessary to retain position and restore function.

3. Teeth of either arch may be elongated and may touch or even indent the mucosa of the opposing edentulous ridge (Fig. 11–17).
4. Alveolar ridges of opposing arches may be in contact or in very close approximation.

VERTICAL DIMENSION

A frequent problem in the vertical dimension is a *decrease* or overclosure, which may occur because of tooth destruction, tilting, or loss (Fig. 11–18). Decreased vertical dimension becomes a problem if it is not recognized at the onset of treatment, because restoration of necessary occlusal height must often be incorporated in the metal framework. If the need to restore the vertical dimension is not recognized until the framework is completed, the casting will have to be remade. The use of a treatment partial denture is imperative in the determination of the correct vertical dimension (Fig. 11–19).

Restoring the vertical dimension may be a problem when the patient has developed an abnormal maxillomandibular relationship that is at the correct vertical dimension, but is not in centric relation. When the casts are mounted on the articulator in centric relation, there is deflective occlusal contact, which separates the jaws beyond an acceptable vertical dimension. Treat this situation with occlusal adjustment. An attempt to achieve equilibration at a later stage may not be possible.

OCCLUSAL PLANE

The occlusal plane is positioned *after* the vertical dimension of occlusion (VDO) is deter-

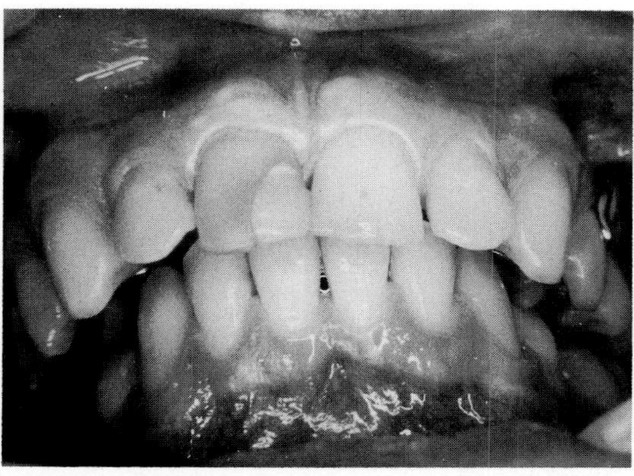

Figure 11–16 ■ An interarch malposition with mandibular posterior teeth completely lingual to the maxillary teeth. Correction can require orthodontic treatment or unusual prosthetic designs.

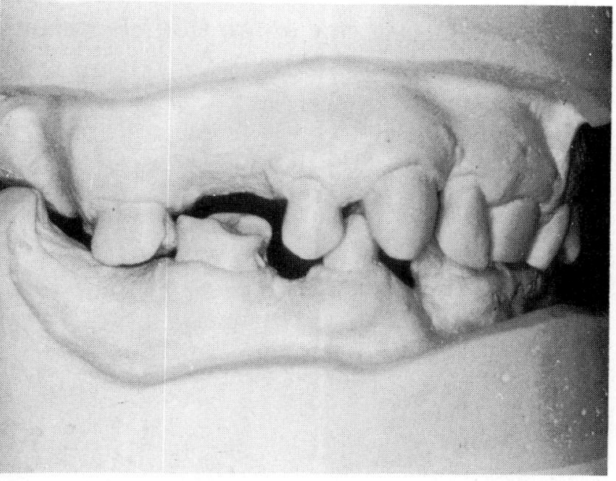

Figure 11–17 ■ Unopposed teeth can elongate over a period of time. When the vertical dimension of occlusion is correct, aggressive restorative or surgical procedures are necessary to establish the proper occlusal plane.

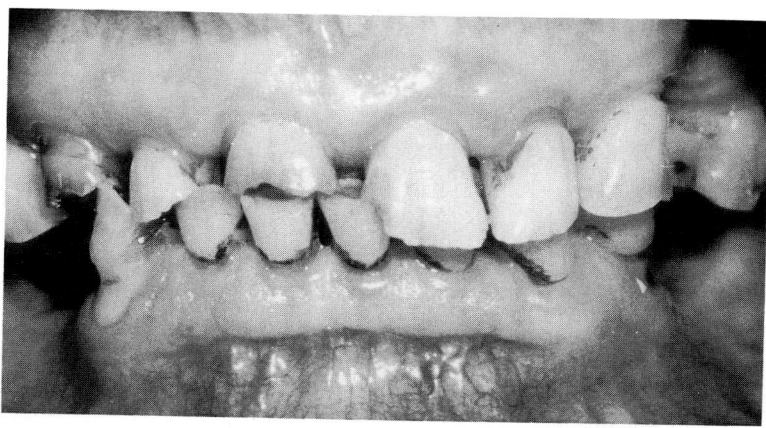

Figure 11–18 ■ Closure or loss of the proper vertical dimension of occlusion is a frequent occurrence due to loss and wear of teeth.

mined. The anatomic landmark for posterior location is the middle third of the retromolar pad; therefore, diagnostic and working casts *must* include the retromolar pad. The anterior position of the occlusal plane is determined by esthetics and phonetics of the maxillary anterior teeth when the arches are positioned at the proper VDO.

1. A posterior molar, standing alone, is usually the greatest offender in the occlusal plane. It may be elongated and tilted, and in such cases, gross modification is required to achieve a satisfactory occlusal plane (Fig. 11–20).

2. Elongation of a single tooth into an open opposing space creates design and equilibration problems. The occlusal plane must be restored. To do so may require gross reduction with restoration (Fig. 11–17) and, in some instances, removal.

3. Elongation of one entire side of the arch (Thielemann's Diagonal Law) (Fig. 11–21): Reduction of the elongated teeth may be required to improve esthetics. The cause is a posterior deflective occlusal contact in excursions in the opposite side of the arch, which allows elongation of the anterior teeth diagonally across the arch from the molar. The posterior deflective contact must be corrected (Fig. 11–22).

OCCUPATION

The patient's occupation must be taken into consideration in preliminary treatment planning, which may vary for patients who are for example, musicians, pilots, or divers. Treatment requires special try-outs of the mouth pieces used by the individual. In some situations it may be necessary to fabricate two prostheses — one for occupational function and another for esthetic and normal functions.

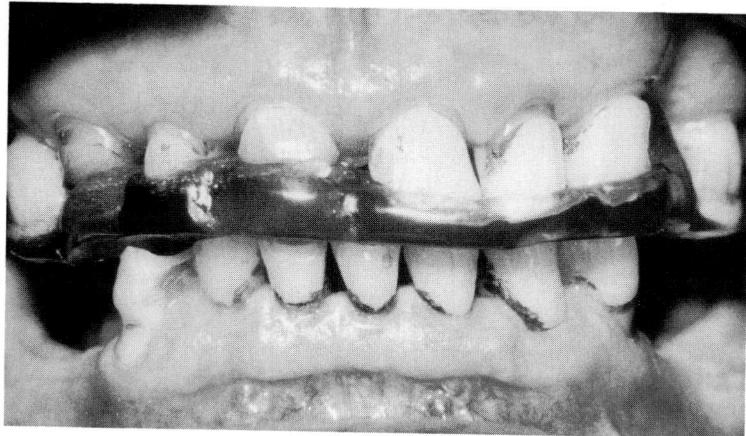

Figure 11–19 ■ A treatment partial denture or occlusal stent is used to assess the restored vertical dimension of occlusion.

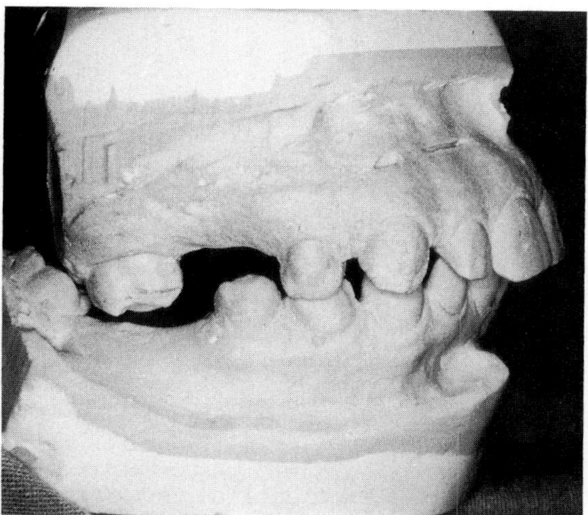

Figure 11–20 ■ One tooth grossly out of position often occurs. Aggressive restoration and occasionally removal are required.

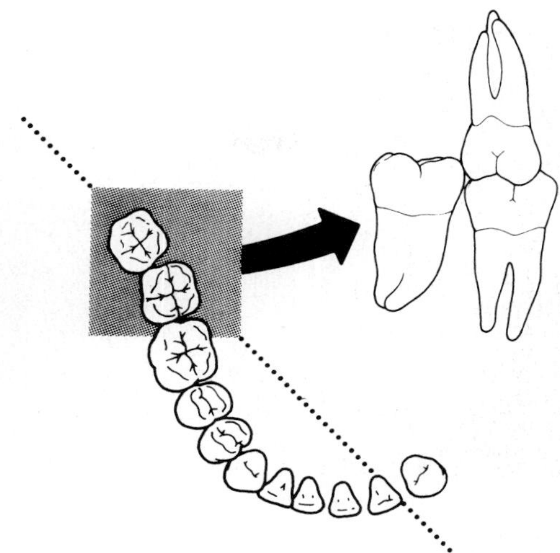

Figure 11–22 ■ The cause of unilateral anterior elongation is usually a hypercontact in excursions of posterior teeth diagonal from the anterior elongated teeth.

RECORDING OF THE FINAL TREATMENT PLAN

The final treatment plan is recorded with

1. Diagnostic casts mounted on the articulator.
2. The partial denture design drawn on the casts in red.
3. Areas of tooth alteration drawn on casts in blue.
4. All other restorative requirements marked as necessary.
5. All restorative procedures marked in proper sequence (Fig. 11–23).

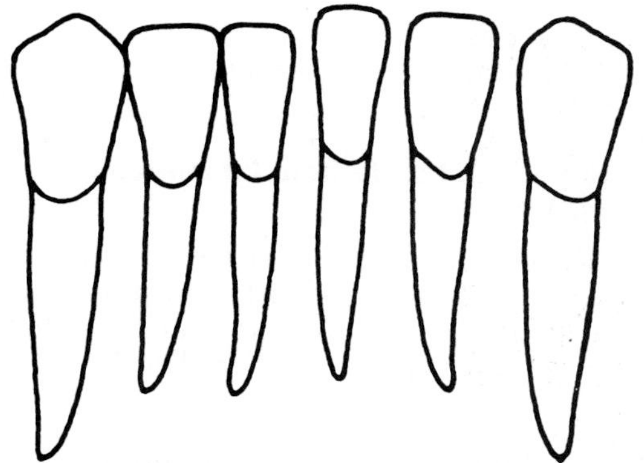

Figure 11–21 ■ Elongated anterior teeth *only* on one side of the arch create esthetic and anterior guidance difficulties.

TREATMENT SEQUENCE

Treatment procedure sequence may vary with the presence of individual problems, but, whenever possible, the following order of treatment should be considered.

Soft Tissue Treatment

In denture base areas where the tissues are irritated or traumatized by a prosthesis that the patient is wearing, treat the irritation until the tissues have recovered. This may be accomplished in either of two ways:

1. Remove the denture completely until the tissues have recovered (this is the best method) (Fig. 11–24).
2. Alter the denture to take it *out of tissue and occlusal contact,* and use a resilient denture treatment liner for treatment before constructing a new denture or relining the present denture, adding occlusal rests if necessary (Fig. 11–25). (Follow this by complete removal of the denture for 24 hours to ensure complete tissue recovery before making final impressions.)

Apply antifungal medication to control infection.

Surgical Preparation

Required surgery (i.e., exodontics, removal of impactions, or tissue and bone alterations)

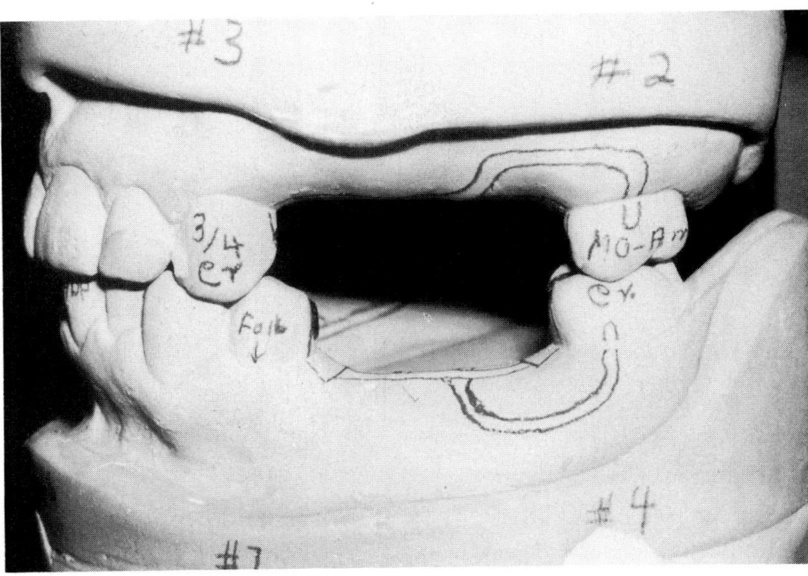

Figure 11–23 ■ Treatment sequence is marked on the diagnostic casts for treatment expediency and organization. It may be necessary to place prosthetic teeth in a diagnostic wax-up at this time for difficult situations.

should be performed as soon as possible. There are exceptions to this procedure; for example, it may be advisable to delay extractions until an immediate treatment partial denture can be fabricated, so that the denture may act as a matrix or bandage during healing. This helps prevent alveolar ridge resorption and loss of bone.

Periodontal Treatment

In many instances there are teeth that require periodontal surgery. Whenever periodontal treatment is indicated, begin it immediately.

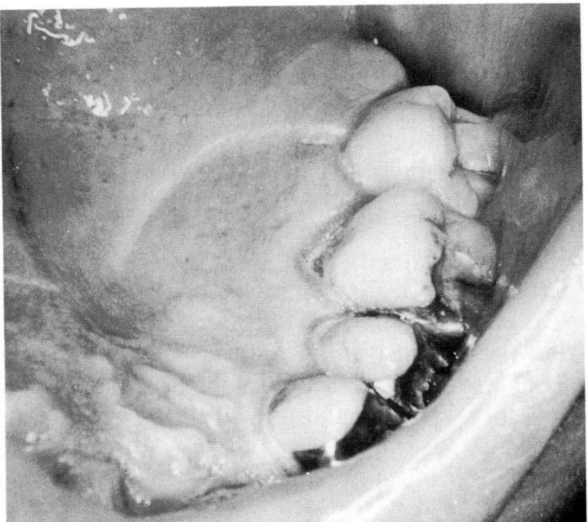

Figure 11–24 ■ Soft tissue disorders are treated immediately by removal or modification of the offending prosthesis.

The position of the healed gingival attachment, the contour of restorations, and the tooth alterations that follow influence partial denture design and mouth preparation.

Restorations of Individual Teeth

Restorative treatment is not limited to treatment of caries and faulty restorations. It must also

1. Contour tooth surfaces to make them compatible with the MAP and to eliminate voids.
2. Provide sufficient strength and bulk for occlusal rest preparations.
3. Provide an acceptable occlusal plane.
4. Reduce excessive interproximal spaces.
5. Provide undercut areas for retention where they are absent or reduce excessive undercut areas.
6. Provide for good esthetics.

Evaluation of the Vertical Dimension of Occlusion

When the vertical dimension of occlusion is to be evaluated or restored, a treatment prosthesis is fabricated, inserted, and evaluated to determine the proper position (Fig. 11–26).

Patient Presentation and Information

1. Written report. This report is sent to the patient detailing all clinical, radiographic, and

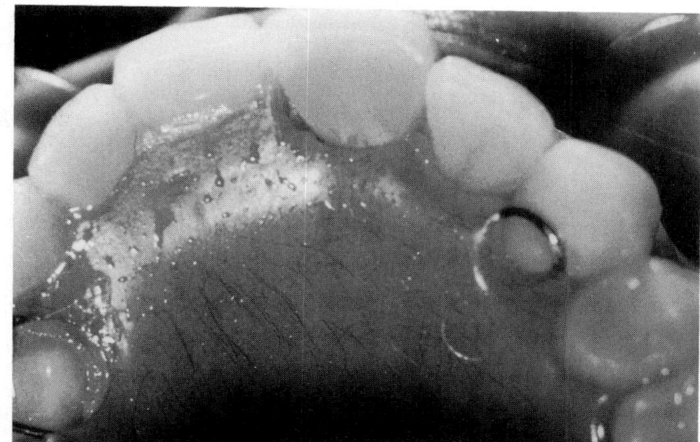

Figure 11–25 ■ The addition of rests to the existing prosthesis helps control tissue irritation.

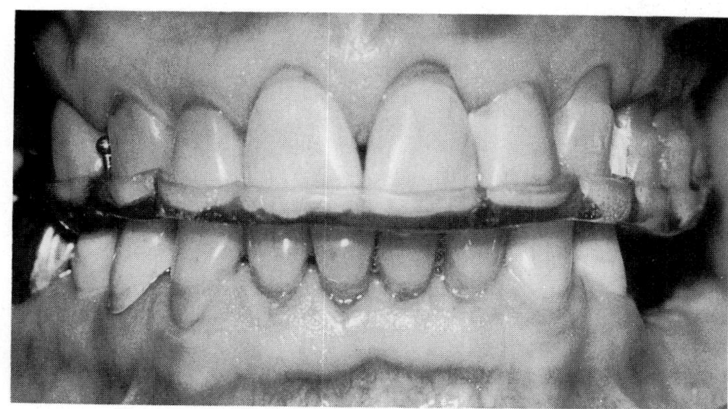

Figure 11–26 ■ Evaluation of the vertical dimension of occlusion is a most important diagnostic procedure and is often necessary for emergency control of discomfort.

diagnostic findings. Difficulties are enumerated, methods of treatment are explained in detail, and cost of treatment is given.

2. A treatment presentation appointment is arranged to explain and discuss treatment procedures and prognosis.

REFERENCES

Applegate OC: Keeping the partial denture in harmony with biological considerations. J Am Dent Assoc 43:409, 1951.

Applegate OC: The interdependence of periodontics and removable denture prosthesis. J Prosthet Dent 8:269, 1958.

Applegate OC: Evaluation of oral structures for removable dentures. J Prosthet Dent 11:882, 1961.

Dail RA and Kopczyk RA: Removable partial dentures and oral health: a literature review. J West Soc Periodontol 25:122–129, 1977.

Fenner W et al: Tooth mobility changes during treatment with partial denture prosthesis. J Prosthet Dent 6:520, 1956.

Girardat RL: History and development of partial denture design. J Am Dent Assoc 28:1399, 1941.

Jordan LG: Treatment of advanced periodontal disease by prosthetic procedures. J Prosthet Dent 10:908, 1960.

Kratochvil FJ: Five year survey of treatment with removable partial dentures. Part I. J Prosthet Dent 48:237, 1981.

Mann AW: Examination, diagnosis, and treatment planning in occlusal rehabilitation. J Prosthet Dent 20:98, 1968.

McCall JO: The periodontist looks at the clasp partial denture. J Am Dent Assoc 43:439, 1951.

McKensie JS: Mutual problems of the periodontist and the prosthodontist. J Prosthet Dent 5:37, 1955.

Miller EL: Systems for classifying partially edentulous arches. J Prosthet Dent 24:25, 1970.

Neurohr FG: Health conservation of the periodontal tissues by a method of functional partial denture design. J Am Dent Assoc 31:54, 1944.

Nevin RB: Periodontal aspects of partial denture prosthesis. J Prosthet Dent 5:215, 1955.

Potter et al: Removable partial denture design. J Prosthet Dent 17:63, 1967.

Pound E: Cross arch splinting vs premature extractions. J Prosthet Dent 16:1058, 1966.

Rudd KD: Making diagnostic casts is not a waste of time. J Prosthet Dent 20:98, 1968.

Schmitz AH: Partial denture planning and designing J Am Dent Assoc 35:562, 1947.

Steffel VL: Fundamental principles involved in partial denture design. J Am Dent Assoc 42:534, 1951.

Steffel VL: Current concepts in removable partial denture service. J Prosthet Dent 20:387, 1968.
Stewart KL and Rudd KD: Stabilizing periodontally weakened teeth with removable partial dentures. J Prosthet Dent 19:475, 1958.
Thayer H and Kratochvil FJ: Periodontal considerations with removable partial dentures. Dent Clin North Am, 1980.
Waerhaug J: Justification for splinting in periodontal therapy. J Prosthet Dent 22:201, 1969.

chapter 12

Intraoral preparation

Preparation of the mouth for final treatment, with the exception of emergency situations, is begun after the completed treatment plan has been prepared and accepted by the patient. *Preliminary intraoral procedures* for treatment are

1. Prophylaxis.
2. Impressions for working and occlusal waxing casts.

Prophylaxis

A complete and thorough prophylaxis is necessary prior to the start of treatment, so that an exact replica of all tooth surfaces can be made. The prophylaxis removes any debris from teeth, so that detailed impressions can be made and to eliminate the possibility of a deposit being left on the impression and casts, which results in rough or vague cast detail.

Working Casts

Accurate, properly extended impressions of both arches are made, which include all teeth and soft tissues that will be involved by the prosthesis as well as anatomical land marks such as (1) retromolar pads, (2) the hamular notch, and (3) tuberosities. Proper lingual and facial extensions are made to record muscle and tissue positions.

Intraoral records are made to record jaw relationship in *centric relation position.* It may be necessary to construct record bases if there are numerous missing teeth (Fig. 12–1).

The *vertical dimension of occlusion* (VDO) is evaluated and recorded for tentative diagnostic evaluation.

The working casts are mounted on the articulator

1. At the proper vertical dimension of occlusion.
2. In centric relation (Fig. 12–2).

THE SEQUENCE OF TREATMENT INTRAORAL PREPARATION PROCEDURE

The usual sequence of procedures is

1. Treatment of abnormal or irritated soft tissues.
2. Surgical intervention to treat teeth, bone, and mucosa, when indicated.
3. Final diagnostic wax-up and occlusal equilibration.
4. Periodontal treatment.
5. Endodontics.
6. Orthodontics.
7. Restorations.
8. Tooth modifications.
9. Procedures for prosthesis fabrication.

Soft Tissue Treatment

Irritation, hypertrophy, or inflammation of the mucosa under an existing prosthesis can be caused by one or more of the following conditions: (1) lack of positive rests (Fig. 12–3); (2) bacterial and fungal organisms (Fig. 12–4); (3) poor adaptation of prosthesis to tissue; (4) hyperocclusion of the prosthesis. The required treatment is often best accomplished by re-

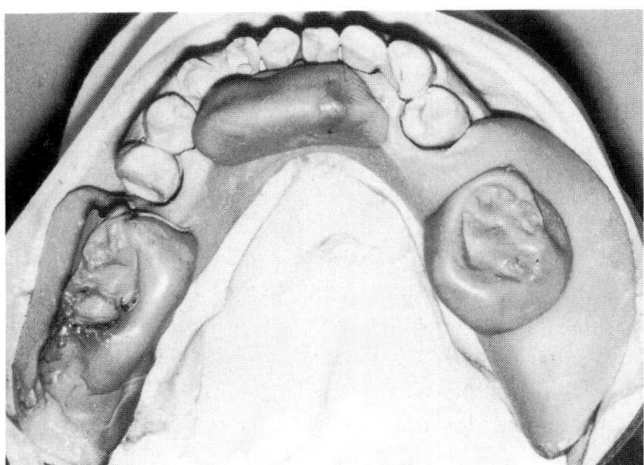

Figure 12–1 ■ Record bases and interocclusal records are necessary for tentative mounting when posterior teeth are missing.

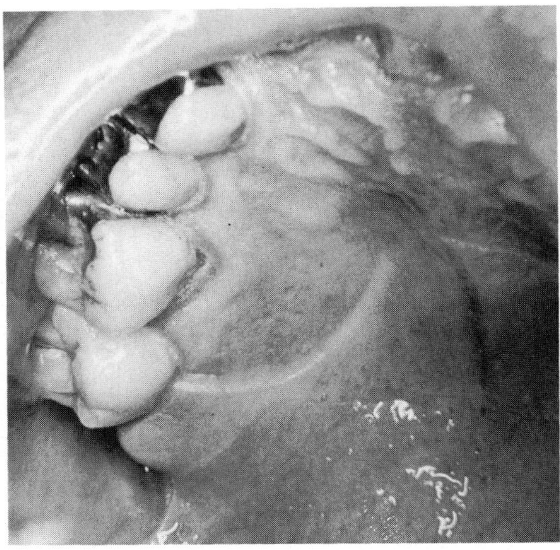

Figure 12–3 ■ Lack of positive rests results in prosthesis displacement, which can destroy mucosa and periodontal attachments.

moval of the offending prosthesis until the tissues are healed or by construction of a treatment prosthesis. If the old prosthesis is to be used during treatment procedure, it may be necessary to (1) add positive rests (Fig. 12–5), which will not allow the prosthesis to be depressed into the mucosa during function, (2) apply a fungicide ointment to the prosthesis-tissue surface, (3) place tissue conditioning material on the tissue side of the prosthesis to ensure good tissue adaptation (Fig. 12–6), (4) equilibrate the prosthesis to ensure that equal, harmonious occlusion is present (Fig. 12–7).

Do not proceed with impressions for the final prosthesis until the mucosa is completely healthy.

Surgical Intervention

Teeth ■ Teeth that are not serviceable should be removed as soon as possible to allow for maximum healing time prior to final prosthesis fabrication. Try to retain impacted and partially erupted teeth whenever possible, since when they erupt they often provide useful abutments and prevent the need for an extension prosthesis.

Bone ■ When bone problems jeopardize the success of prosthetic treatment, surgical procedures are necessary. Examples are gross maxillary and mandibular tori that interfere with prosthetic design and function (Fig. 12–8), lack of space between tuberosity and retromolar pad, and bony undercuts that prevent insertion and removal of the prosthesis (Fig. 12–9).

In situations of severe Class 2 and Class 3 jaw relations, surgical repositioning of one or both

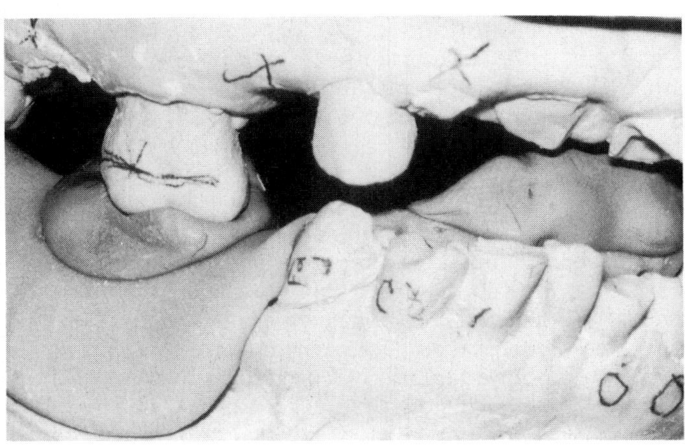

Figure 12–2 ■ Evaluation casts are mounted in centric relation at the estimated vertical dimension of occlusion.

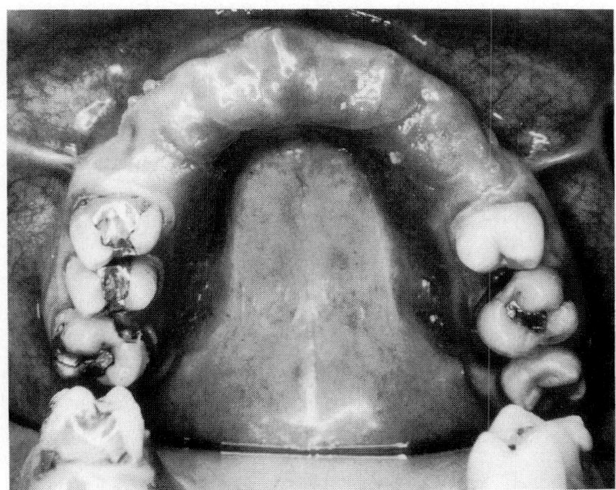

Figure 12–4 ■ Bacterial and fungal infections increase tissue irritation.

arches may be required (Figs. 12–10 through 12–12).

Mucosa ■ The most common site for soft tissue surgery is the maxillary tuberosity area. A wedge of tissue may need to be removed to give space for the denture base material (Fig. 12–13).

Soft tissue surgery may be required to remove redundant tissue or to reposition muscle and tissue attachments.

Surgical intervention may be necessary when there are residual infections, and to remove cysts, root fragments, and foreign bodies. Be most conservative when roots are present. They usually erupt after the denture is inserted and can then be removed more easily and with less bone loss. Inform the patient of the presence of a root, and make an entry about it in the chart.

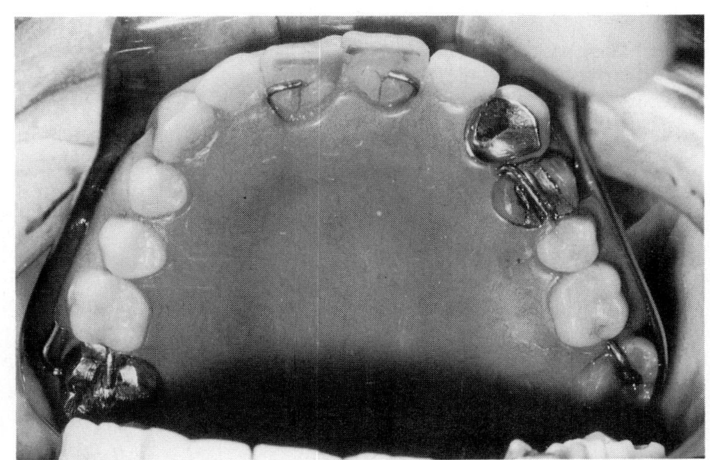

Figure 12–5 ■ Adding positive rests to old prostheses controls the relationship of prosthesis to mucosa during the tissue treatment period.

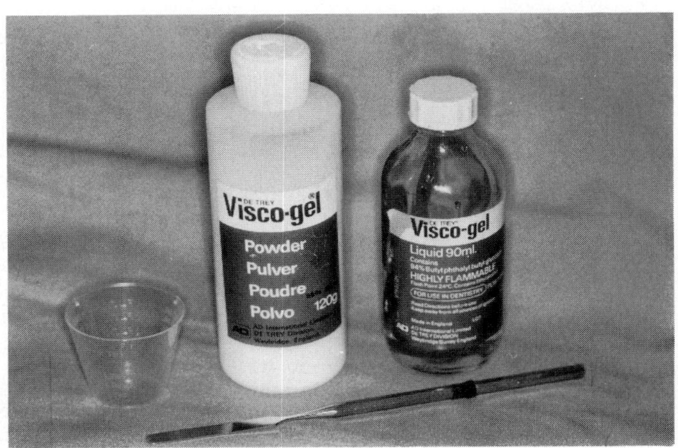

Figure 12–6 ■ A treatment liner provides proper mucosa-prosthesis contact during the tissue treatment period.

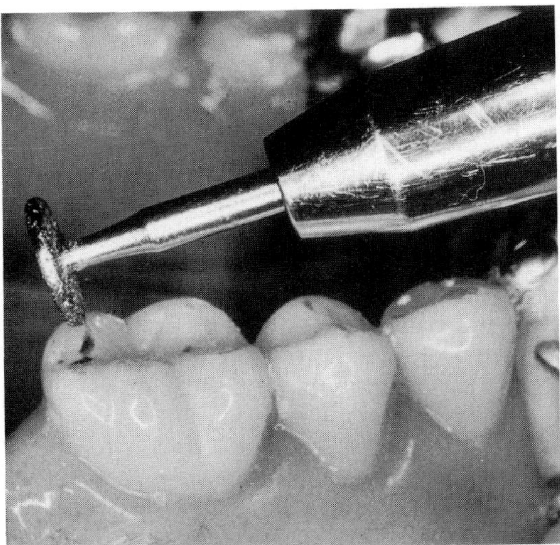

Figure 12–7 ■ Equilbration for proper occlusal contacts is necessary *after* the addition of rests and the placement of a treatment liner.

Final Diagnostic Wax-up and Occlusal Equilibration

A diagnostic wax-up is often necessary for treatment planning and can be modified or refined prior to treatment. This procedure helps to identify and solve complications of tooth modification, preparations for restorations, development of occlusion, and coordination with partial denture design.

Deflective occlusal contacts are adjusted and equilibrated before teeth are modified and before rests are prepared. Equilibration can alter the position and depth of rest preparations and removes interferences in centric closure and lateral excursions. Equilibration can be accomplished on the mounted diagnostic casts and gives advance information on final tooth and jaw positions.

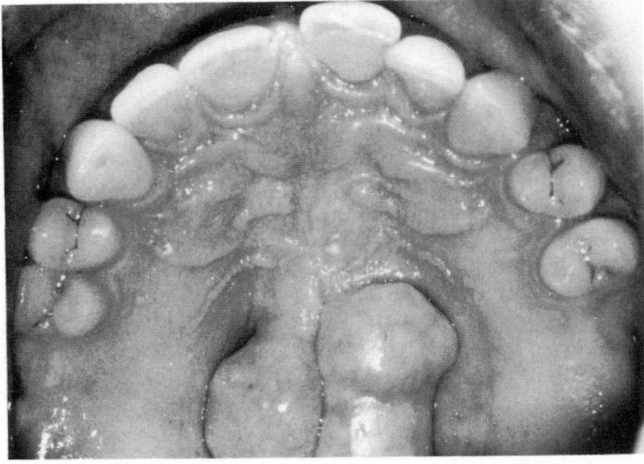

Figure 12–8 ■ Maxillary tori may have to be removed if there is interference with partial major connectors, especially in the placement of the posterior palatal connector.

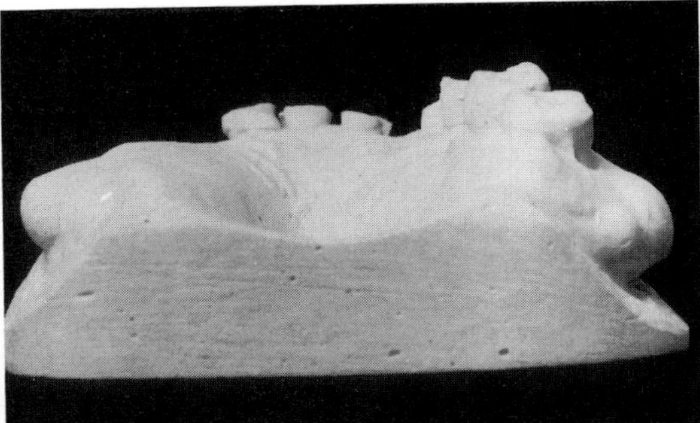

Figure 12–9 ■ Gross bone undercuts that interfere with placement of the prosthesis or the peripheral seal may have to be surgically altered.

Periodontal Treatment

Oral hygiene is evaluated beginning with the first appointment and is an important consideration in partial denture diagnosis. Personal care is a *must.* If it is not adequate, the patient may be better off without a partial denture.

Pocket depth of mucosa surrounding all teeth is evaluated and recorded (Fig. 12–14). Of particular significance is the type and topography of mucosa in any area that will be touched or be in close proximity to the partial denture casting. Teeth with pockets too deep to be cleaned may have to be treated with surgical repositioning for the proper guiding plane contacts, tissue contours, and reduction of pocket depth.

Mobility of teeth may be caused by a combination of factors: (1) inflammation, (2) occlusal problems, (3) insufficient bone support, and (4) loss of arch integrity. Inflammation and occlusal problems can be treated in the first phases of oral preparation. The loss of arch integrity can be rectified with a treatment prosthesis (Fig. 12–15) and a final prosthesis, which will unite and utilize all remaining teeth and ridges to stabilize the teeth and reduce mobility. Appropriate treatment of loss of bone support and resultant tooth mobility becomes a clinical judgment decision. If mobility can be kept to an acceptable level by treatment, the tooth should be retained if at all possible. In instances of a borderline clinical decision to retain a tooth, it is advantageous to design the metal casting so that loss of the tooth at a later time will not

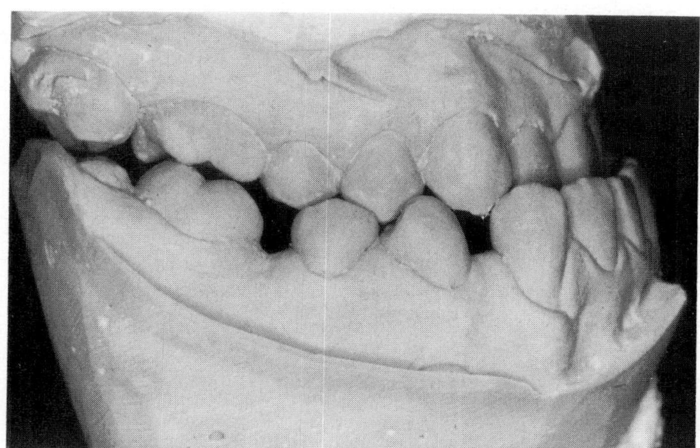

Figure 12–10 ■ Gross malposition of the arches may require surgical repositioning for function and esthetics.

necessitate remake of the prosthesis; the tooth can be removed when necessary and a prosthetic tooth added to the existing prosthesis (Fig. 12–16).

The periodontal attachment is a major consideration in mouth preparation for a removable partial denture (RPD). Very narrow or thin attached mucosa can cause difficulties in areas where the prosthesis touches the teeth or under infrabulge retainers. Adequate attached tissue can be provided in these areas by tissue repositioning or by free mucosa grafts (Fig. 12–17).

The patient's conditioning and instruction in mouth care should begin immediately in preparation for receiving the denture.

Endodontics

Wherever it is possible to provide endodontic treatment, it is indicated for partial denture patients. The root provides the stimulus to conserve and retain bone. Saving the root results in additional periodontal ligament support for the prosthesis, which is far superior to support that can be provided by the partial denture base placed directly on the mucosa. Many times an overdenture above a remaining root is the treatment of choice because it greatly reduces the crown : root ratio and enhances the prognosis of the remaining root (Fig. 12–18).

If it is necessary to place a post and crown on any *endodontically* treated tooth, that tooth *should not* be used as a *rotation rest* or as an axis for an extension partial denture. The torquing forces of the extension prosthesis on the crown and post can cause root fracture.

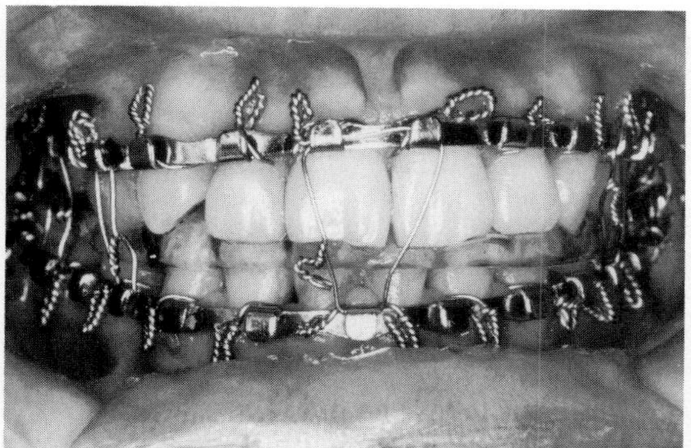

Figure 12–11 ■ Careful analysis of the structural position of the arches and the extent of reconstruction required are essential, as is rigid interarch fixation during healing.

Orthodontics

When orthodontic procedures are used, the treatment is accomplished before definitive restorative procedures, such as crowns, are started. Contours of crowns and restorations are determined by the final position of the teeth, so that guiding surfaces and occlusal planes can be properly positioned (Fig. 12–19).

Restorations

The primary prerequisite before beginning *any* restoration is to *prepare the guiding surfaces* on all teeth. This establishes the *path of insertion* for the removable partial denture. After the teeth have been prepared for the guiding surfaces, the preparation for the restoration can be made. If this sequence is not followed, it may not be possible to prepare the proper path of insertion without jeopardizing the restoration.

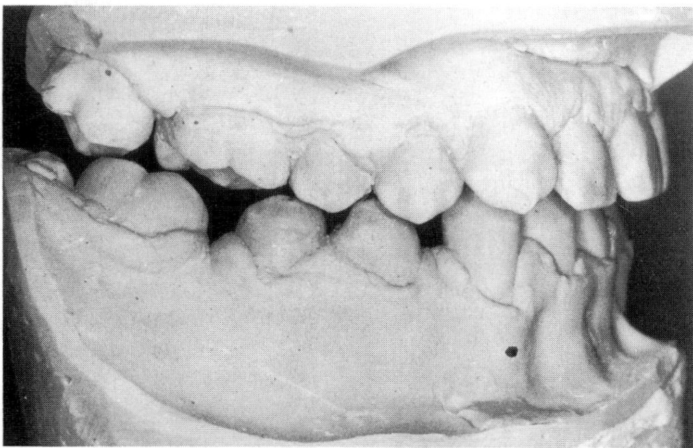

Figure 12–12 ■ Prosthetic treatment is usually necessary to establish occlusal control following surgical repositioning.

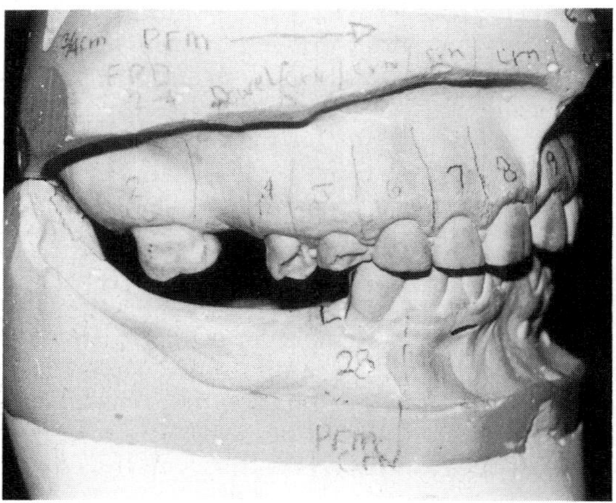

Figure 12–13 ■ Tissue contact in the retromolar pad area may require a surgical procedure to provide space for the prosthetic coverage of the retromolar pad.

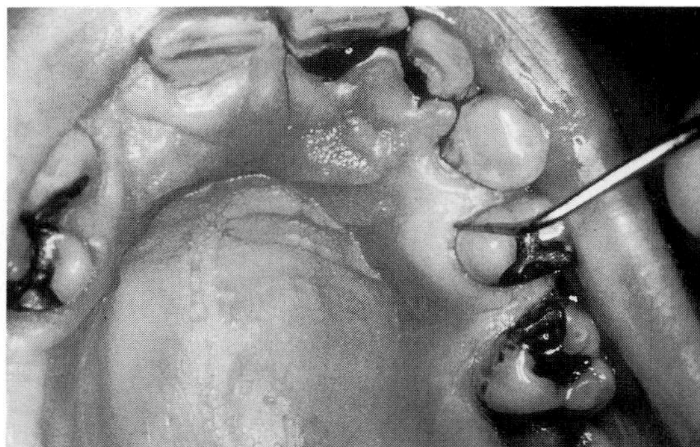

Figure 12–14 ■ Complete periodontal evaluation and consultation is a primary step in treatment.

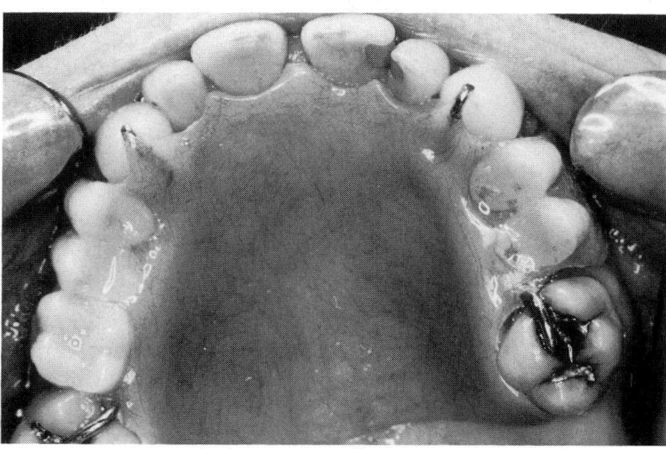

Figure 12–15 ■ A treatment prosthesis can stablize the remaining teeth, restore occlusion, and evaluate the vertical dimension of occlusion.

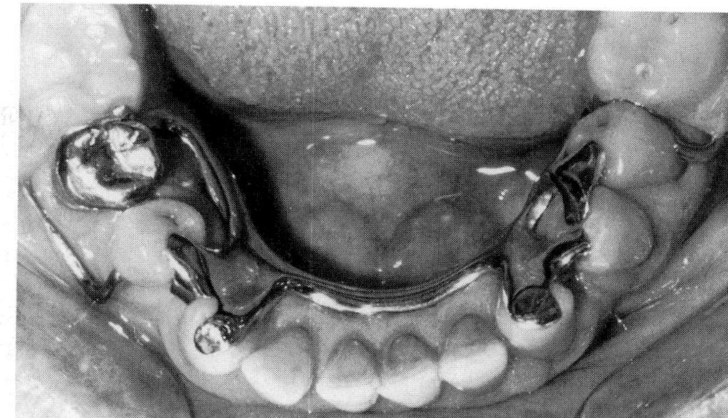

Figure 12–16 ■ Periodontally weak or compromised teeth can be retained by designing *around* them. Their responsibility to support the prosthesis is minimal.

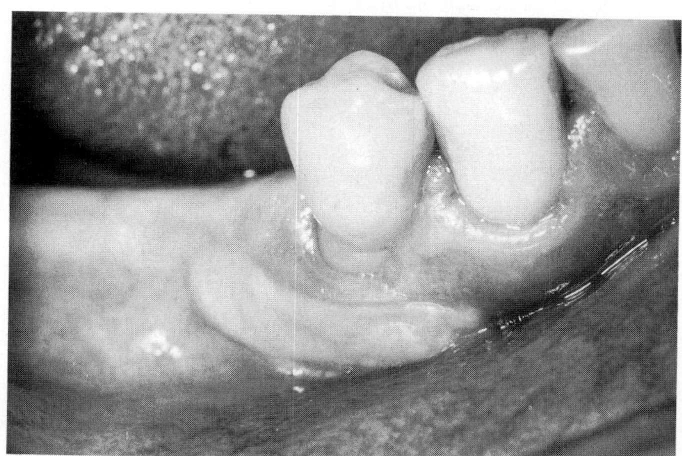

Figure 12–17 ■ Free gingival grafts can provide attached mucosa in an area critically associated with the prosthesis.

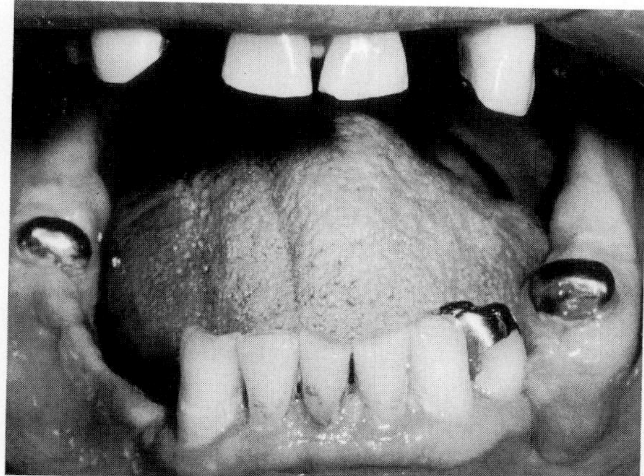

Figure 12–18 ■ Roots serve as excellent abutments for overdentures and provide periodontal ligament support for the prosthesis.

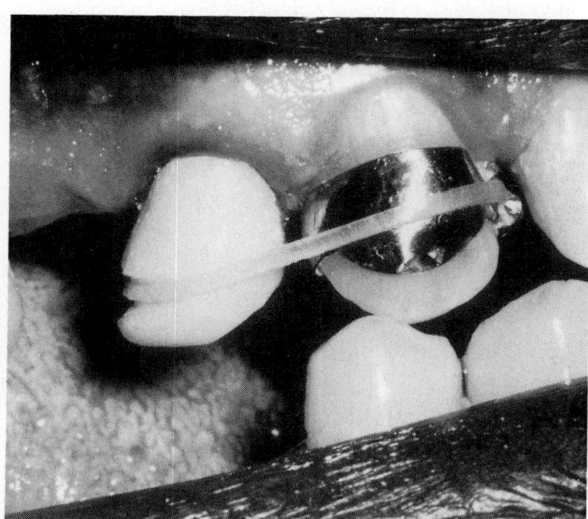

Figure 12–19 ■ Minor orthodontic tooth movements can greatly enhance tooth positions for improved prosthetic results.

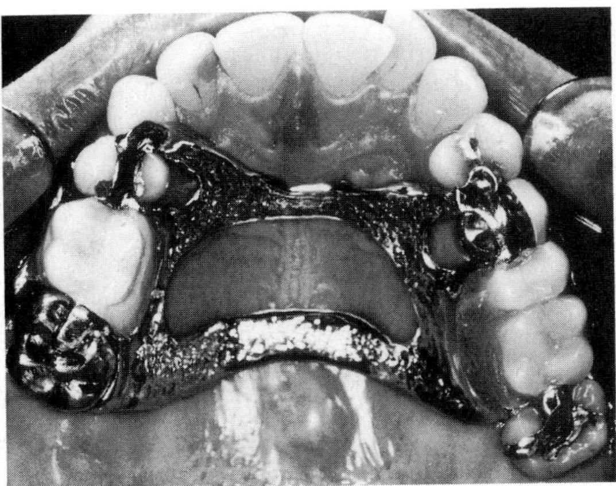

Figure 12–20 ■ Amalgam restorations are satisfactory for partial denture abutments if they fulfill basic restorative requirements.

Amalgam restorations are satisfactory for partial denture abutments if there is sufficient bulk of tooth structure for proper amalgam support. Adequate bulk is the basic consideration in rest and guiding surface areas (Fig. 12–20).

Castings on individual teeth may be necessary when full crowns, inlays, onlays, or partial veneers are to be used. Full crowns are necessary to (1) restore badly broken down clinical crowns, (2) reposition the occlusal plane, (3) reposition the clinical crown, and (4) provide proper rests, especially on anterior teeth (Figs. 12–21 through 12–24). Inlays, onlays, and partial veneers are more conservative treatments, and their use is preferred whenever possible (Fig. 12–25).

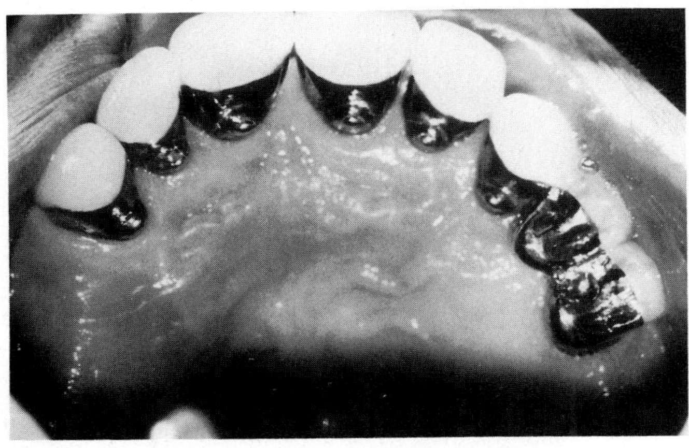

Figure 12–21 ■ Complete crowns to restore remaining teeth are often necessary and are contoured to accommodate and coordinate with removable partial denture treatment. Note positive lingual rests.

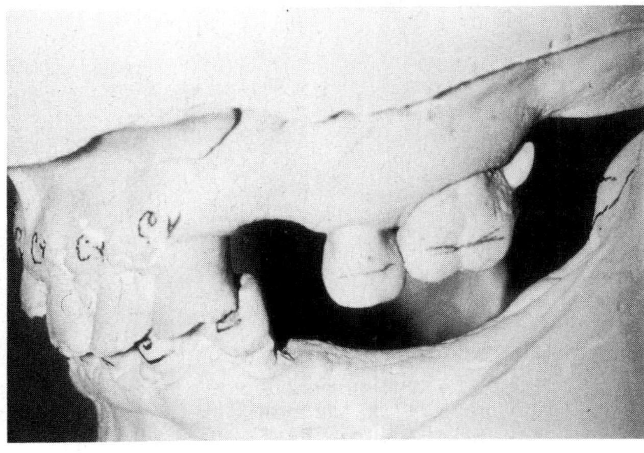

Figure 12–22 ■ Extruded teeth may need to be reduced to the proper occlusal plane and treated with crowns.

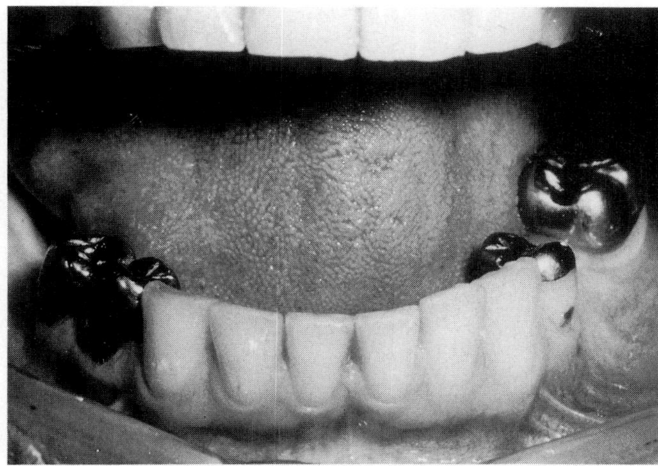

Figure 12–23 ■ Restoration of the occlusal plane often requires treatment with crowns or onlays.

The clinical crown that is restored by a casting will not have the contours of the original tooth. With the loss of contacting teeth and surrounding supporting structures, it is usually necessary to remove the mesial and the distal curvatures so that the guiding surfaces of the RPD casting can slide into position without a space being left between the prosthesis and the remaining mouth structures. The existing condition is not the same as a normal tissue-tooth situation such as originally existed when all tissues were intact. The tooth form is altered for greater compatibility with the current situation (Fig. 12–26).

Partial veneer crowns are the treatment of choice whenever possible, since tooth structure is conserved, facial esthetics remain unchanged, and the normal tooth-tissue junction is left intact on the facial surface (Fig. 12–27).

Complete arch impressions for wax-up and fabrication of crowns and onlays are required; they record all guide surfaces that influence the path of insertion (Fig. 12–28). The crown wax-up and final casting can then be fabricated parallel to all other guide surfaces and with proper retention contours (Figs. 12–29 and 12–30).

Tooth Modifications

Guiding surfaces are prepared first, as determined and outlined by the path of insertion on the diagnostic cast. The guiding surfaces need not be flat planes; the objective is to eliminate tooth undercuts.

Usually, the prepared surface is rounded, following the curvature of the tooth (Fig. 12–31).

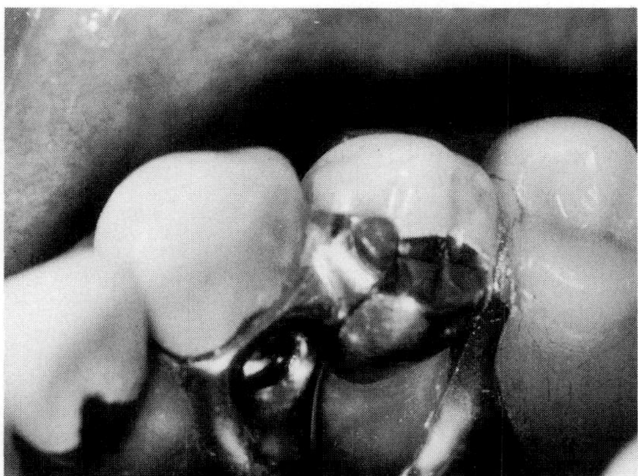

Figure 12–24 ■ A cuspid crown with a positive lingual rest to unite with the partial casting. The premolar crown with a recess on the mesial side receives the partial casting, restoring contour.

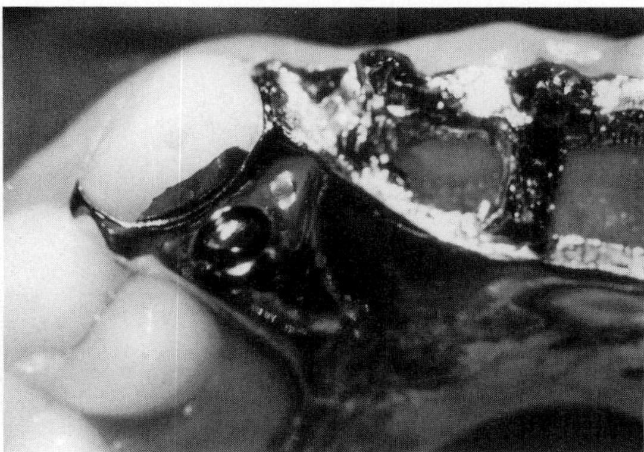

Figure 12–25 ■ A conservative lingual inlay provides a maxillary anterior rest. The central portion of the partial casting is open to ensure proper seating.

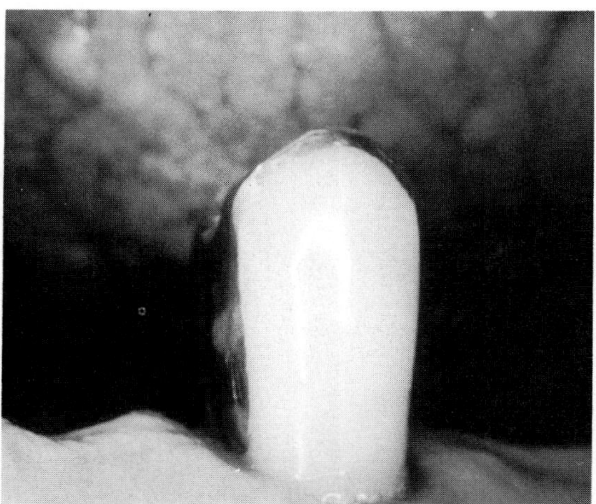

Figure 12–26 ■ Parallel guiding surfaces and elimination of voids require reduction of the mesial-distal contour of restorations.

A large, cylinder-shaped diamond stone, together with water and air spray, are used in much the same grinding and shaping procedure used to establish parallelism in abutment preparation for fixed partial dentures (Fig. 12–32). A larger-diameter diamond does not have the tendency to produce an uneven or a wavy surface, as does a smaller-diameter diamond.

Interproximal surfaces may need reshaping to provide space for the metal casting to keep it within the tooth contours (Figs. 12–33 and 12–34).

Lingual tooth surfaces may require reduction if the teeth are tilted and interfere with the path of insertion of the lingual bar.

Excessive undercuts in the facial retainer placement areas may need to be removed so that retainers do not stand away from the mucosa and cause cheek interference (Fig. 12–35A and B).

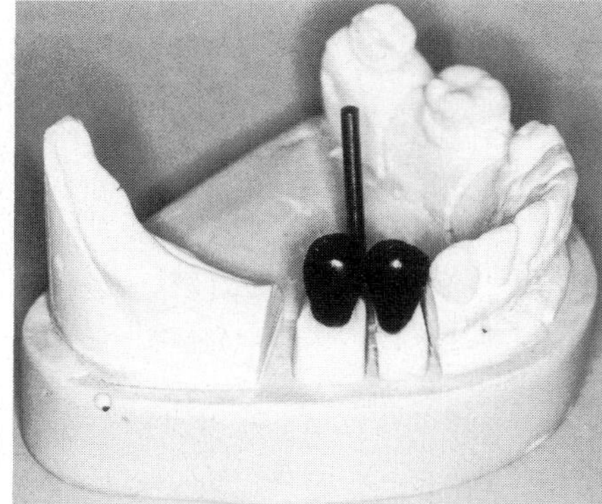

Figure 12–28 ■ Complete arch impressions are essential when crowns are fabricated for abutment teeth to assure parallel guide surfaces with other teeth.

Rests are prepared *after* the guiding surfaces are completed. This ensures the proper placement of marginal ridges and rest contours. Basic requirements for rest preparations are as follows:

1. All surfaces must be rounded and smoothed with no sharp angles (Fig. 12–36).
2. A minimum thickness of 1mm is essential.
3. The seat should be lower in the middle of the tooth than at the marginal ridge (Fig. 12–37).
4. The rest preparation should be wider at the marginal ridge area than toward the center of the tooth (Fig. 12–35).
5. Junctions with other parts of the casting must be rounded to reduce fracture possibilities.

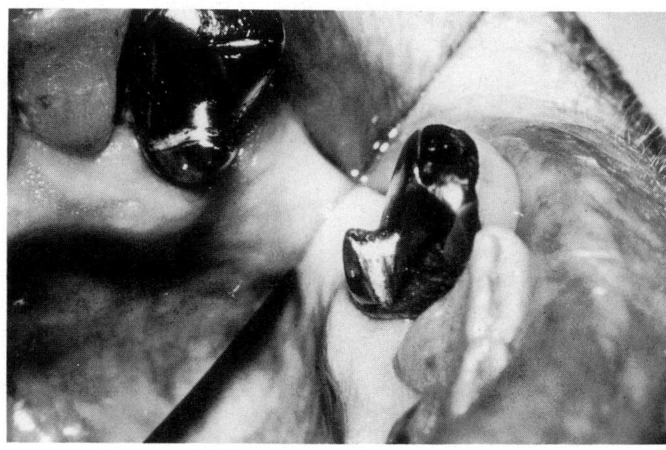

Figure 12–27 ■ Partial veneer crowns provide for ideal placement of rests and preserve facial esthetics. Note that the rest is circular and is aligned with the residual ridge.

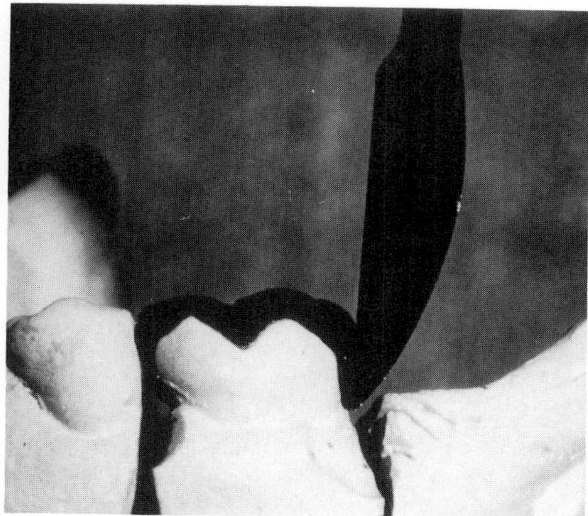

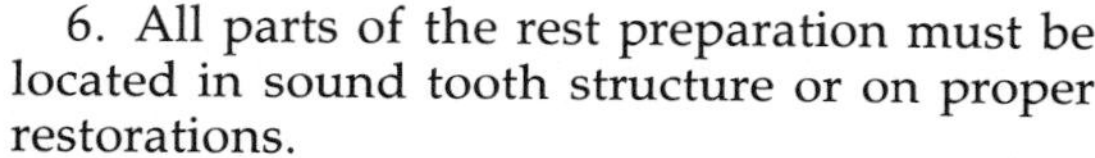

Figure 12–29 ■ Parallel guide surfaces are produced in the wax crown pattern with the cast on the surveyor in the MAP.

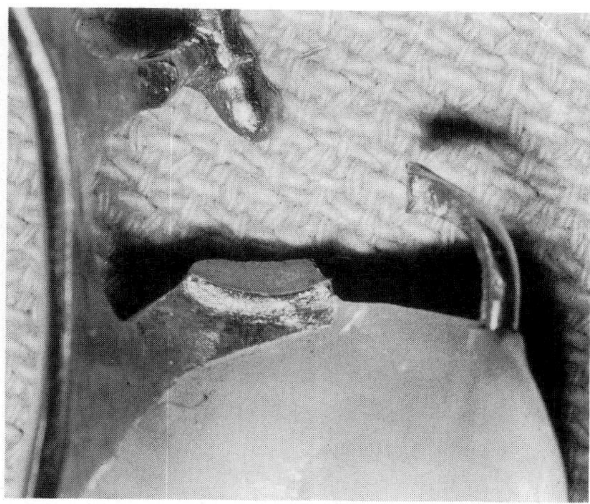

Figure 12–31 ■ The guiding surface is usually curved from buccal to lingual aspects, and demonstrated by this partial casting.

6. All parts of the rest preparation must be located in sound tooth structure or on proper restorations.

Instruments used for rest preparation on posterior teeth are a round number 6 or 8 diamond stone or carbide bur, with water and air spray. If the rest is part of an extension prosthesis associated with a rotation axis, the portion of the rest *closest* to the edentulous area will become the rotation point. This part of the rest is prepared as a half circle so that it will form a *ball and socket* joint, allowing a pure axis of rotation (Fig. 12–38). If the rest is prepared as a slope at the rotation point, the partial rest may tend to slide down the slope, producing lateral or torquing forces on the tooth.

Anterior rest preparation in natural tooth structure is limited because of tooth anatomy and enamel thickness (Fig. 12–39). Attempts to prepare anterior rests in enamel can result in (1) inadequate preparation that will not provide a positive rest seat and stabilization or (2) penetration of the enamel-dentin junction with the possibility of decay. If the dentin is entered, it is

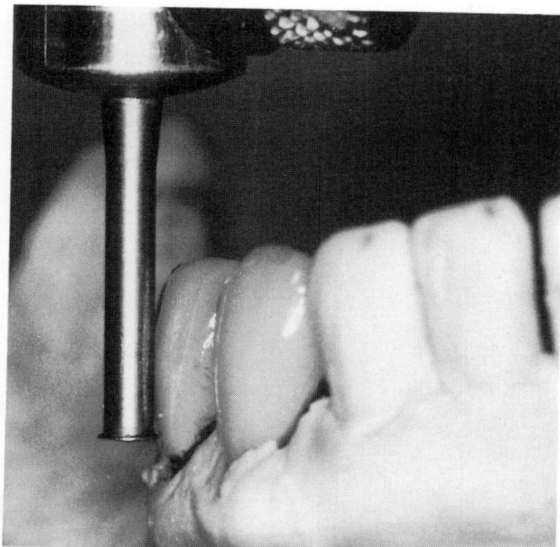

Figure 12–30 ■ Retention areas are checked for proper position and depth of undercut in relation to the MAP.

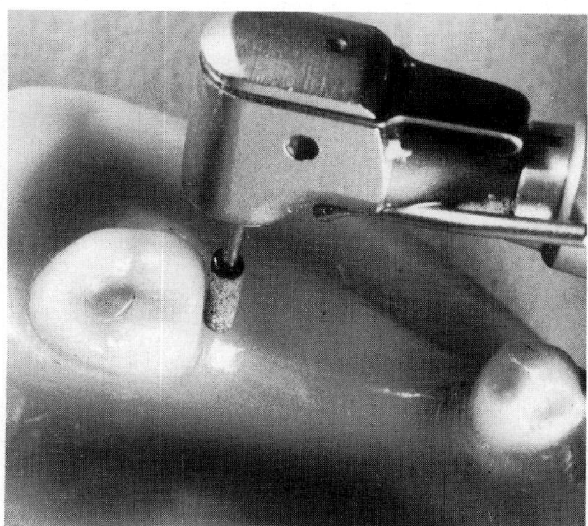

Figure 12–32 ■ A large, straight or slightly tapered diamond stone is the instrument of choice to prepare guide surfaces.

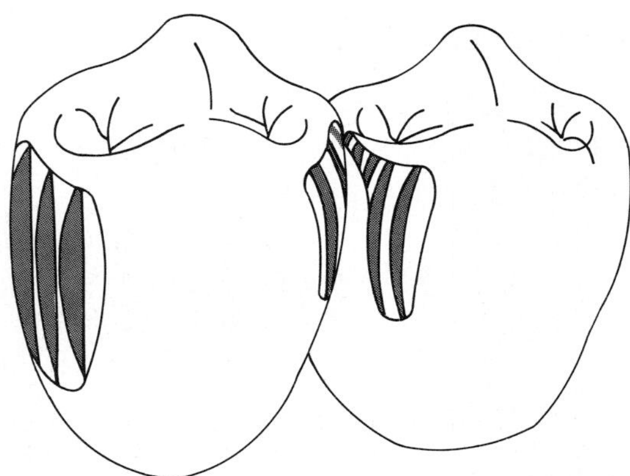

Figure 12–33 ■ A recess is prepared on the lingual surfaces of teeth at the place where the major connector will join with the occlusal rest.

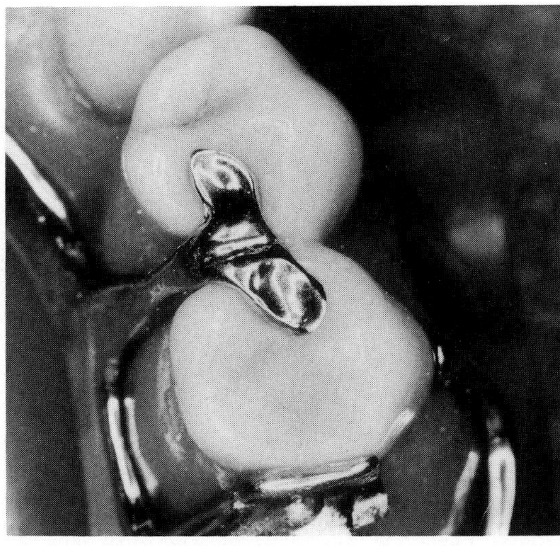

Figure 12–34 ■ The major connector is recessed between the teeth to minimize interference with the tongue.

possible to seal the junction with amalgam or gold foil (Fig. 12–40). It is imperative that a *positive, definite* rest seat be provided, which usually requires placement of a restoration.

Preparation in natural tooth structure is accomplished by use of a small tapered diamond, which is positioned at a 45-degree angle to the long axis of the tooth. The greater part of the rest is prepared in the thick enamel of the marginal ridge (Fig. 12–41).

Acid-etched bonding of metal rests to enamel can be a solution for providing anterior rests. Bonded composites to provide bulk for the preparation of the positive anterior rest is another solution.

The placement of anterior rests is determined by examination of the mounted diagnostic casts, which demonstrate the relationship of the anterior teeth. The rest preparations must be located so that they do not interfere with the planned scheme of occlusion in centric and eccentric positions (Fig. 12–42). In some situations the rests may serve to restore vertical dimension and anterior guidance.

Preparation of anterior incisal rests can be minimal since there is often extensive wear of the incisal surface and reduction of the vertical dimension of occlusion. The rest is designed and prepared to cover most of the mesial-distal width of the tooth and to restore the diagnosti-

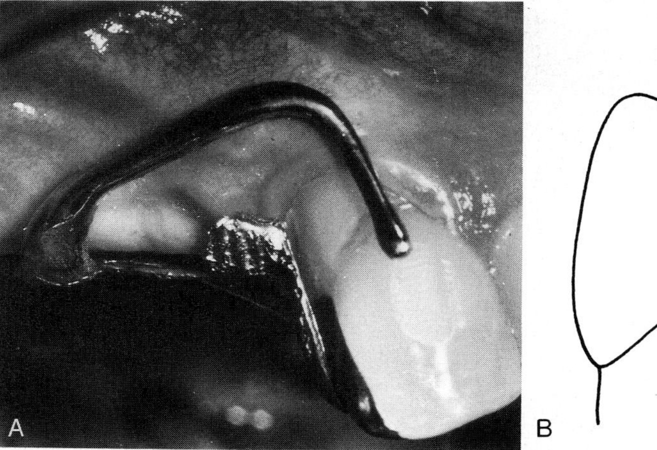

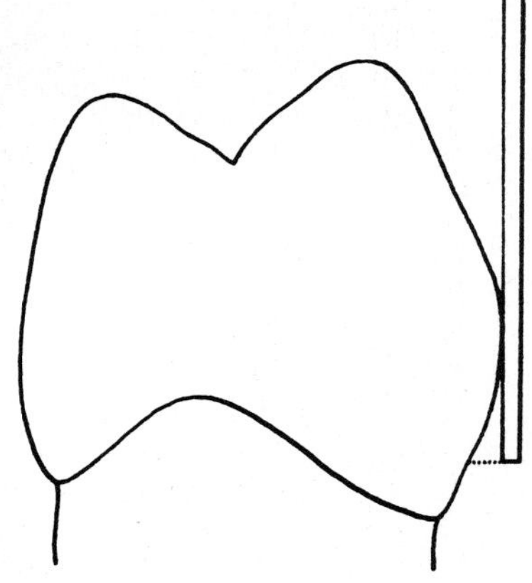

Figure 12–35 ■ *A* and *B*, Excessive facial tooth bulk may require recontouring to change the retention area and to move the retainer closer to the mucosa.

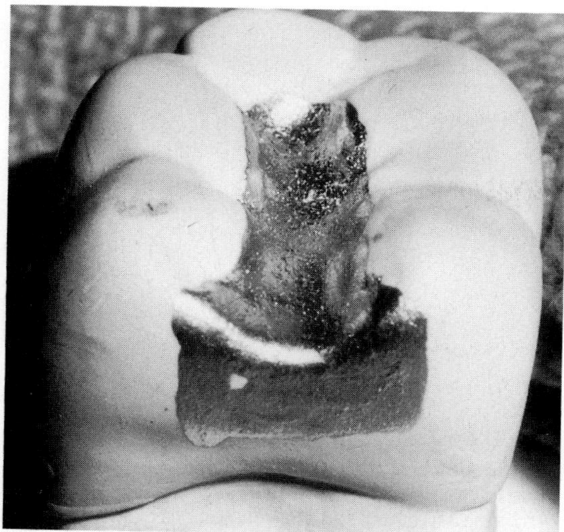

Figure 12–36 ■ All surfaces involved with the rest are rounded, with *no* sharp line angles.

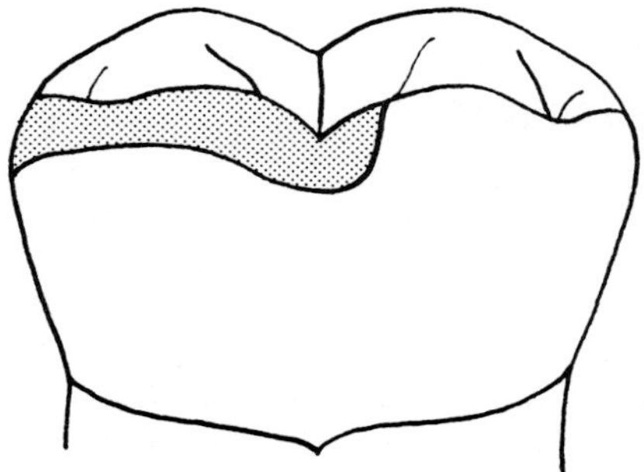

Figure 12–37 ■ Rests are made lower in the center of the tooth. The minimum interocclusal space for metal thickness is 1 mm.

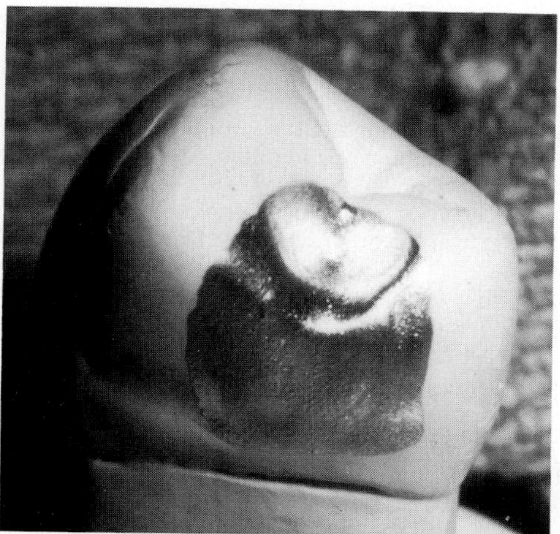

Figure 12–38 ■ Rest areas that are axes of rotation for extension situations are rounded to form a *ball and socket* joint.

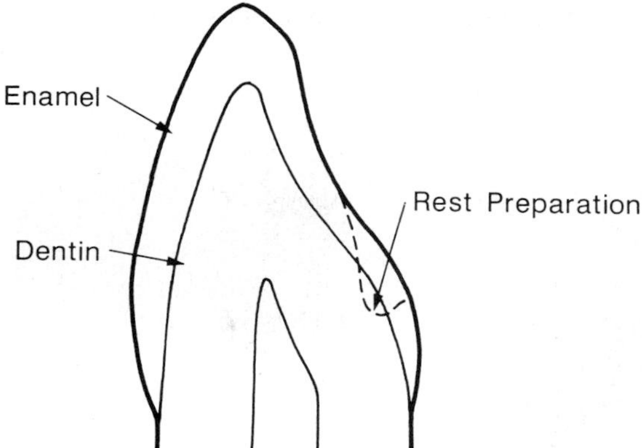

Figure 12–39 ■ Preparation of a *positive* rest in the natural structure of anterior teeth usually involves the enamel-dentin junction.

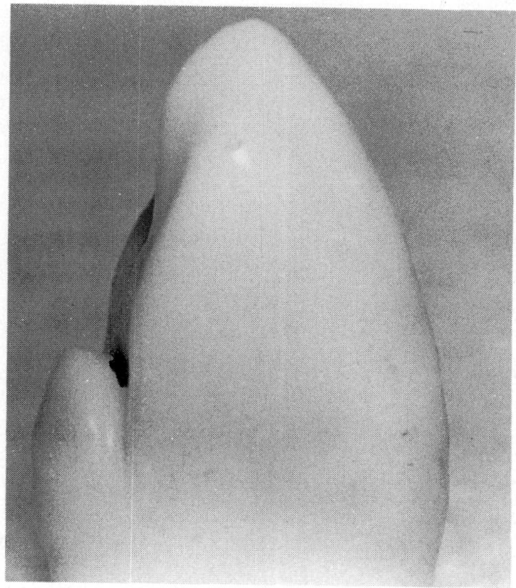

Figure 12–40 ■ Penetration of the enamel-dentin junction can be sealed with amalgam or gold foil.

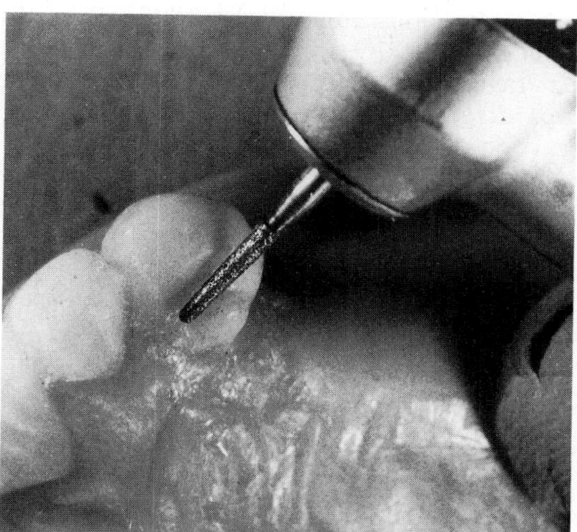

Figure 12–41 ■ Rests in anterior teeth are prepared with a small tapered diamond instrument positioned at a 45-degree angle.

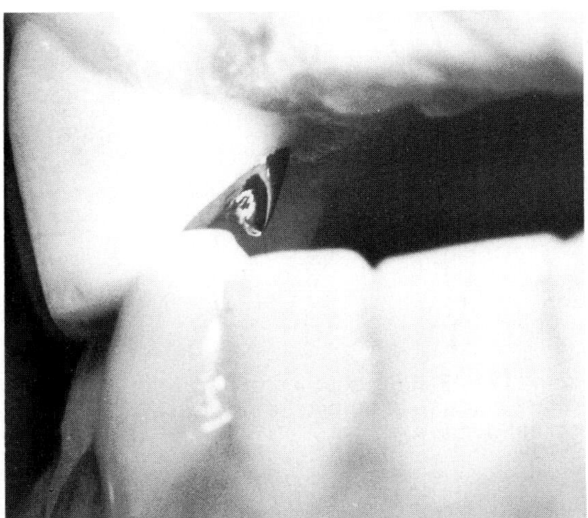

Figure 12–42 ■ The location of opposing occlusion is a major consideration in the positioning of anterior rest restorations. Study of mounted working casts is necessary.

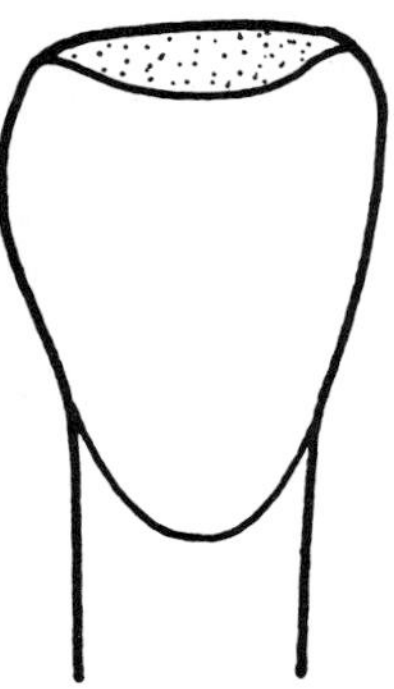

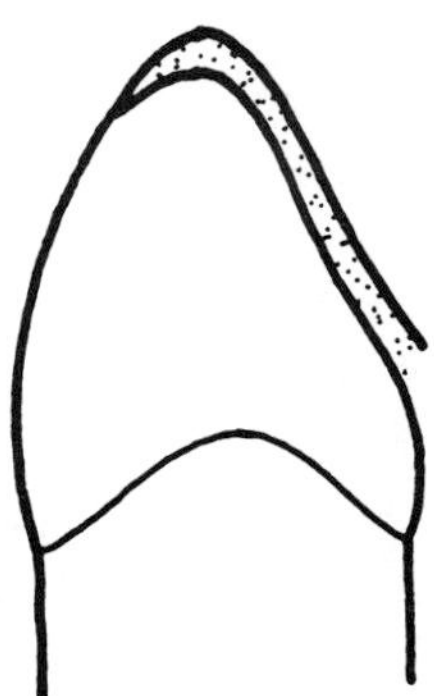

Figure 12–43 ■ Incisal rest preparations must slope to the facial side for positive position and must extend from mesial to distal surfaces to restore guidance in all excursions and for better esthetics.

cally determined occlusal height. The appearance from an anterior view is similar to the appearance of a $\frac{3}{4}$ crown, which is much more esthetic than a thin, narrow incisal rest. It is imperative that the facial portion of the rest extend onto the facial surface of the tooth so that it forms a positive positional seat (Fig. 12–43). In many instances, all that is necessary to prepare the incisal rest is a sandpaper disk to smooth and remove the sharp lingual-incisal angle.

All prepared surfaces are rounded and smoothed to provide bulk and strength for the casting and for ease of fabrication and cleaning. The surfaces are smoothed and polished with medium and fine sandpaper disks, followed with rubber polishing wheels and, finally, with pumice.

If the integrity of any of the teeth has been jeopardized by the preparations, it may be necessary to place restorations.

If there are any questions concerning the mouth preparation, a diagnostic cast can be made and evaluated with the surveyor. The cast can demonstrate parallelism of guiding surfaces, proper tooth contours, retention, and rest preparation.

REFERENCES

Applegate OC: Keeping the partial denture in harmony with biological considerations. J Am Dent Assoc 43:409, 1951.

Applegate OC: The interdependence of periodontics and removable denture prosthesis. J Prosthet Dent 8:269, 1958.

Fenner et al: Tooth mobility changes during treatment with partial denture prosthesis. J Prosthet Dent 6:520, 1956.

Holmes JB: Preparation of abutment teeth for removable partial dentures. J Prosthet Dent 20:396, 1968.

Jordan LG: Treatment of advanced periodontal disease by prosthetic procedures. J Prosthet Dent 10:908, 1960.

Lythe RB: Soft tissue displacement beneath removable partial dentures. J Prosthet Dent 12:34, 1962.

McCall JO: The periodontist looks at the clasp partial denture. J Am Dent Assoc 43:439, 1951.

McKensie JS: Mutual problems of the periodontist and the prosthodontist. J Prosthet Dent 5:37, 1955.

Neurohr FG: Health conservation of the periodontal tissues by a method of functional partial denture design. J Am Dent Assoc 31:54, 1944.

Nevin RB: Periodontal aspects of partial denture prosthesis. J Prosthet Dent 5:215, 1955.

Smith FW: Roentgenographic study of bone changes during exercise stimulation of edentulous areas. J Prosthet Dent 11:1086, 1961.

Thayer H and Kratochvil FJ: Periodontal considerations with removable partial dentures. Dent Clin North Am, 1980.

Waerhaug J: Justification for splinting in periodontal therapy. J Prosthet Dent 22:201, 1969.

chapter 13

Impressions

The making of impressions and the fabrication of a cast to replicate the oral tissues are sensitive to technique and materials procedures. The results can be affected by patient's actions and facial muscle activity; quantity, setting time, and temperature of the materials; and the operator's dexterity.

The Impression material can be any type that produces an accurate impression of the oral tissues. The most commonly used material for partially edentulous arches is *irreversible hydrocolloid (alginate).* Other materials that can be used are

1. Reversible hydrocolloid agar
2. Rubber base
3. Polysulfides
4. Silicones

These materials are all acceptable from the standpoint of *accuracy.*

Factors that influence the selection of impression materials are

1. Convenience of use.
2. Time of manipulation and set.
3. Cost.
4. Need for special trays.
5. Operator training and preference.

A primary factor in accurate impression-making is the tray that carries the impression material and positions it in place. The tray must carry the impression material to proper extension without distorting movable tissues and must provide uniform thickness of the material. If the impression material between tissues and tray is too thin, it may be distorted on removal and when poured. If too thick, it may displace or distort movable tissues (Fig. 13–1).

Metal Trays for Alginate Impressions

Stock metal trays of the rim lock type are excellent for use in making alginate impressions because they are quite rigid and strong yet adjustable to mouth anatomy (Fig. 13–2). If the material should separate from the tray at removal, it can be detected and repositioned with this type of tray.

SELECTION OF TRAY SIZE

1. If a cast is available, size the tray to the cast (Fig. 13–2).

2. Test the tray in the patient's mouth by moving it from anterior to posterior and from side to side to ensure the presence of at least 2 mm of space between tray and all tissues to be recorded.

3. Check tray length for coverage of teeth and relevant soft tissues.

TRAY ALTERATION

Mandibular Tray

Posterior extension ■ Proper extension is 1 to 2 mm short of the posterior border of the retromolar pad, when the mouth is closed. Wax or composition extensions in this area may be necessary.

The flanges or overall contour of the tray ■ This may be adjusted and contoured to adapt the tray to within 2 mm of the peripheral tissues.

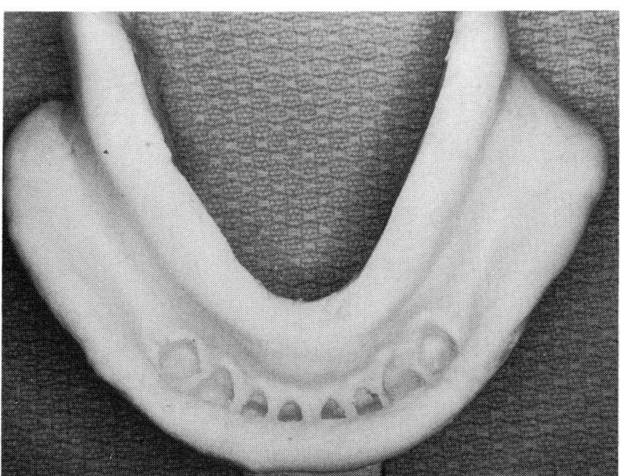

Figure 13–1 ■ Alginate impression. Correct tray size and contour produce an even thickness of impression material in all areas.

Periphery wax ■ Place periphery wax on the lingual surface of the tray, especially from the premolar to the posterior border. This assists in proper placement of the tongue so that it will not intrude between the tray and the lingual side of the mandible. Position this wax at right angles to the border of the tray (Fig. 13–3). (*Do not* obliterate the rim lock). The patient will be instructed to position the tongue on this lingual wax shelf before the tray is completely seated. In edentulous areas with extensive tissue loss, where excessive space exists between tray and tissues, it is advisable to fill in the space with wax or composition.

Maxillary Tray

1. Establish the posterior length to the hamular notch. Add wax or composition to extend the posterior border of the tray into the hamular notch area, and establish positive contact with posterior palatal tissues (Fig. 13–4). This posterior seal ensures positive contact of impression material with the palate and prevents the impression material from escaping out the back of the tray. Check that the palatal portion of the tray is built up to ensure that the impression material is carried into positive contact with the entire palate (Fig. 13–5).

2. Trays with wax additions are warmed in the water bath and molded in the patient's mouth to ensure correct contact and extension and to eliminate excess space.

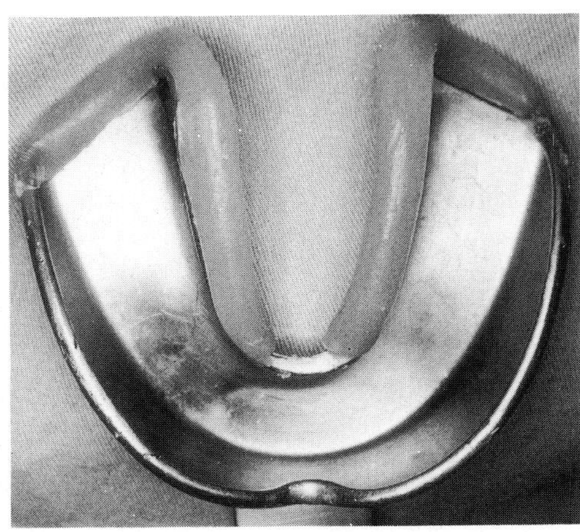

Figure 13–3 ■ Wax on the lingual and posterior portion of the mandibular tray assists in tongue control and in obtaining proper lingual impression detail. Do not obliterate the rim lock.

CUSTOM TRAYS

In some situations, extensive anatomical anomalies make the adaptation of stock metal trays most difficult, and construction of an indi-

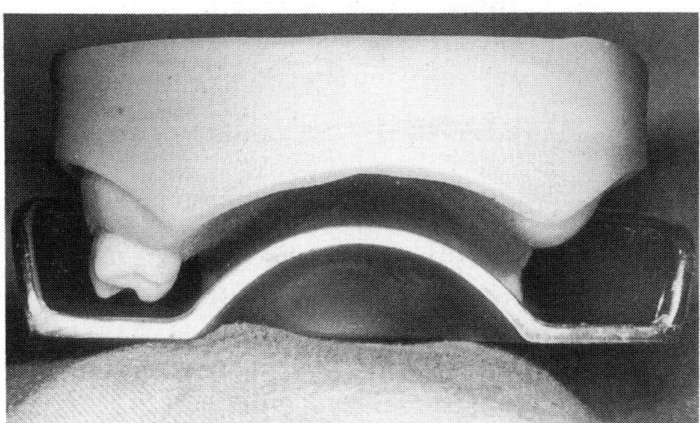

Figure 13–2 ■ The tray must be strong and rigid to minimize distortion. Evaluation of proper tray size and adaptation can be done if a cast of the patient's mouth is available.

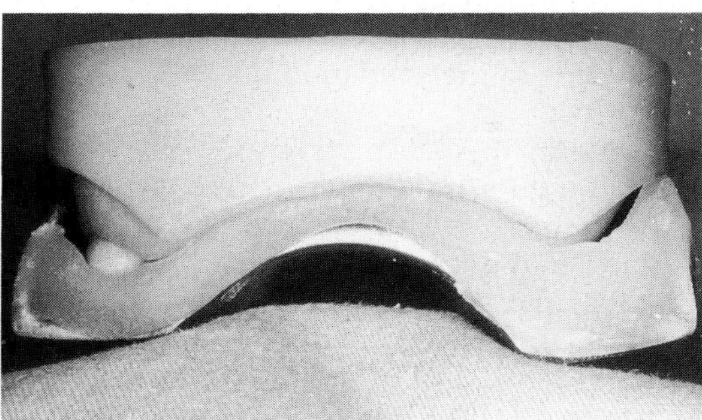

Figure 13–4 ■ Impression material is contained in the posterior palate area with a post-dam to ensure adaptation to the palate and prevent escape into the throat.

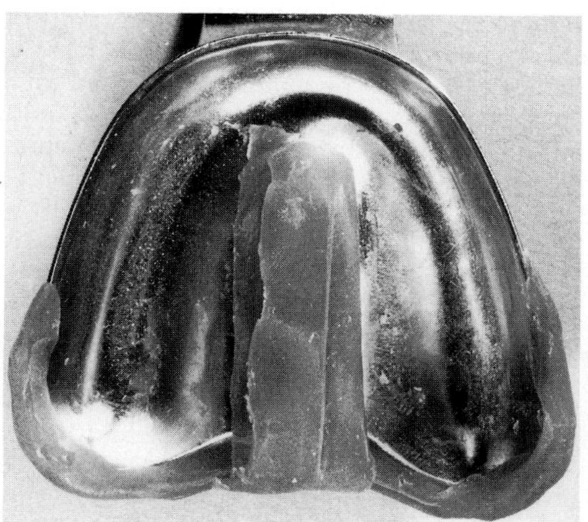

Figure 13–5 ■ Positive contact of impression material to the center of the palate requires the addition of wax in this area.

vidual plastic tray may be necessary. Individual trays are usually used for impression materials such as rubber bases, polysulfides, and silicones.

When constructing individual trays, ensure that

1. There is uniform and adequate space for impression material in all directions (for sufficient relief, before applying plastic).
2. The tray is rigid.
3. The tray does not warp (from dimensional change or moisture).
4. There is adequate retention for impression material.

Impression Materials

ALGINATE

Provide precisely the powder:water ratio set by the manufacturer. They are set by ADA specifications for the most acceptable results. A common cause of difficulties is measurement of the powder and of the amount of water (Fig. 13–6). Powder by measure can vary up to 30 percent of the required weight; the water must also be measured, at room temperature, to produce an impression of the proper dimensions.

The application of an adhesive material to all parts of the tray that will be contacted by the alginate helps prevent separation of the material from the tray (Fig. 13–7). The impression must be kept in the patient's mouth for the proper time, as specified by the manufacturer, and removed in a single, positive movement to minimize distortion.

Pour the cast immediately to prevent

1. Imbibition: If placed in contact with water, the alginate impression will absorb the water, swell, and distort.

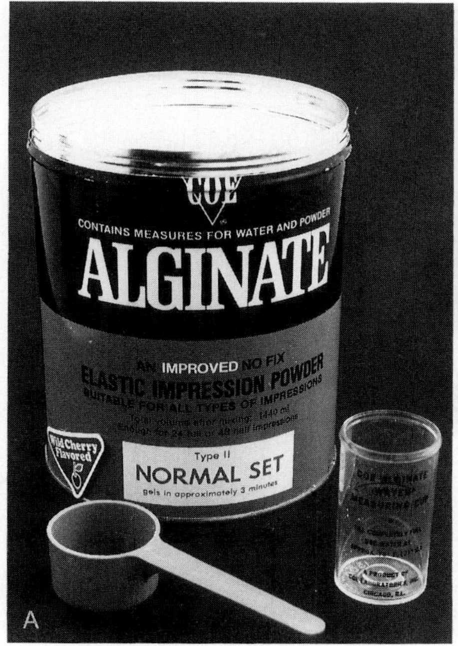

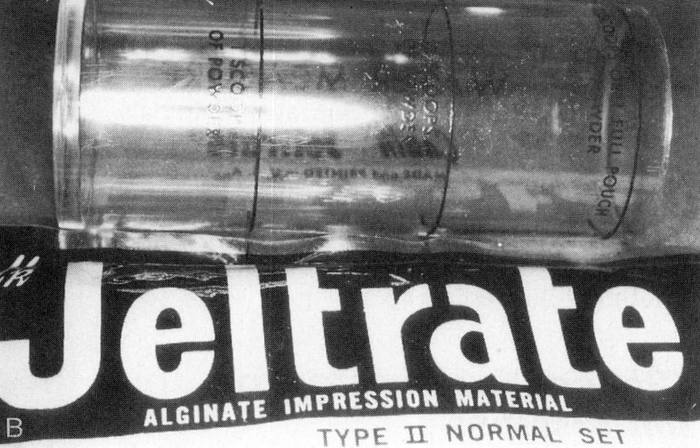

Figure 13–6 ■ *A*, Bulk alginate must be completely mixed or tumbled before use. The powder by measure can have considerable variation in weight. *B*, Alginate by weight or by individual package provides a more accurate amount. Water is measured at room temperature for recommended amount.

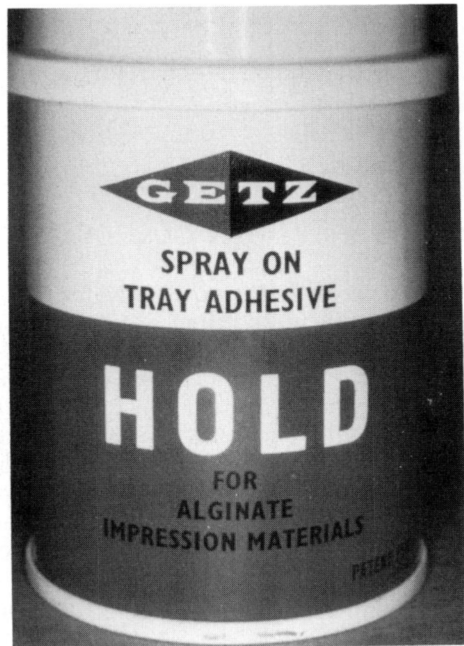

Figure 13–7 ■ Adhesive material is applied to the tray surface to minimize separation of impression material from the tray at removal, producing distortion.

2. Syneresis: If the impression is left in open air, it will lose water and shrink.

OTHER IMPRESSION MATERIALS

Other materials that are used for removable partial denture impressions are the mercaptan materials (rubber base or polysulfide rubber), polyether rubber, silicon, and agar materials. All of these materials meet the necessary accuracy requirements and may be preferred for strength, stiffness, or working time, or as a result of personal experience. With all impression materials, it is imperative that the directions be carefully followed.

Clinical Procedures for Impressions

PATIENT PREPARATION

As in all patient procedures, it is important that the patient be informed of the procedure and instructed as to the nature of his or her participation. Instructions should include position of the jaw, tongue, head, and cheeks, as well as breathing involvement and time required to complete the procedure. It is *most* important to inform the patient of the need for all muscles and tissues to be relatively relaxed so that these tissues are not recorded in a tensed, distorted position, which would affect the fit of the finished prosthesis. A trial "run through" of the impression procedure can greatly improve the final impression results.

Prophylaxis

Use flour of pumice in a rubber cup to remove any debris from the tooth surface and to help produce a smooth, clean surface. Rinse the mouth very thoroughly.

Instructions to the patient

1. Keep the cheeks, lips, and tongue as relaxed as possible.
2. Open the mouth only enough to insert the tray. When the tray is in the mouth, close just short of tooth-tray contact.
3. Place the tongue gently forward on top of the lingual wax flange adapted to the tray (this refers to the mandibular impression) (Fig. 13–8).
4. Instruct the patient to breathe through the nose during the making of the maxillary impression and to concentrate on breathing. Remind the patient that he or she has a second complete airway through the nose and that it is well posterior to where the impression material will be placed.

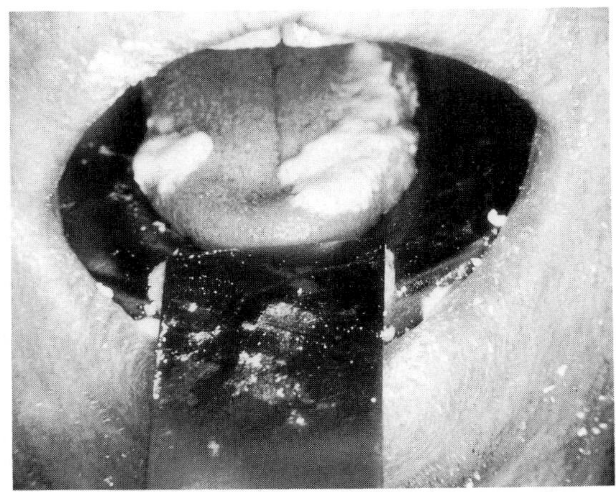

Figure 13–8 ■ When an impression is being made, the jaw is slightly open, the tongue is gently forward, and the muscles are relaxed *prior to final seating* of the tray.

Place a 4 × 4 gauze pad over the occlusal surface of the teeth to remove excess saliva. (Do not dehydrate the mouth. This could remove the water from the impression material.)

MATERIAL PREPARATION

1. Mix the powder and water in the correct ratio at room temperature; mix for 45 sec.
2. Place the alginate in the tray, without bubbles or voids in the material.
3. Smooth the surface of the material with a moist finger. Do not add material or water to the smoothed surface.

TRAY PLACEMENT

1. Remove the gauge from patient's mouth; instruct the patient not to moisten the teeth.
2. Spread a very *thin* layer of alginate on the occlusal surfaces and other difficult access areas using your finger.
3. Place the tray in the basic position and have the patient close the mouth just short of tray contact.
4. Instruct the patient to place the tongue on the lingual wax shelf (in the mandibular impression) (Fig. 13–8).
5. When the patient's mouth is closed with the tongue in position and he or she is completely relaxed, gently vibrate the tray into place.
6. Always hold the tray in position until the impression is completed.
7. Do not allow the tray to contact tooth cusps or impinge on soft tissues.
8. Gently massage the peripheral areas with the fingers for better adaptation. Always massage the impression material toward the tissues and in an anterior–posterior direction. (Never pull the tissues up or away from the bone, since this can produce a space between the impression material and the tissues, which would be reproduced in the finished prosthesis).

TRAY REMOVAL

1. Hold the tray in one position for the setting time recommended by the manufacturer. Use a timer to check the interval (Fig. 13–9).
2. Remove the tray with a quick, positive movement.

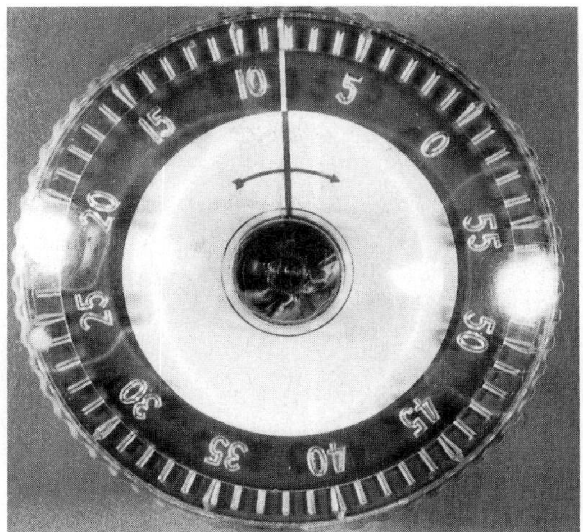

Figure 13–9 ■ The tray is held in position for the period of time recommended for the material.

3. Check to ensure that the alginate has not separated from the tray.
4. Carefully examine all areas to be sure that details are reproduced and that no voids are present. If the alginate between the teeth has been displaced, carefully reposition it. Cover the impression with moist gauze or towel and place in a humidor.
5. Do not set the tray down in a position that will displace the alginate from the tray.
6. Pour the impression *immediately*.

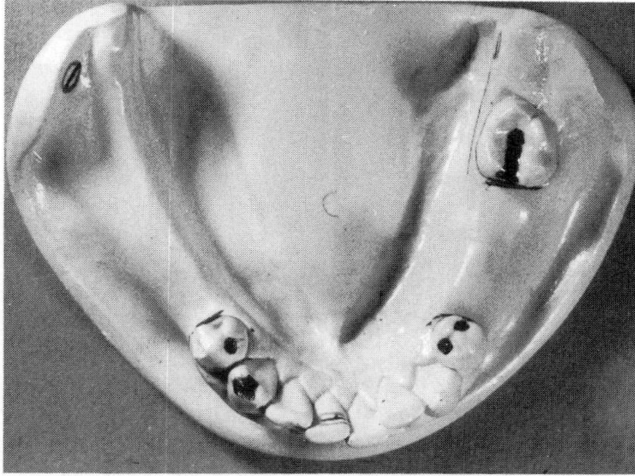

Figure 13–10 ■ The casts are an exact reproduction of the oral situation and include all areas involved with the prosthesis. The peripheral border is evenly trimmed at right angles to the cast base.

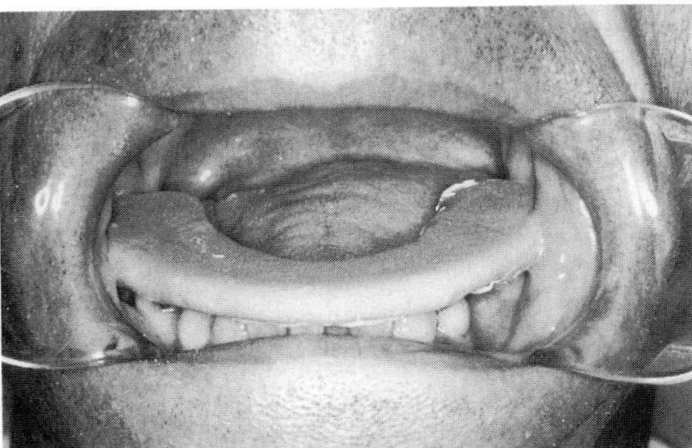

Figure 13–11 ■ Cast accuracy can be verified by use of an occlusal index made of the occlusal surfaces in the patient's mouth.

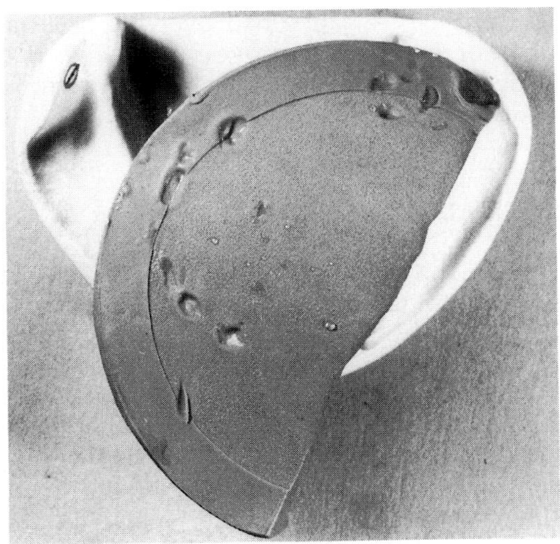

Figure 13–13 ■ An alternative method of providing an occlusal index is the use of a cake of modeling composition.

POURING THE IMPRESSION

1. Clean saliva and debris from the impression with air or light water spray. Remove any water with air spray.
2. Prepare the yellow dental stone to the correct water : powder ratio, according to the manufacturer's directions. Use a mechanical spatulator if available.
3. Place a small amount of stone at one end of the impression. With low vibration against the handle of the tray, watch to ensure the complete flow of stone into every part of the impression. Too great vibration produces bubbles on the cusp tips. Slowly add the stone until the impression is filled to the periphery.
4. Invert the tray into a circle of stone placed on the workbench top. Take care not to distort or displace the alginate, which may extend beyond the tray. Use light pressure to prevent distortion.

Note: An alternative procedure is to complete the cast in two pours. The first pour fills the impression to the periphery; it is allowed to set and is then inverted into a second base pour.

5. When the initial set has taken place, trim the outline of the cast with a knife and place the base in $\frac{1}{4}$-in water for the final set.
6. Allow the cast to set for 1 hour before separation.
7. Trim the cast, being careful to preserve the peripheral roll. The flange beyond the peripheral roll is trimmed at right angles to the base and is made 2–3 mm wide (Fig. 13–10).

Occlusal Index

To ensure accuracy of the cast, an occlusal index is made of the occlusal surfaces of the

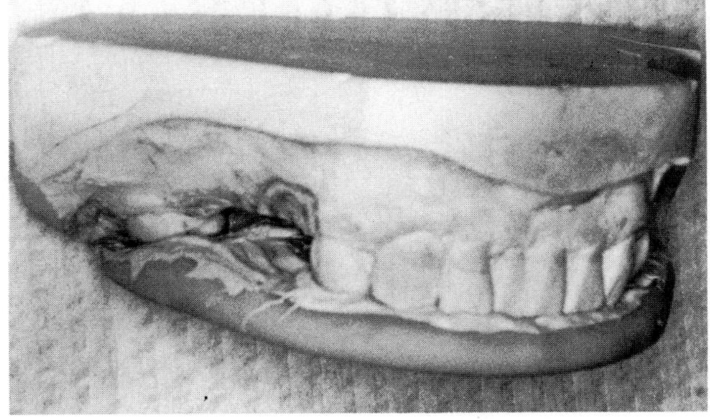

Figure 13–12 ■ The occlusal index of plastic and registration paste is tested against the occlusal surfaces of the finished cast to ensure accurate reproduction.

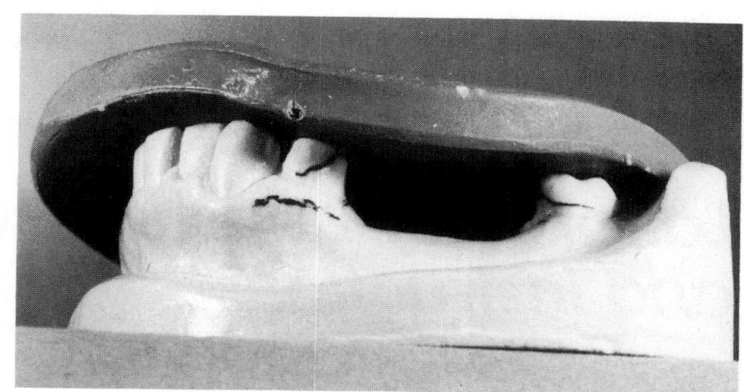

Figure 13–14 ■ The occlusal index is used in the laboratory to verify accuracy of working casts and the refractory cast at duplication.

patient's teeth and is checked for accuracy of fit to the stone cast. The procedure is as follows:

1. A preformed plastic or metal matrix is used to carry the registration paste onto the occlusal surface of the remaining teeth in the patient's mouth (Fig. 13–11).
2. Modeling composition can be added to the matrix to ensure contact with occlusal surface of the teeth.
3. Registration paste is placed on the matrix and reseated on the occlusal surface of the teeth in the patient's mouth. (A thin layer of petroleum jelly on the patient's teeth prevents adhesion of the registration material).
4. The registration material is trimmed to shallow cusp exposure. This occlusal index can be fitted to the occlusal surface of the stone master cast to check for accuracy, since the index must fit onto all cusp tips with no discrepancies (Fig. 13–12).

An alternate method of producing an occlusal index is the use of a cake of modeling composition, which is slightly softened in a water bath, adapted to the occlusal surface of the patient's teeth, and chilled. The composition is trimmed to the shallow cusp indentations and is used to check cast accuracy, as described above (Figs. 13–13 and 13–14).

REFERENCES

Bailey LR: Acrylic resin tray for rubber base impression materials. J Prosthet Dent 5:458–462, 1955.

Fusayama T and Nakazato M: The design of stock trays and the retention of irreversible hydrocolloid impressions. J Prosthet Dent 21:136–142, 1969.

Harris WT Jr: Water temperature and accuracy of alginate impressions. J Prosthet Dent 21:613–617, 1969.

Heartwell CM et al: Comparison of impressions made in perforated and non-perforated rimlock trays. J Prosthet Dent 27:494–500, 1972.

Kramer HM: Impression technique for removable partial denture. J Prosthet Dent 11:84–92, 1961.

Mitchell JV and Damele JJ: Influence of tray design upon elastic impression materials. J Prosthet Dent 23:51–57, 1970.

Morrow RM et al: Compatibility of alginate impression materials and dental stones. J Prosthet Dent 25:556–566, 1971.

Rudd KD, Morrow RM, and Bange AA: Accurate casts. J Prosthet Dent 21:545–554, 1969.

Rudd, KD, Morrow RM, and Strunk RR: Accurate alginate impressions. J Prosthet Dent 22:294–300, 1969.

Rudd KD et al: Comparison of effects of tap water and slurry water on gypsum casts. J Prosthet Dent 24:563–570, 1970.

chapter 14

Laboratory communications and instructions

Design of the removable partial prosthesis is a critical factor for proper treatment. It is the major factor in diagnosis and treatment planning. Since the design is entirely dependent upon the amount, type, and condition of the remaining oral anatomic structures of the patient, it is the doctor's complete responsibility to control all of the procedures. Ethically, the design cannot be delegated to an individual other than the treating doctor.

The dental laboratory technician is a trained, skilled individual, who is capable of producing a prosthesis that can successfully replace a missing part of the oral cavity, if he or she is given complete information, instructions, and proper casts. A most important factor is the transfer of complete clinical information and instructions from the doctor to the laboratory. *Communication* must be complete, precise, and in three dimensions: The only way that this information can be transmitted is by a three-dimensional replica of the patient's oral anatomy—the *diagnostic cast.*

The diagnostic casts that were prepared and used for treatment planning procedures (Fig. 14–1) are sent to the laboratory along with the master casts. These diagnostic casts show the exact placement of all parts of the removable prosthesis and how it will be positioned in the mouth. This information is also necessary in the fabrication of crowns and in other restorative procedures.

Partial designs, which are drawn directly on the master casts, are not as useful as the diagnostic cast information, since (1) drawings on the master cast may damage the cast surface, (2) portions of the design are covered with wax in preparation for duplication, with resulting loss of detail, and (3) when the relief wax is removed from the master cast, the design is removed; therefore, it is impossible to compare the finished casting with the original design.

Master Cast Preparation

All parts of the master cast are inspected for smooth, accurate reproduction of the anatomy of the mouth. Special attention is directed to those places that the partial casting will contact, such as rest areas, guide surfaces, retention areas, and interproximal contact areas. Artifacts and bubbles are removed.

The trimmed and dried master cast is checked for dimensional accuracy by placing the occlusal index, which was recorded from the patient, on the occlusal surfaces of the cast (Fig. 14–2). If there are spaces between the index and the cast or if there is a "rocking" of the index on the occlusal surface, it is an indication that there are inaccuracies in the cast, and a new impression must be made. The technician can also use this index to ensure accurate duplication of the refractory cast.

The master cast is placed on the survey table, and the same procedure used with the diagnostic casts is repeated to establish the *most advantageous position* (MAP) (Fig. 14–3). When the

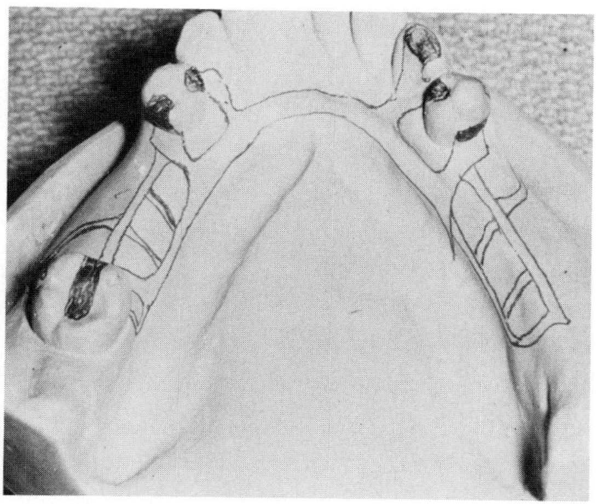

Figure 14–1 ■ The diagnostic cast contains information for treatment planning, mouth preparation, and *laboratory communication* and *instructions.* It provides detailed three-dimensional information.

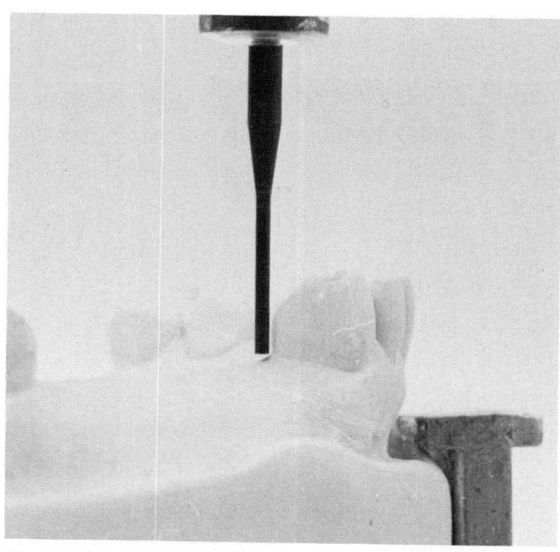

Figure 14–4 ■ Parallelism of the guiding surfaces is the primary factor to be checked. Mouth preparation will have eliminated as many voids as possible.

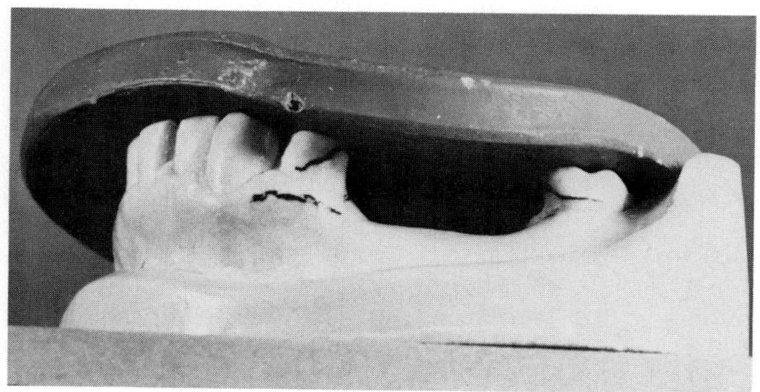

Figure 14–2 ■ The accuracy of the master cast is checked with the occlusal index made in the patient's mouth. Impression and pouring errors are immediately identified.

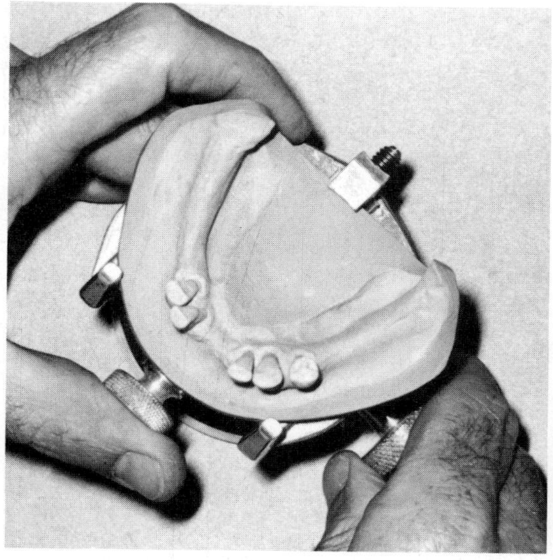

Figure 14–3 ■ The *most advantageous position* (MAP) for the master cast is located as originally planned with the diagnostic cast.

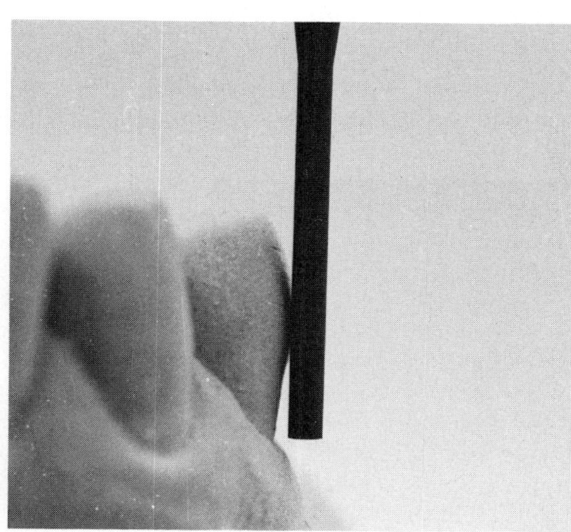

Figure 14–5 ■ The amount and position of retention areas are checked for compatibility with planned treatment.

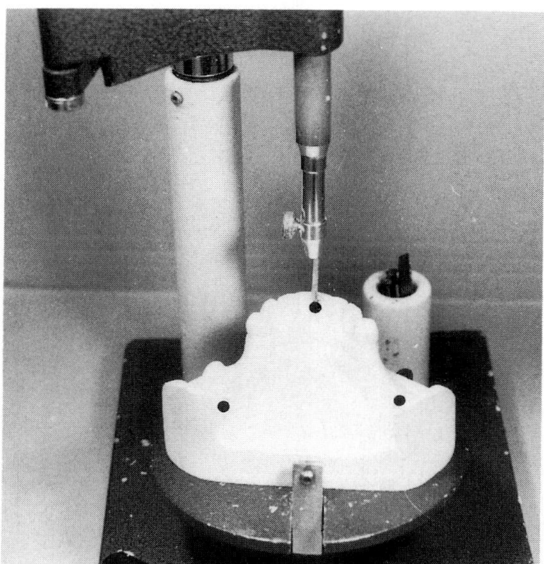

Figure 14–6 ■ The MAP is recorded on the cast by *tripoding*. This procedure enables reproduction of the exact position at any time.

MAP appears by eye survey to be correct, proceed with the following checks, using the surveyor.

1. The guiding surfaces must be parallel to each other—use the diagnostic rod (Fig. 14–4).
2. There must be proper retention undercuts as planned—use the diagnostic rod, then measure with the undercut gauge (Fig. 14–5).

TRIPOD THE MASTER CAST

In order to be able to fabricate a casting according to the doctor's planned prescription, the laboratory must be able to reproduce the identical MAP that the doctor developed. This position can be easily reproduced by the laboratory if the cast has been tripoded. To accomplish this procedure, the diagnostic rod is placed in the upper, movable arm of the surveyor. The upper member is then *fixed* in position, so that the tip of the diagnostic rod touches the master cast in three widely separated places (Fig. 14–6), as the survey table with the cast in

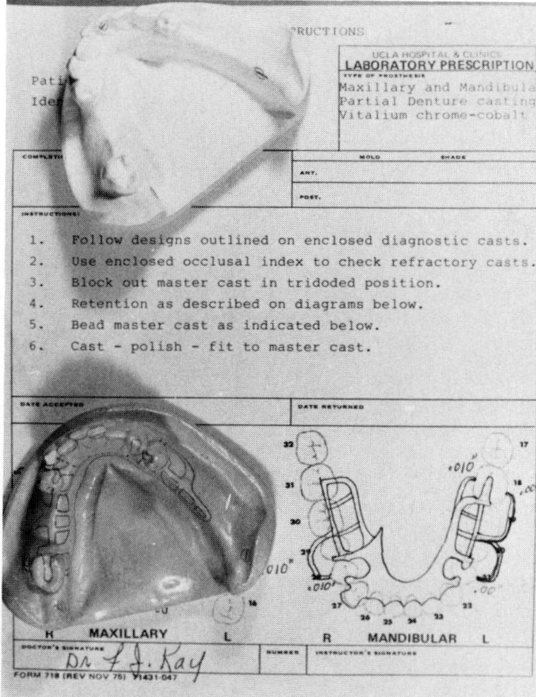

Figure 14–8 ■ The written laboratory prescription or work authorization is a required document. It gives precise instructions that augment the diagnostic cast information.

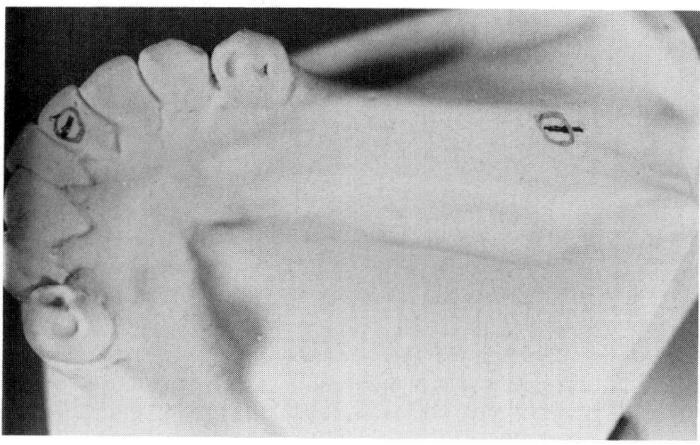

Figure 14–7 ■ Tripod marks are outlined in red for easy identification later and especially for use in laboratory procedures.

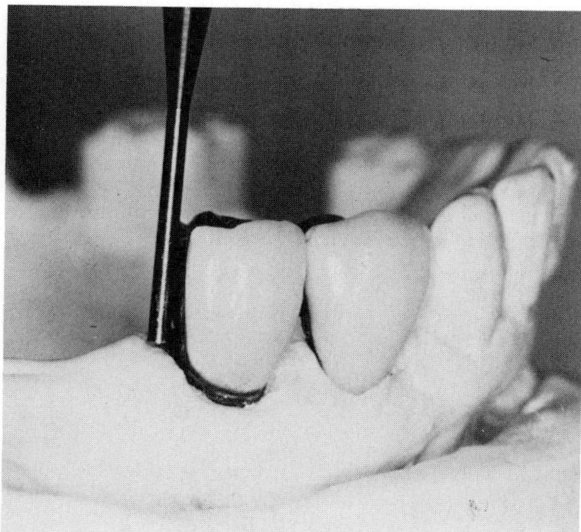

Figure 14–9 ■ Complete and detailed information can be communicated between doctor and technician if properly prepared and enclosed along with the cast. A complete arch impression is necessary if a crown is to be coordinated with other guide surfaces.

place is moved around the base table of the surveyor. *Without changing the position of the upper arm,* the doctor places a mark on the master cast at these three points and circles them in red for easy identification (Fig. 14–7). The exact position can now be reproduced by the laboratory by repeating the procedure with their surveyor.

Written Instructions

Basic information and additional instructions are written on the laboratory prescription that accompanies the master and diagnostic casts (Fig. 14–8). The following information is included:

1. Patient identification.
2. Type of prosthesis requested.
3. Type of metal to be used.
4. Design instructions.
5. Retention instructions.
6. Specific individual requests, such as measurements for the placement of connectors.
7. Doctor's signature and license number.

Crowns and Fixed Prostheses

In many situations requiring removable partial denture (RPD) treatment, it is necessary to provide fixed prosthetic treatment that must coordinate with the removable design. A common situation is the placement of a crown on an abutment tooth, where guiding surfaces must be parallel with the guiding surfaces of other crowns or natural teeth.

It is necessary to send the diagnostic cast with the RPD design along with the master cast of the crown preparations, so that the technician can properly position rests, retention areas, and guide surfaces (Fig. 14–9). If occlusal contacts are involved, especially in the anterior rest area, *articulated* diagnostic casts or working casts may be necessary for proper placement of rests on the crown and to provide space for the RPD casting (Fig. 14–10).

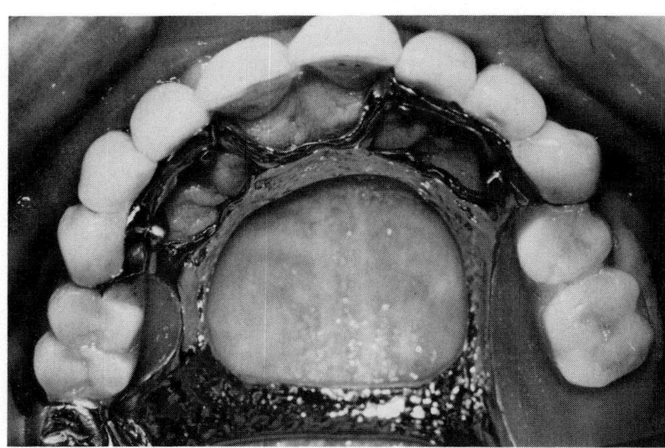

Figure 14–10 ■ Special instructions or information can require articulated diagnostic casts. Examples are in the restoration of anterior guidance by the partial casting and in the critical placement of rests in the anterior area.

REFERENCES

Brown ET: The dentist, the laboratory technician, and the prescription law. J Prosthet Dent 15:1132–1138, 1965.

Dutton DA: Standard abbreviations for use in dental laboratory work authorizations. J Prosthet Dent 27:94–95, 1972.

Enright CM: Dentist-dental laboratory harmony. J Prosthet Dent 11:393–394, 1961.

Gehl DH: Investment in the future. J Prosthet Dent 18:190–201, 1968.

Grunewald AH: Dentist, dental laboratory and the patient. J Prosthet Dent 8:55–60, 1958.

Henderson D: Writing work authorizations for removable partial dentures. J Prosthet Dent 16:696–707, 1966.

Hickey JC: Responsibility of the dentist in removable partial dentures. J Ky Dent Assoc 17:70–87, 1965.

Quinn I: Status of the dental laboratory work authorization. J Am Dent Assoc 79:1189–1190, 1969.

chapter 15

Physiologic adjustment of the casting and altered cast impression procedures

Inspection of the Casting

The metal partial denture casting, as returned from the laboratory, is carefully inspected for compliance with prescription design, adaptation to the master cast, and overall quality.

DESIGN

The finished casting is compared with the design prescribed on the diagnostic cast (Fig. 15–1), which has the advantage of being detailed and precise. The technician can use the diagnostic cast design during fabrication, and the doctor can make a comparison of casting to design on the cast to ensure proper placement of all parts of the finished casting. This procedure provides excellent design control and communication between doctor and technician during all procedures.

ADAPTATION

The adaptation or fit of the metal casting to the master cast is carefully evaluated. It is advantageous to develop a systematic check procedure.

1. Inspect the underside and tissue side of the casting for bubbles or roughness. Any discrepancies that occurred during duplication or on the refractory cast are manifested on the underside of the metal casting. This inspection is done with magnifying loupes or with a laboratory magnifier, which can dramatically reveal any irregularities present (Fig. 15–2). Irregularities are removed with high speed handpieces and carbide fissure burs (Fig. 15–3).
2. All rests must be well adapted and in intimate contact with the rest preparations on the master cast. Excess metal beyond the actual rest preparation must be removed (Fig. 15–4).
3. Check for movement or rocking action of the metal casting on the stone cast.
4. Retention areas must be properly positioned and must contact the prescribed amount of tooth undercut in order to provide retention (Fig. 15–5).
5. Check the metal guiding surface for contact with the tooth and with 2 mm of the mucosa covered. There should be no space or voids between the metal guiding surface and the tooth or tissue (Fig. 15–6).

Careful fitting and adjustment of the finished casting to the master cast ensures the best possible adaptation and fewer adjustments in the mouth. The technician adjusts the casting to the master cast, taking care not to scrape the stone cast with the first seating of the casting. To prevent interference in seating, the retention areas on the stone cast are first removed (these are planned undercut areas and interfere with placement of the casting). The casting is adjusted in place on the master cast until there is no resistance and areas of interference are lo-

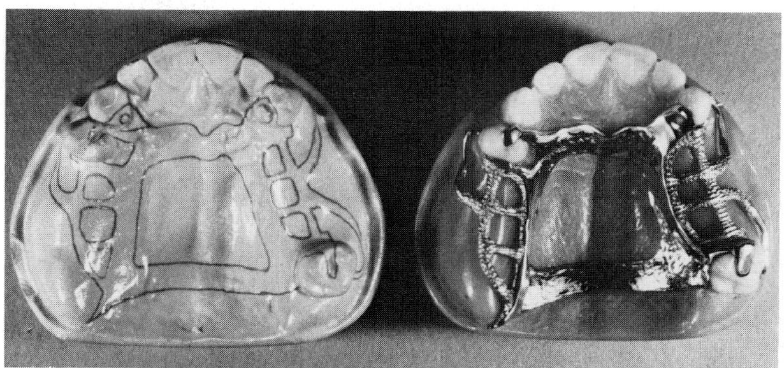

Figure 15–1 ■ Complete, precise design on the diagnostic cast is compared with the finished casting to ensure accuracy.

cated and relieved. Care is taken not to force the casting, since this would scrape stone off the master cast and distort the tooth replication. The casting is adjusted until it smoothly comes on and off the master cast. Careful adjustment of the cast results in excellent adaptation in the mouth without binding or the need for time-consuming adjustment in the operatory.

QUALITY

Evaluation of the quality of a casting includes the following areas: overall assessment for continuity, reproduction of normal anatomical contours, blending of the casting into existing tissues, and smoothness and polish. Specific areas to evaluate are:

1. Porus areas.
2. Rough or irregular surfaces.
3. Sharp edges, which may cause irritation.
4. Position of the casting where it crosses tooth-tissue junctions.
5. Contour of connectors, to reduce food impaction.
6. Proper bulk and thickness, for strength.

Physiologic Adjustment of the Casting

The final procedure in evaluating the metal partial denture casting *interorally* is to ensure that all rests are completely seated. This is demonstrated when there is no rocking of the casting on the teeth or lack of intimate rest contact. Improper seating may be due to artifacts on the

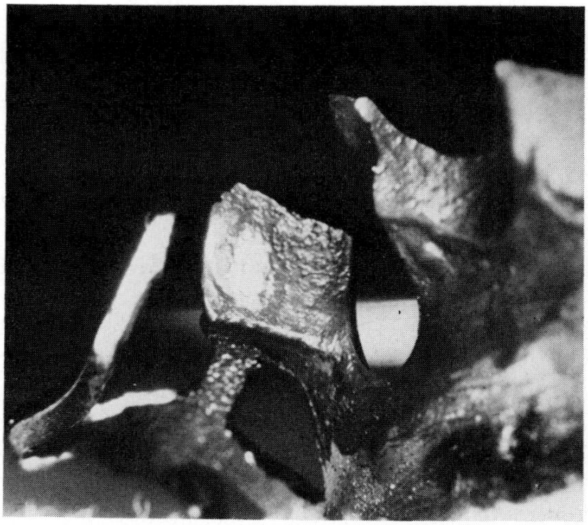

Figure 15–2 ■ The tissue surface of the casting is inspected for nodules, roughness, and imperfections.

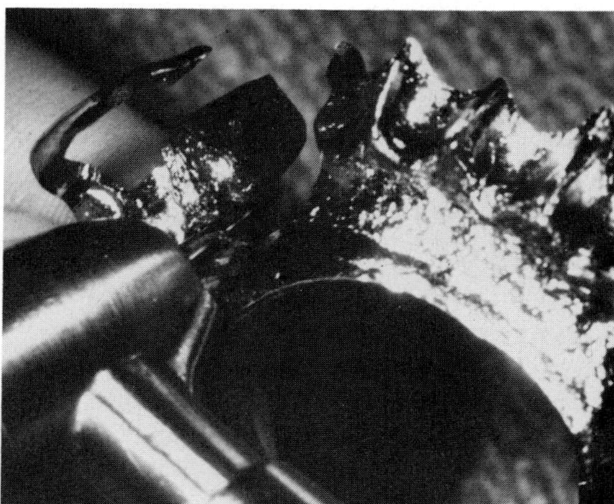

Figure 15–3 ■ Surfaces are smoothed and contoured as necessary with carbide burs in high-speed handpieces.

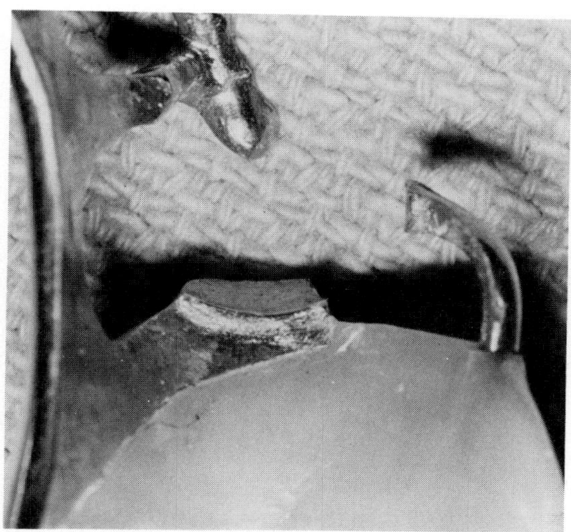

Figure 15–4 ■ Rests are viewed from the undersurface to check for metal flash that might extend beyond the actual rest preparation.

underside of the casting, to errors in fabrication, or to movement of teeth since the time that the impression was made. Interference areas can be located with the use of a disclosing medium such as *gold rouge* and *chloroform* (as described in Chapter 8), *disclosing wax,* or other disclosing materials. Errors in fabrication or movement of teeth can require remaking of the casting.

When the prosthesis is an extension partial denture, it is necessary to *physiologically adjust* the casting to allow for the movement of the prosthesis. This adjustment prevents undue lateral forces and torquing of the abutment teeth and keeps the axis of rotation within the *planned rest rotation axis,* with forces in the long axis of the abutment teeth and horizontal to the edentulous mucosa. (A complete description of the physiologic adjustment procedure is given in Chapter 8.)

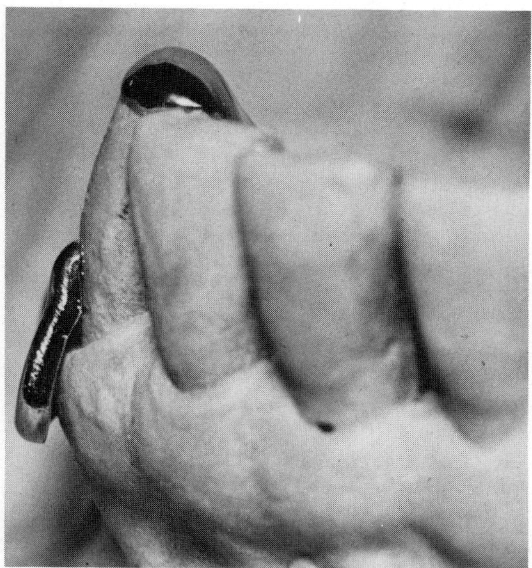

Figure 15–5 ■ The position and location of the retainer is checked.

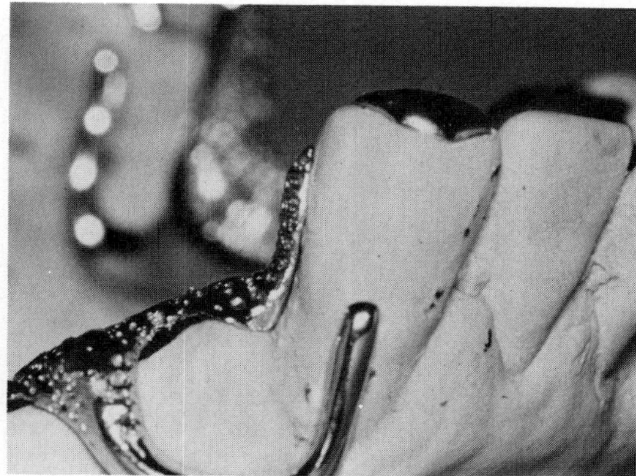

Figure 15–6 ■ Minor connectors are positioned at least 2 mm onto the mucosa, with no space or voids between tooth and mucosa.

Altered Cast Procedure

The purpose of the altered cast procedure is to obtain the maximum support possible from the edentulous area of the extension partial denture. A detailed description of this procedure has been provided by Leupold.

The increase in support provided in extension partial dentures by the altered cast procedure has been documented by Holmes, who compared three impression procedures: (1) stock metal tray, (2) individual resin tray, and (3) altered cast. The results demonstrated that the *altered cast impression procedure* provided two to three times *greater support* and allowed *less movement* than the other two methods.

The altered cast procedure applies the principle of recording the edentulous tissues in a form that provides proper denture base extension and maximum support without distortion or displacement of tissues.

The objective is to ensure the best possible relationship between the casting framework,

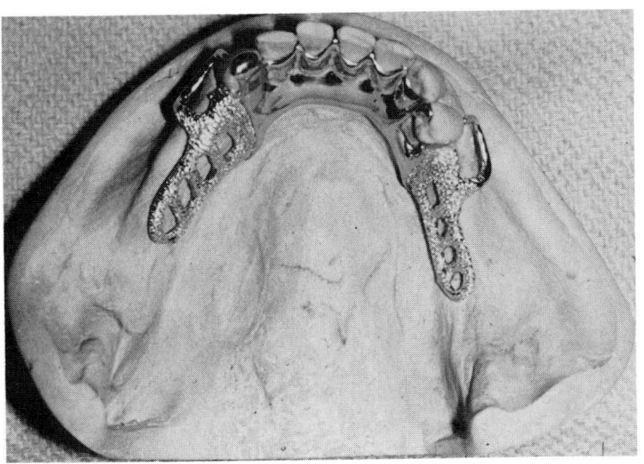

Figure 15–7 ■ When the casting is returned from the laboratory, it is adjusted on the master cast, inspected for accurate fit, contours, and design and physiologically adjusted in the patient's mouth. It is then ready for attachment of the altered cast impression tray.

properly fitted on the teeth, and the denture base, thereby deriving the greatest support potential from both teeth and edentulous areas.

IMPRESSION TRAY PROCEDURES

1. The casting, which has been physiologically adjusted, is placed on the master cast (Fig. 15–7).

2. A single layer of base plate wax is placed over the edentulous area to provide a space for the impression material. Warm the metal casting and reseat on the master cast, ensuring that all rests are well in place (Fig. 15–8). Remove the wax from the denture base retention area to provide for a mechanical lock of the acrylic to the metal (Fig. 15–9).

3. Prepare the tray. The purpose of the tray is to carry a uniform thickness of the final impression material to within 1 mm of the peripheries, without exerting pressure on the mucosa. Adapt autocuring acrylic resin to the metal casting over the edentulous area to form an impression tray (Figs. 15–10 and 15–11). When the resin has cured, place it in warm water and remove the wax spacer from under the tray. Check to be sure that the tray is firmly secured to the casting (Figs. 15–12 and 15–13).

4. The cast with tray attached is checked in the patient's mouth, and overextensions are relieved (Fig. 15–14).

5. The border extensions are refined with gray stick, low-fusing modeling composition or comparable border molding material. The modeling composition is heat-conditioned in a

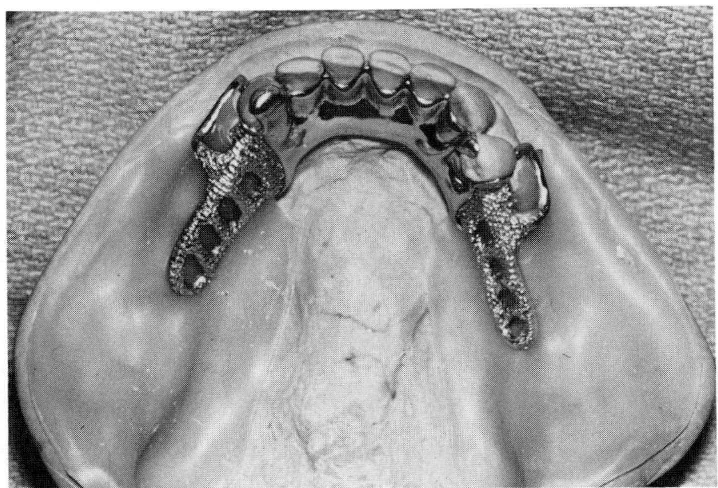

Figure 15–8 ■ A layer of base plate wax is placed over the edentulous area of the master cast to provide space for the final impression material, and the metal casting is heated and seated in place on the cast.

water heater at 140°F; it is removed from the interior side of the tray to provide space for the final impression material (Fig. 15–15).

6. A number 8 bur is used to prepare relief holes in the acrylic next to the metal finish line to allow for escape of excess final impression material (Fig. 15–16).

7. Use of the tray, held in position over the edentulous area by the metal casting, is the ideal method for recording the tissues in an undistorted position. There is equal space between tissue and tray in all areas. The border extensions are in the exact position at which they were recorded.

IMPRESSION MATERIALS

Original work by Holmes concluded that the altered cast procedure produced the best support results. In addition, he tested four types of

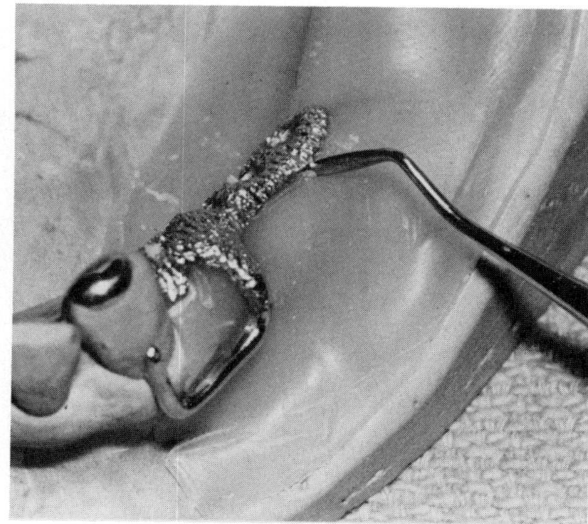

Figure 15–9 ■ Wax is removed from under the metal base connector to ensure good retention for the plastic impression tray.

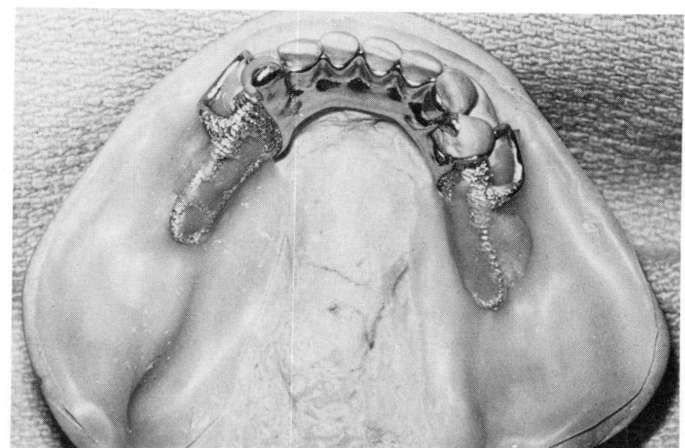

Figure 15–10 ■ A small amount of fluid autocuring acrylic resin is applied to the metal to ensure secure attachment of the plastic.

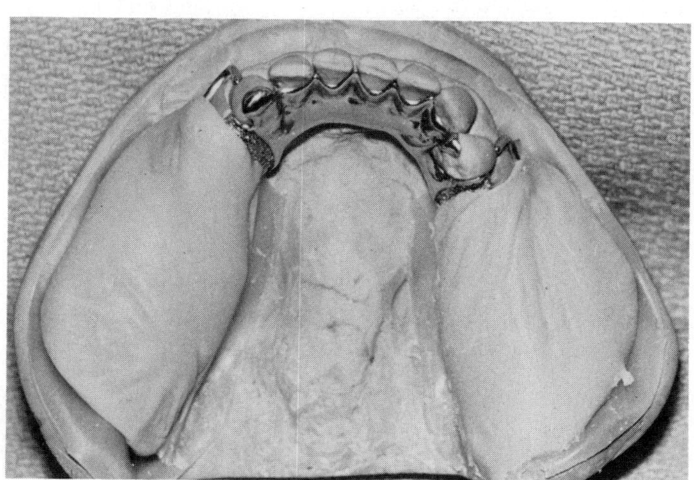

Figure 15–11 ■ Plastic tray material in the "dough" stage is adapted to the edentulous area to form the extension impression tray.

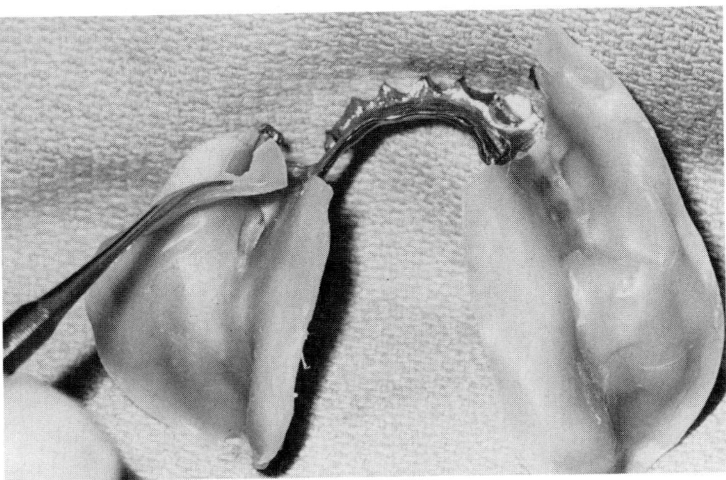

Figure 15–12 ■ When the plastic tray material is cured, the entire cast with tray is submerged in a warm water bath at 140° F for a few seconds for easy separation. The wax spacer is removed.

final impression materials in the altered cast tray. These materials were irreversible hydrocolloid, rubber base (injection type), metallic paste, and wax. Of these four materials, the last three produced relatively similar results, with the wax impression providing the least movement. A further study by Muller found that wax produced more distortion or displacement of the mucosa than the other impression materials.

All of the previously described impression materials, used in conjunction with the altered cast procedures, provide good edentulous area stability.

The *metallic paste* is used for the following reasons:

1. It produces excellent edentulous area support, with minimal partial movement.
2. It sets to a hard, rigid state that is difficult to distort during laboratory procedures.
3. It causes minimal tissue displacement.
4. It records good tissue detail.
5. It sets quickly in clinic use.

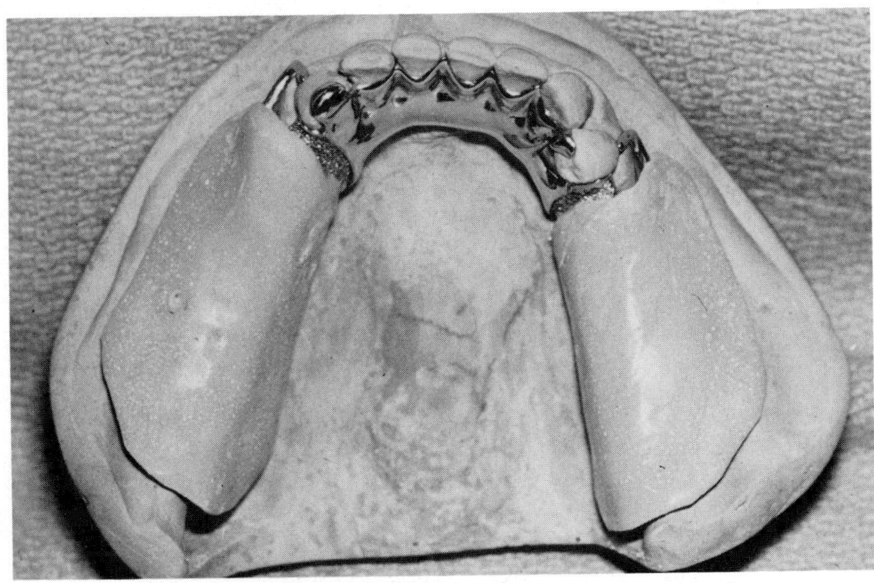

Figure 15–13 ■ The plastic tray is trimmed and polished.

IMPRESSION PROCEDURE

The patient is informed of the steps in the procedure, and a rehearsal is performed.

1. Petroleum jelly is placed on the metal casting for ease of removal of the paste, which may contact structures beyond the edentulous areas.
2. Petroleum jelly is placed on the abutment teeth to facilitate the removal of excess paste.
3. The impression material, in the proportions given by the manufacturer, is mixed and placed in the tray.
4. The tray is placed in the patient's mouth, *short of complete seating.* The patient is instructed to place the tongue in a forward position (for the mandibular impression) and to almost close the mouth, short of touching teeth or prosthesis. The casting and tray are then seated with the patient's masticatory muscles in a relaxed position. The metal casting is firmly seated on the teeth and is held in position over the rests until the material is completely set. *Do not place force or allow movement* on the edentulous area.
5. When the material is set, check to see that the rests are completely seated on the teeth. Remove the impression, check for discrepancies (Fig. 15–17), and trim the impression material exactly to the metal finish line on the tissue surface (Fig. 15–18).

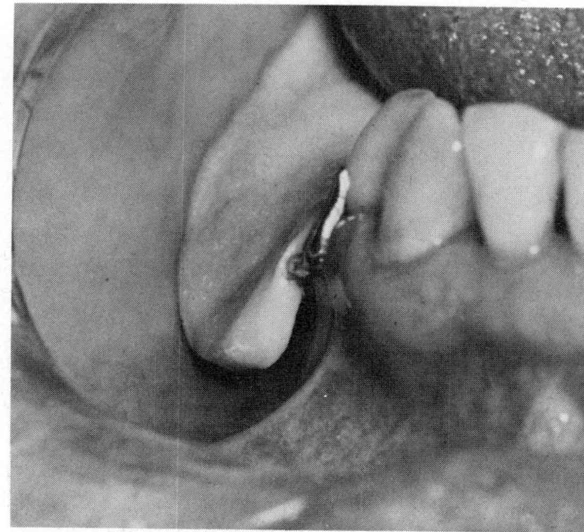

Figure 15–14 ■ The tray is checked in the patient's mouth for proper peripheral extension. The impression trays are held in ideal position by the metal casting seated on the remaining teeth.

CAST ALTERATION

The edentulous portion of the master cast is removed (Fig. 15–19), and retention grooves are prepared. Position the metal framework with the attached impression on the master cast, ensuring that all rests and metal portions are completely seated (Fig. 15–20). The casting is secured to the stone cast with sticky wax.

The impression is beaded and boxed before the stone is poured into the area. *All* surfaces must be sealed to prevent the stone from flowing onto the occlusal surfaces of the cast (Fig. 15–21). When the stone is set, place the impression in a water bath at 140°F prior to removal of the casting and the tray.

This cast accurately reproduces the edentu-

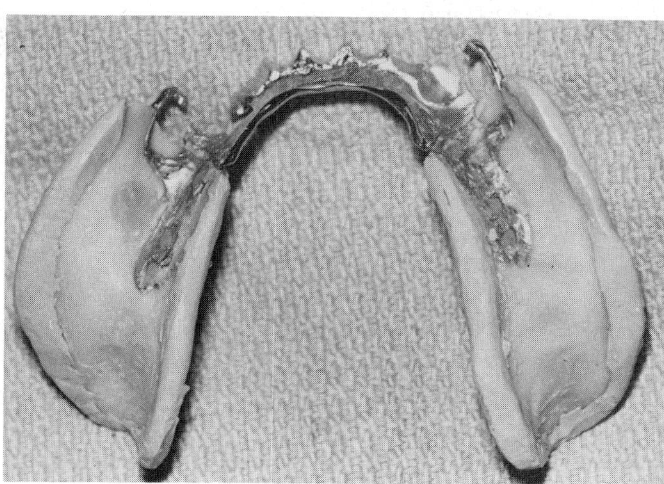

Figure 15–15 ■ The extensions of the peripheral borders are refined with border molding material. The inner surface of the molding material is relieved to provide space for the final impression material.

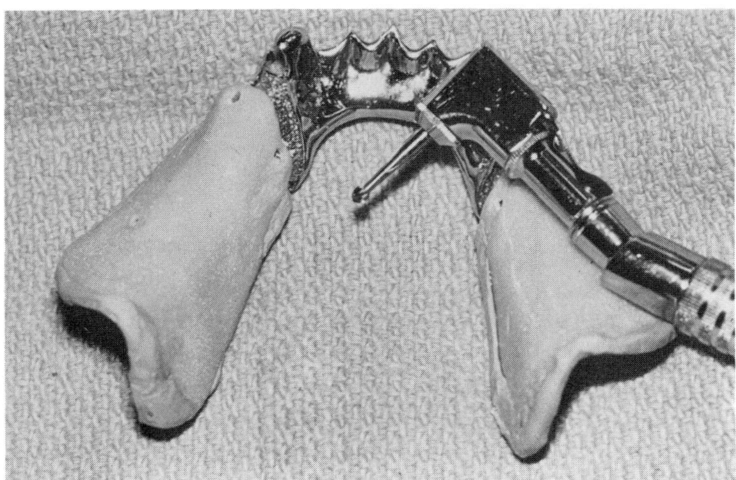

Figure 15–16 ■ Holes for escape of excess final impression material are made in the plastic tray next to the finish line (a number 8 bur is used).

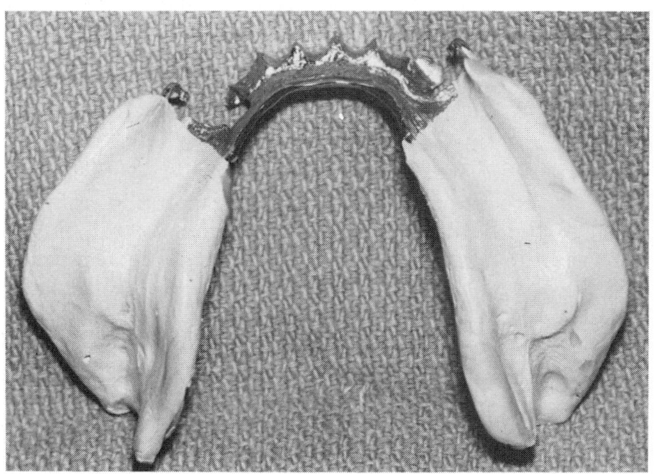

Figure 15–17 ■ The finished impression is inspected for accuracy of the tissue recording and of the extension.

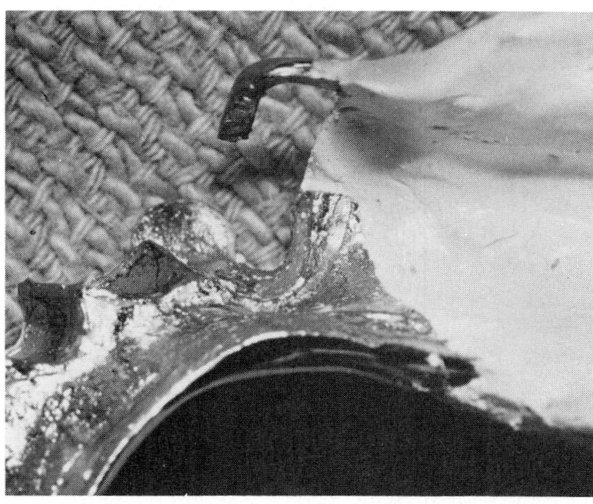

Figure 15–18 ■ Excess impression material is removed up to the metal finish line. Metal and impression material should form a smooth continuous surface.

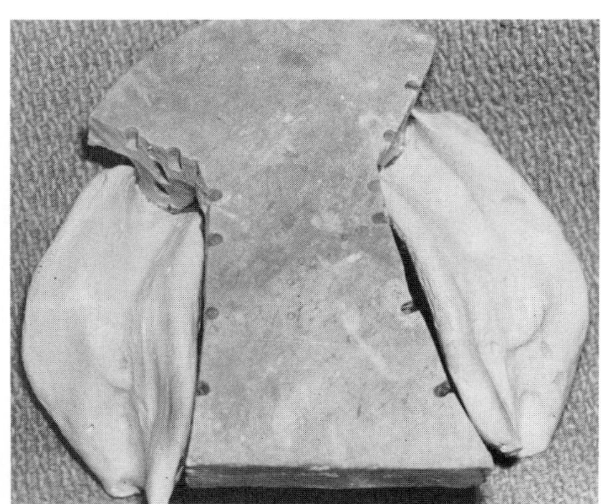

Figure 15–19 ■ The edentulous area of the master cast is removed with a plaster saw and the metal casting seated in place on the teeth. (Note that *only metal* will touch the cast—all impression areas must be *out of contact*).

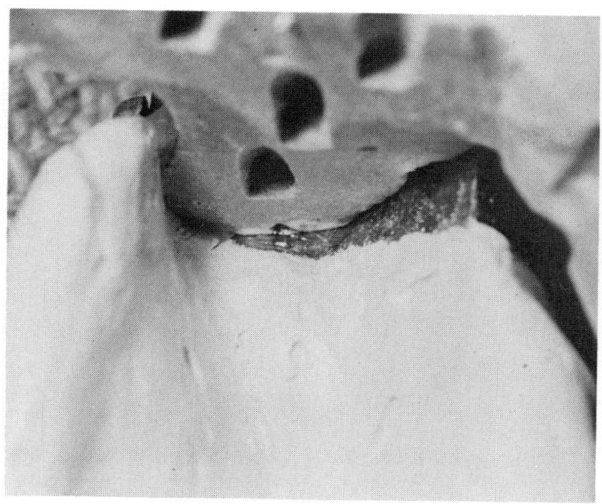

Figure 15–20 ■ The metal of casting is in intimate contact with the crest of the cast ridge. Retention grooves are placed in the cast.

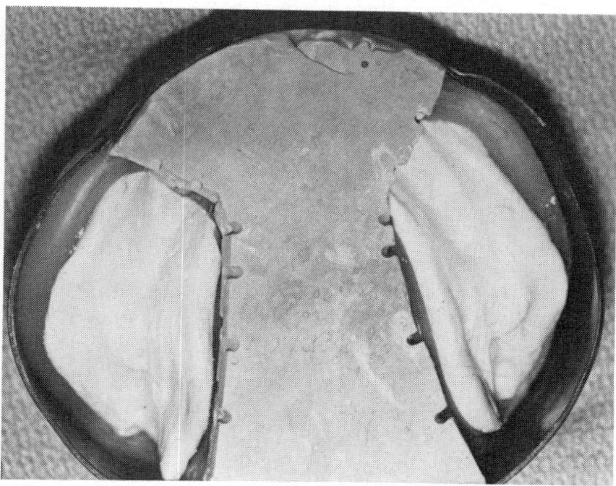

Figure 15–21 ■ The impression, beaded and boxed, ready to replace the edentulous area. All areas must be sealed with wax to prevent stone from leaking through onto the occlusal surface of the original master cast.

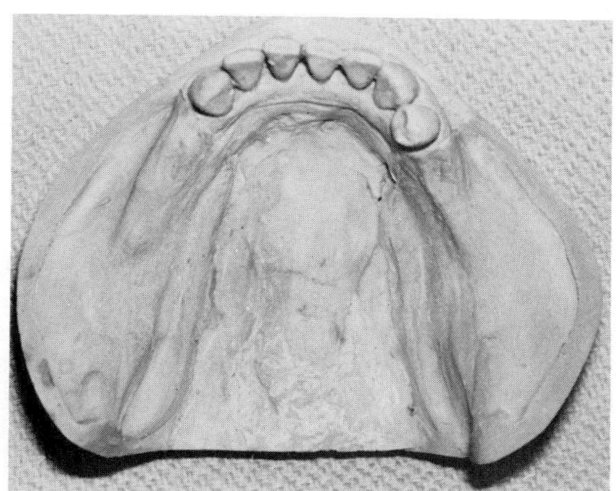

Figure 15–22 ■ The altered cast with the edentulous area repoured, producing the best possible support and orientation to the metal casting and to the remaining teeth.

lous area in a form that provides maximum support in conjunction with ideal position of the casting in relation to the remaining teeth (Fig. 15–22).

All maxillary extension prostheses have the altered cast impression procedure completed at this stage, using the same procedure.

REFERENCES

Applegate OC: The partial denture base. J Prosthet Dent 5:636–648, 1955.

Applegate OC: An evaluation of the support for the removable partial denture. J Prosthet Dent 10:112–123, 1960.

Hindels GW: Load distribution in extension saddle partial dentures. J Prosthet Dent 2:92–100, 1952.

Holmes JB: Influence of impression procedures and occlusal loading on partial denture movement. J Prosthet Dent 15:474–481, 1965.

Leupold RJ: A comparative study of impression procedures for distal extension removable partial dentures. J Prosthet Dent 16:708–720, 1966.

Leupold RJ and Kratochvil FJ: An altered cast procedure to improve support for removable partial dentures. J Prosthet Dent 15:672–678, 1965.

Rapuano JA: Single tray dual-impression technique for distal extension partial dentures. J Prosthet Dent 24:41–46, 1970.

Smith RA: Secondary palatal impressions for major connector adaptation. J Prosthet Dent 24:108–110, 1970.

chapter 16

Maxillomandibular relations and registrations

Maxillomandibular relations are variable, and therefore it is necessary to decide upon the position of the mandibular arch relative to the maxillary arch, at which the prosthesis will be fabricated. This decision is influenced by individual philosophies of jaw relations, coordinated with a diagnostic evaluation of the patient. Factors of prime influence are the vertical dimension of occlusion, occlusion, the centric relation record, and the protrusive record.

Vertical Dimension of Occlusion

First, it is necessary to evaluate contact of remaining occluding teeth, in order to confirm proper vertical dimension of occlusion. The need to *restore* or *reduce* vertical dimension must be determined (Fig. 16–1).

There are many methods of evaluating vertical dimension of occlusion. All methods agree on one major principle: In physiologic functions (speaking and swallowing), there should be *little or no contact of opposing teeth*—thus, the factor of greatest importance is *absence of occlusal interference in physiologic function.*

When there is a suspected loss of vertical dimension of occlusion between opposing teeth (Fig. 16–2) or absence of opposing teeth, it is necessary to provide a treatment prosthesis to evaluate the vertical dimension at which the final treatment will be accomplished (Fig. 16–3). Evaluation with the treatment prosthesis is continued until the patient is comfortable and without temporomandibular joint, muscle, or periodontal symptoms. A minimum diagnostic trial period is 3 to 4 weeks, when vertical dimension of occlusion needs to be restored.

Occlusion

Decisions regarding treatment with respect to maxillomandibular positional relationship are determined by the individual philosophy of the doctor providing the treatment. There are *two basic philosophies* of jaw relationships:

1. Centric occlusion *coincident with centric relation.*
2. Occlusion established by *positional* contact of existing opposing teeth or by muscles.

CENTRIC OCCLUSION COINCIDENT WITH CENTRIC RELATION

This jaw relationship is a combination of *centric occlusion* (the relation of opposing occlusal surfaces that provides the maximum planned contact or intercuspation) at *centric relation* (the most retruded relation of the mandible to the maxilla at a given degree of vertical opening). A strong rationale for use of this relationship is that the position can be repeated and reproduced by duplicate records. This factor is advantageous, since it provides a check of clinical procedures and laboratory transfers to ensure reproducibility and removes the possibility of interocclusal interference if the jaw moves to the retruded position.

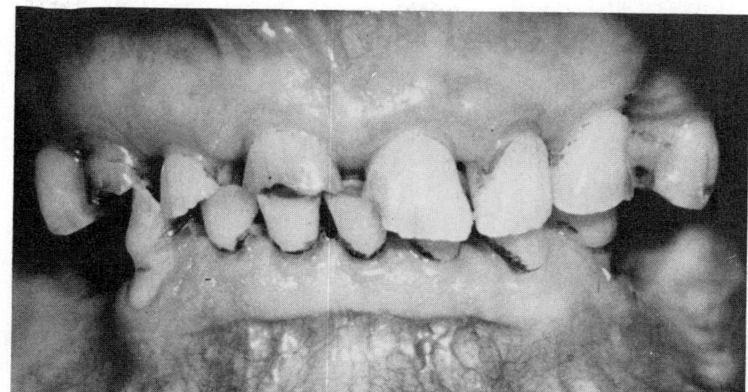

Figure 16–1 ■ Assessment of the correct vertical dimension of occlusion is the first requirement when establishing maxillomandibular relations.

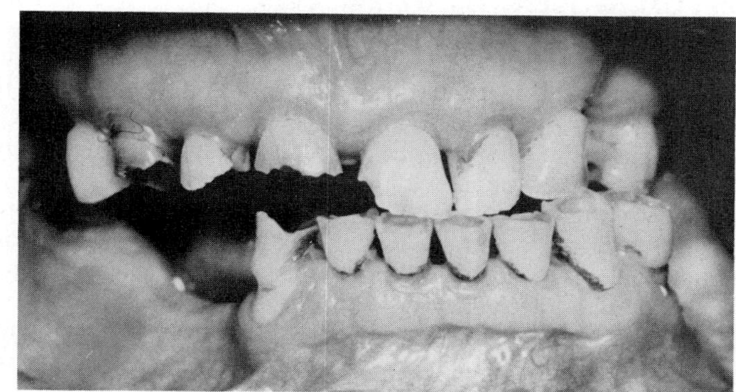

Figure 16–2 ■ Tentative location of the vertical dimension of occlusion is determined by the use of phonetics and by observing swallowing positions.

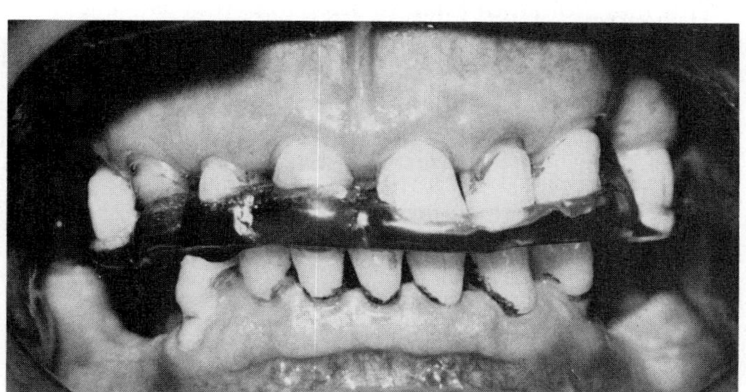

Figure 16–3 ■ The vertical dimension of occlusion is evaluated with a stint or treatment prosthesis before the treatment position is accepted.

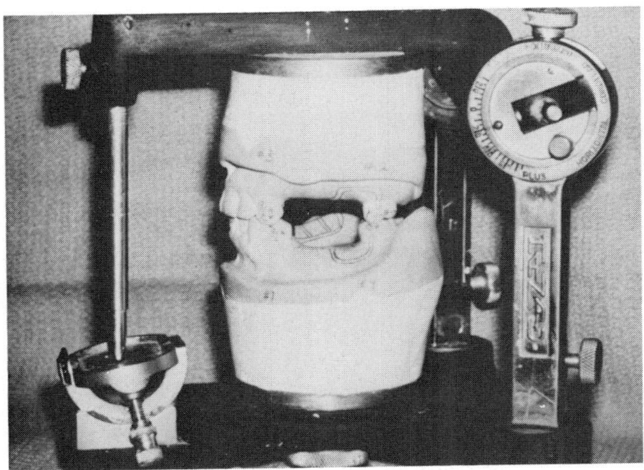

Figure 16–4 ■ An intermediate or semiadjustable articulator is acceptable for fabrication of a removable partial denture prosthesis.

OCCLUSION ESTABLISHED BY POSITIONAL CONTACT OF EXISTING OPPOSING TEETH OR BY MUSCLES

This philosophy of jaw relationship for treatment is predicated on the theory that functional activities and muscle action and development have established this jaw position. If diagnostic evaluation determines that no disease or adverse symptoms are occurring within the entire supporting masticatory system, the existing jaw relationship is considered acceptable.

It is important to evaluate the presence of occlusal discrepancies when the patient is in centric relation, when this jaw position is accepted for treatment with a prosthesis.

RECOMMENDED JAW RELATIONSHIP

The maxillomandibular relationship that is *recommended* is *centric occlusion coincident with centric relation* because it is a repeatable position that can be checked and proven with duplicate records and allows jaw movement to an outer or terminal position if so desired or required.

MAXILLOMANDIBULAR REGISTRATIONS

The purpose of maxillomandibular registrations is to record or register the relation of the mandible to the maxilla so that this relationship can be transferred to an articulator or reproduced in a laboratory situation.

Instruments

The articulator ■ This instrument can reproduce the exact position of the patient's oral anatomy for replicas (casts) in a laboratory situation. The articulator can be

1. A basic instrument that can reproduce only one position.
2. A completely adjustable instrument that can reproduce all mandibular positions.
3. An intermediate instrument that can reproduce two or more selected or arbitrary positions.

The accurate reproduction by the articulator of the patient's jaw movements is entirely dependent upon the information and registrations that are used and the preciseness with which the instrument is programmed. Clinical, laboratory, technical, and material errors can interfere

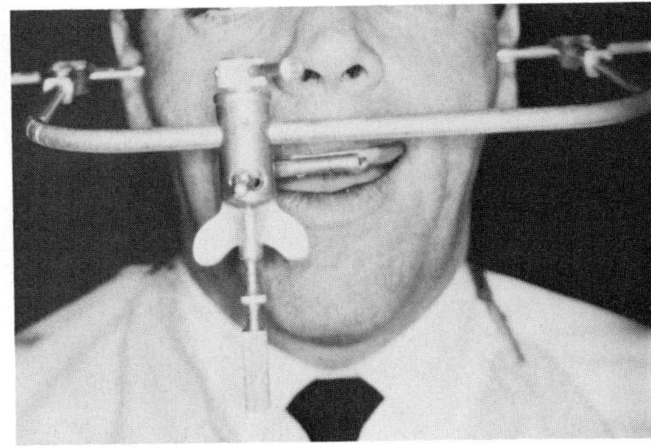

Figure 16–5 ■ The face bow registration records the exact position of the maxillary arch in relation to the head.

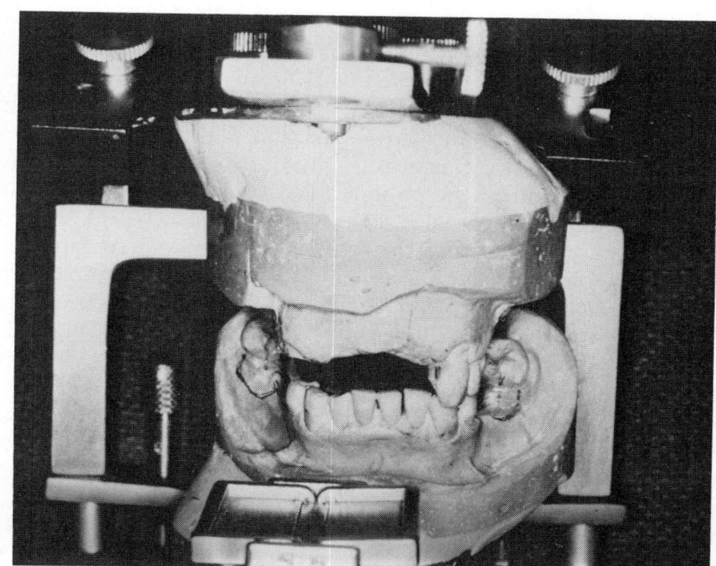

Figure 16–6 ■ Patients often present asymmetries of arches in relation to the condyles; these measurements must be transferred to the articulator to reproduce actual jaw movement.

with proper reproduction of the patient situation. It is imperative that a second set of registrations be taken to eliminate the potential for errors and to check all transfers.

The *intermediate articulator* is an acceptable instrument for use in fabricating removable partial prostheses. An example of this type of instrument is the Hanau (Fig. 16–4) articulator. The records used in conjunction with this type of instrument are the

1. Face bow record.
2. Centric relation record.
3. Protrusive relation record.

Face bow registration ■ The face bow record or registration orients the occlusal arch in its exact position in reference to the head (Fig. 16–5). If the exact position is not recorded, there is a possibility of error in three dimensions when the casts are mounted on the articulator. These errors result in occlusal contacts of the prosthesis developed on the articulator, which will not be compatible with movements in the patient's mouth.

The face bow registration must orient the maxillary cast in three planes:

1. Anterior-posterior location.
2. Superior-inferior orientation (sagittal).
3. Horizontal orientation.

Anterior position ■ The articulator must reproduce the anatomic distance from the hinge axis to all occlusal contacts. If this distance is not a faithful duplication (i.e., if the radius of the articulator's arc of closure is different from the patient's radius of arc of closure), there is the

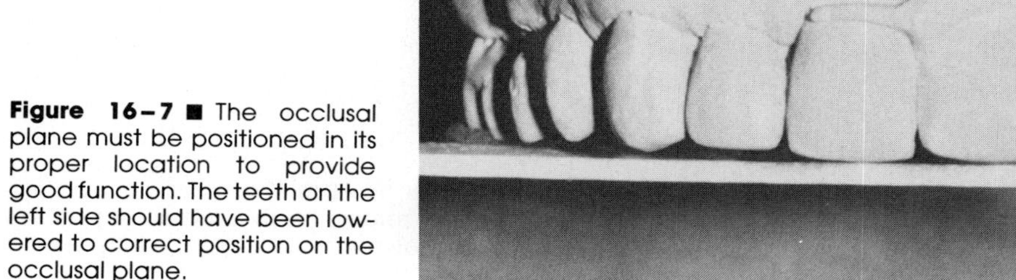

Figure 16–7 ■ The occlusal plane must be positioned in its proper location to provide good function. The teeth on the left side should have been lowered to correct position on the occlusal plane.

possibility of traumatic contact of teeth as the patient opens and closes the jaw.

Superior-inferior orientation ■ From the side (lateral) view, the maxillary cast must duplicate the proper up-and-down position. If the anterior or posterior position of the cast does not duplicate that of the patient's anatomy on the articulator, the prosthesis will not reproduce correct occlusal contacts in movement when it is placed in the patient's mouth.

Horizontal orientation ■ When viewed from the front, the maxilla of most patients is located to the right or left of a center point between the axis of rotation or the heads of the condyles. In some situations, the discrepancy is quite marked (Fig. 16–6). Also, one side of the occlusal plane may be lower than the other side in the patient's mouth (Fig. 16–7). Measurements of these discrepancies must be properly recorded and transferred to the articulator to produce a duplication of the patient's jaw movement.

The face bow is an essential registration that records these three *base line* anatomic positions of the patient's oral anatomy and allows transfer of these anatomic positions to an instrument—*the articulator.*

Clinical Procedure for Face Bow Registration

1. *Establish the hinge axis point.* Arbitrary location—Locate a straight line from the canthus of the eye to the center of the tragus of the ear. Mark a point 13 mm forward on this line from the posterior border of the tragus of the ear. (If a face bow with ear positioners is used, it is not necessary to mark the hinge axis location.)

2. *Adjust the condylar rods of the face bow* until they just touch the skin over the hinge axis marks. (With ear positioners, adjust the plastic rods within the external auditory meatus until they are secure but comfortable to the patient—have the patient hold both sides for support and security.)

3. *Prepare the bite fork.* Cover the occlusal surface of the bite fork with modeling composition or hard base plate wax. Seat the softened index material on the maxillary occlusal surfaces and have the patient hold it firmly in position with the thumbs of both hands.

4. *Place the face bow onto the bite fork and secure it.* Check for the correct position of the bow over the hinge axis mark, just touching the skin.

5. *Note and record the numerical settings on the axis extension pins* in case they come loose or move. (Note: With self-centering caliper style face bows, it is not necessary to record the setting.)

6. *A third point of reference may be recorded* to position the cast on the articulator as if the patient were in an upright head position. The inferior bony border of the orbit is located, and the orbital pointer tip is positioned at this border and secured to the face bow by means of the toggle. (Note: The end of the orbital pointer is rounded and blunt; however, the eye must be protected with the finger during placement of the pointer and during removal of the face bow.)

7. *Adjust the axis extension pins of the articulator equally on both sides* to accept and hold the face bow. If the condylar rods of the face bow must be moved, always move both an equal distance inward or outward as required.

8. *Prepare the remount notches in the base of*

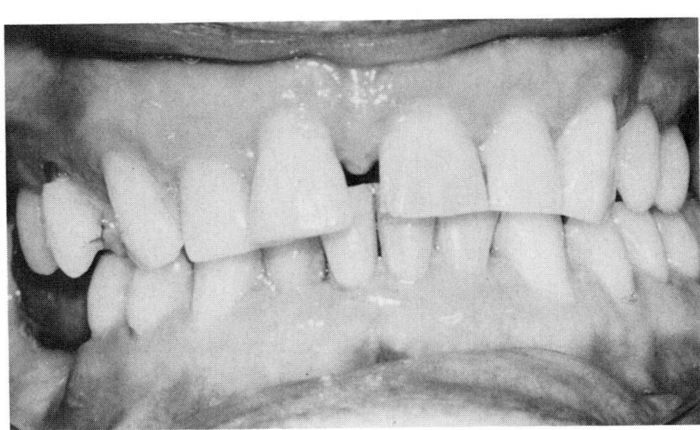

Figure 16–8 ■ When sufficient natural teeth remain to give a positive position, the interarch relationship can be recorded by tooth-to-tooth contact.

the cast, coat them with petroleum jelly, and place the maxillary cast onto the occlusal index of the face bow. Position it on the articulator, and mount the maxillary cast onto the superior member of the articulator.

Centric Relation Record

The purpose of this registration is to record the exact position of the maxilla to the mandible in centric relation. *Centric relation* is defined as "the most retruded relation of the mandible to the maxilla, when the condyles are in the most posterior unstrained position in the glenoid fossa, from which lateral movement can be made at any given degree of jaw separation."

Methods of recording centric relation are greatly influenced by the teeth and tissues remaining. When there are enough remaining occluding teeth to establish a positive interarch position, it is possible to determine the proper position by tooth-to-tooth contact (Fig. 16–8). When an edentulous situation is present, it may be necessary to use a record base in conjunction with interocclusal registration material to properly record centric position and to effect a transfer to the articulator (Fig. 16–9).

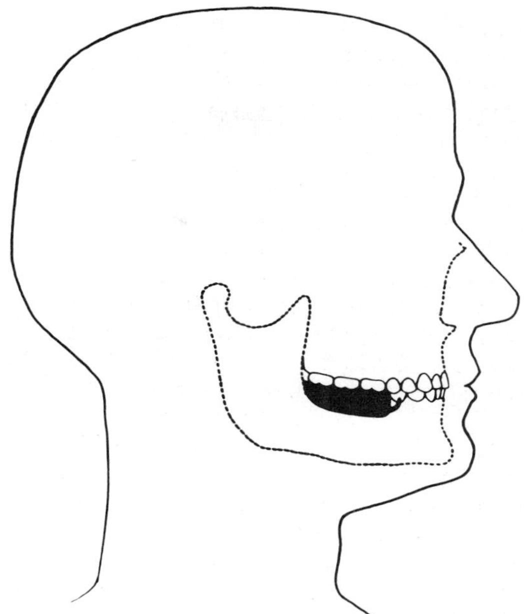

Figure 16–9 ■ A record base is needed to record interarch relationship when there are edentulous areas.

ORIENTATION WITH REMAINING NATURAL TEETH

The method of choice when sufficient teeth remain is to orient the mandibular cast to the mounted maxillary cast, since this method eliminates the interposed record material having to be placed between the teeth, which increases the potential for errors (Fig. 16–10).

When *casts used to fabricate a prosthesis* are oriented by this method, it is imperative that any *interocclusal interferences be removed* in the centric relation position, and that the casts be made *after* these adjustments are completed.

RECORD BASES AND OCCLUSAL RIMS

In most cases involving removable partial dentures, extensive edentulous areas are present (Fig. 16–11). There can be a single

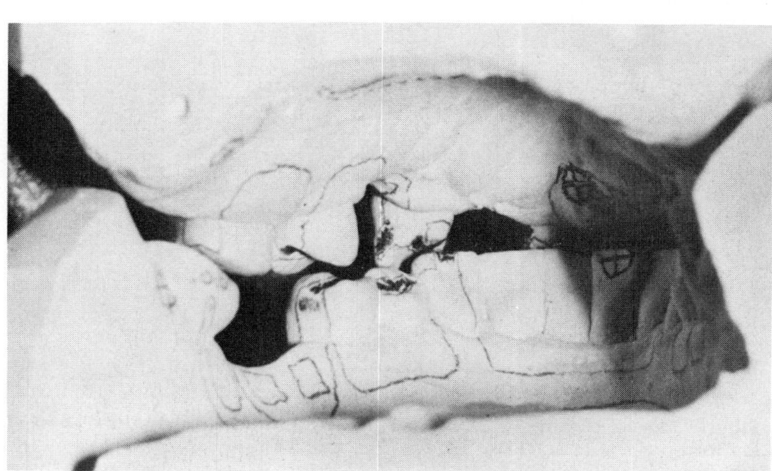

Figure 16–10 ■ Orienting the mandibular cast to the maxillary cast by tooth-to-tooth contact should be done when there are sufficient teeth to contact.

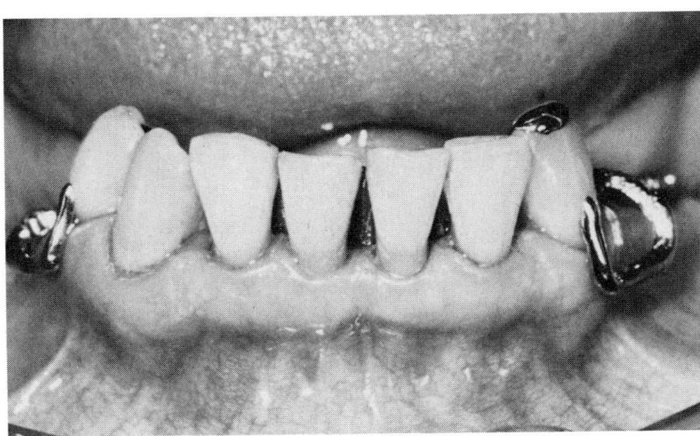

Figure 16–11 ■ A posterior record base must be attached to the metal casting to record the interarch position.

edentulous area in one arch or the extreme situation of a complete maxillary denture opposing six or fewer mandibular anterior teeth.

Positive recording of the centric relation position under these conditions requires

1. Record bases that are *well adapted* to the tissue surface.
2. Occlusion rims that are *positive* and *nonchanging*.
3. Interocclusal registration material that is *positive* and *nonchanging*.

Record Bases

The centric registration reliability depends on support from the edentulous mucosa being equal to the support provided by the finished prosthesis (Fig. 16–12). The record base is fabricated on the surface of the altered cast, which will form the tissue surface of the final prosthesis. This record base is attached to the denture base retainers of the metal casting that hold the base in proper position (Fig. 16–13).

The record base is fabricated by blocking out undercuts on the altered cast, applying a separating medium, sprinkling a thin layer of self-cure plastic onto the support surface, and attaching it to the casting.

Occlusion Rims

The occlusion rim is a ridge of material that fills the space between the record base and the opposing occlusion. This rim should be as stable and as unchanging as possible. A simple yet positive occlusion rim can be constructed at the same time the record base is fabricated. A thin, V-shaped ridge of plastic is formed on the

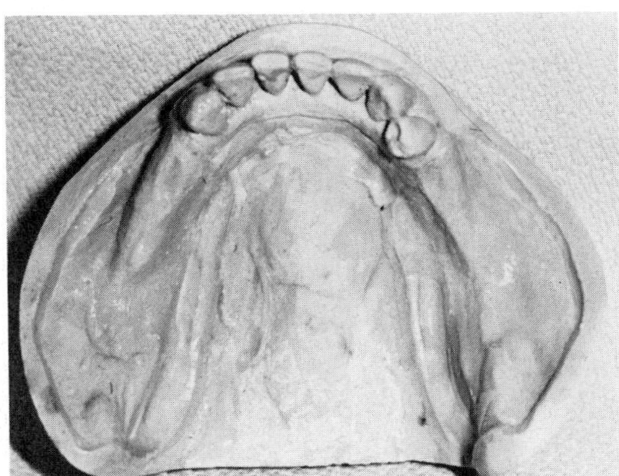

Figure 16–12 ■ A more accurate registration can be made if the record base is well adapted to the altered cast surface.

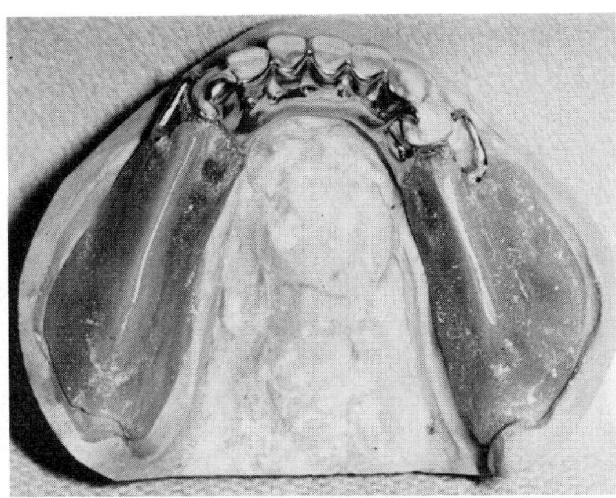

Figure 16–13 ■ Autocure acrylic is sprinkled or adapted to the surface of the altered cast and attached to the metal casting.

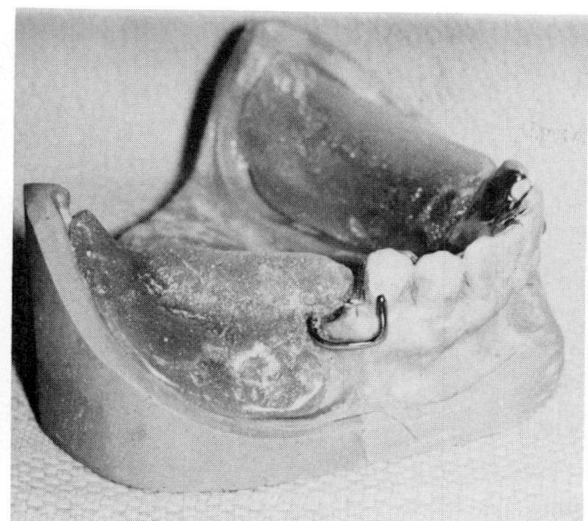

Figure 16–14 ■ The occlusion rim can be formed with a thin V-shaped ridge of autocure acrylic, providing a stable, adjustable record platform.

record base up to the approximate position and height of the opposing occlusal surface (Fig. 16–14). This provides a firm, rigid, unchanging rim and is easily adjusted for height.

Material such as hard waxes are often used for occlusal rims. Exceptional care must be exercised in their use, since they can be changed and distorted by changing temperatures and pressure.

INTEROCCLUSAL REGISTRATION MATERIALS

The purpose of the registration material is to provide the finite, positive, unchanging key to record the relationship of maxillary and mandibular occlusal surfaces. The material should exert little or no opposition to closure. The primary requirement for the material is that when set it undergo no dimensional change with variations of pressure or temperature. Materials that fulfill these requirements are registration pastes, modeling composition, plaster, and auto-cure plastics.

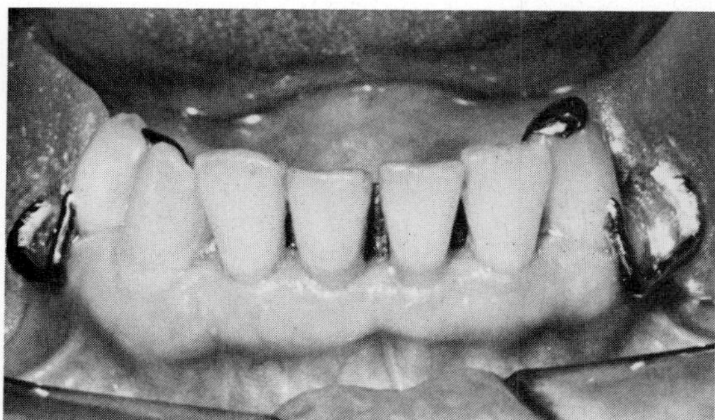

Figure 16–15 ■ Instruct the patient and practice centric relation closure with the record base in place in the mouth.

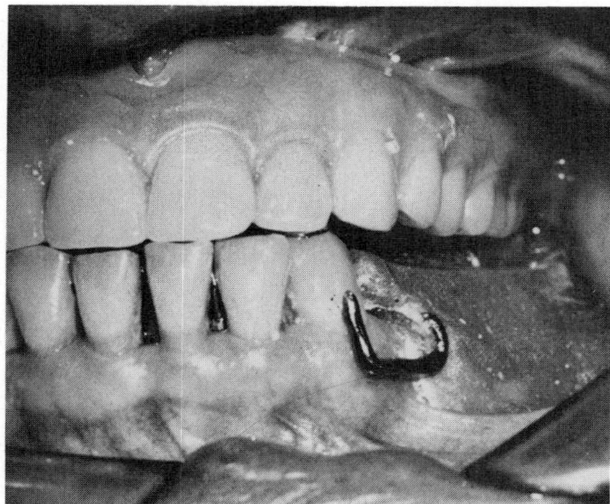

Figure 16–16 ■ Ensure consistent closure in centric position with no interference before attempting registration.

Clinical Procedure — Centric Registration

Patient conditioning and cooperation are of the utmost importance. Explain to the patient what the procedure will be; practice together until there is complete patient relaxation and complete control by the operator (Fig. 16–15).

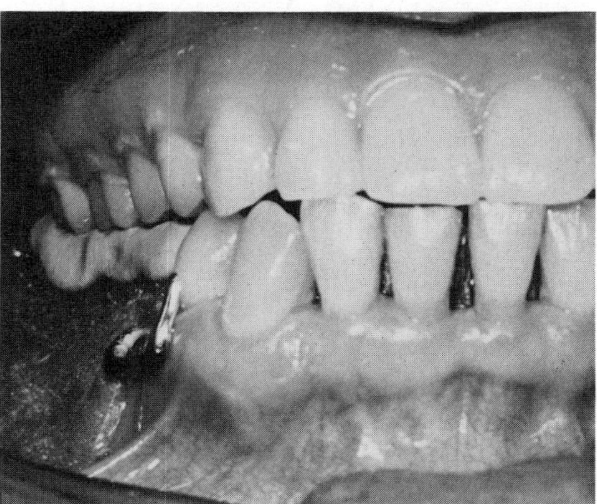

Figure 16–17 ■ Registration material is placed on the occlusion rim, and the centric relation position is recorded *without* tooth contact.

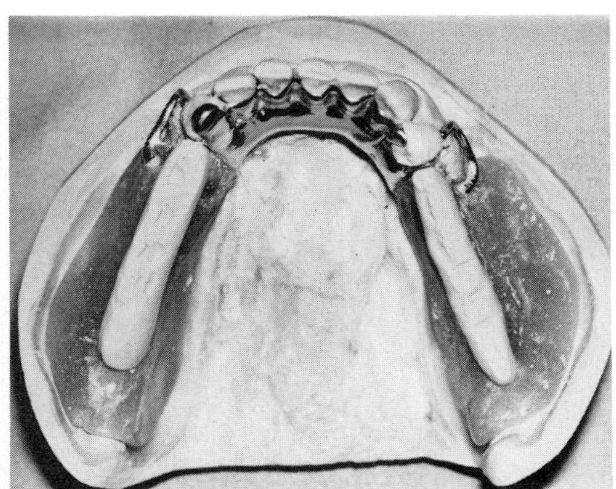

Figure 16–18 ■ The occlusal indentations are trimmed to shallow index records for close observation, and the record base is placed on the master cast.

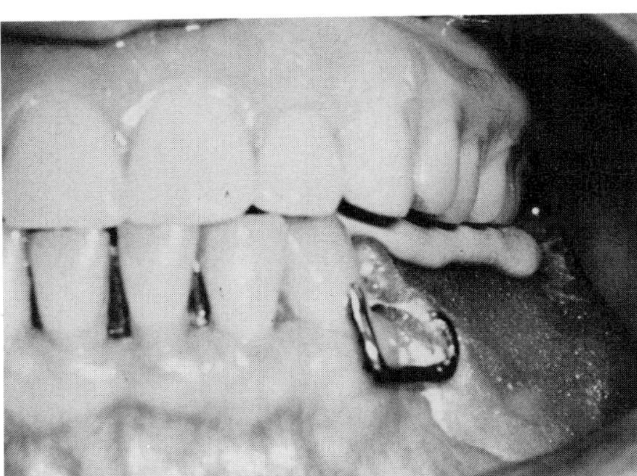

Figure 16–20 ■ A protrusive record is made in the patient's mouth and transferred to the articulator, and the condyle inclinations are adjusted.

Do not attempt a recording until the patient can demonstrate a consistent centric relation position (Fig. 16–16). Close observation is necessary to ensure that there is no movement of the jaw while the registration material is setting.

When the material has set, check the accuracy of the record by having the patient open and close in centric relation and observe the repeatability of the jaw closure into the recording material record (Fig. 16–17).

The casting with record base and interocclusal record intact is removed from the patient's mouth and placed on the master cast (Fig. 16–18), and the interocclusal record is fitted to the opposing cast. Remount notches are cut in the base of the cast, and a thin coat of petroleum jelly is applied. The two casts are secured firmly together with hard, sticky wax, and the mandibular cast is mounted on the articulator (Fig. 16–19). If the vertical dimension of occlusion has been increased during the recording of centric relation, the amount of increase must be measured.

It is advisable to take a second set of interocclusal records in the patient's mouth and to check the mounted articulator casts to confirm the correctness of the transfer against the possibility of error in mounting.

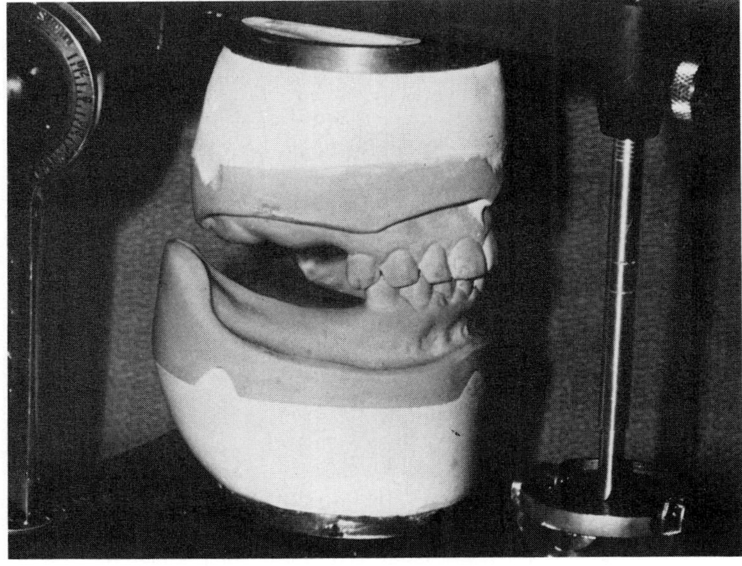

Figure 16–19 ■ Casts mounted on the articulator in centric relation using face bow and record base records. Note the remount index in cast bases and in the articulator mounting.

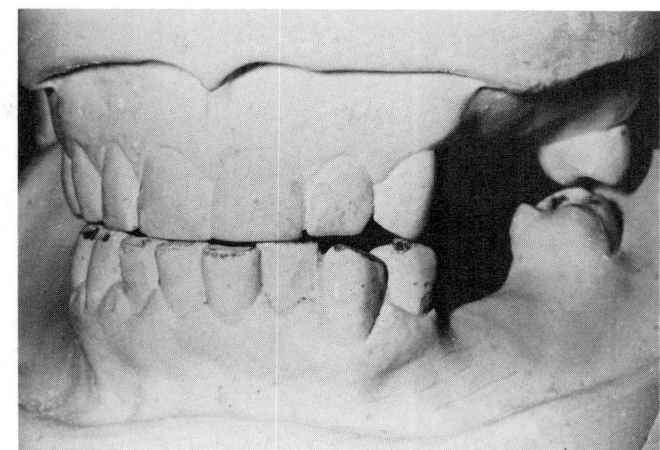

Figure 16–21 ■ Casts mounted on the articulator duplicate the patient's jaw movements and tooth contacts in eccentric positions.

Protrusive Record

The purpose of the protrusive record is to record the forward position of the mandible in relation to the maxilla, when the anterior teeth are edge to edge or approximately 6 mm forward of the centric relation position, and to reproduce this position on the articulator.

Interocclusal records are made with the patient's jaw in this forward position (Fig. 16–20). These records are removed from the patient's mouth, placed on the casts, which have been mounted on the articulator, and the condyle elements of the articulator are adjusted to this position. The casts on the articulator can now duplicate the same position that exists in the patient's mouth at that position (Fig. 16–21).

The actual anatomic position that this registration records is the anterior and lower location on the glenoid fossa, where the head of the condyle is located when it moves forward and down with the anterior teeth at an edge-to-edge position.

REFERENCES

Beck HO: Selection of an articulator and jaw registration. J Prosthet Dent 10:878–886, 1960.

Beckett LS: Accurate occlusal relations in partial denture construction. J Prosthet Dent 4:487–495, 1954.

Block LS: Preparing and conditioning the patient for intermaxillary relations. J Prosthet Dent 2: 599–603, 1952.

Emmert JH: A method of registering occlusion in semi edentulous mouths. J Prosthet Dent 8:94–99, 1958.

Hughes GA and Rigli CP: What is centric relation? J Prosthet Dent 11:16–22, 1961.

Lauritzen AG and Bodner GH: Variations in location of arbitrary and true hinge axis points. J Prosthet Dent 11: 224–229, 1961.

Reitz PV: Technique for mounting removable partial dentures on an articulator. J Prosthet Dent 22:490–494, 1969.

Silverman MM: Determination of vertical dimension by phonetics. Dent Abst 6:465–471, 1957.

Teteruck WR and Lundeen HC: The accuracy of an ear facebow. J Prosthet Dent 16:1039–1046, 1966.

Weinberg LA: An evaluation of the face bow mountings. J Prosthet Dent 11:32–42, 1961.

Weinberg LA: An evaluation of basic articulators and their concepts. Parts I and II. J Prosthet Dent 13:622–663, 1963.

chapter 17

Developing occlusion and esthetics

The objectives in developing occlusion are to

1. Preserve and control remaining oral structures.
2. Organize occlusion for correct vertical dimension, centric relation, and excursions.
3. Provide masticating surfaces.
4. Restore, preserve, and improve esthetics.

Preserve and Control Remaining Structures

Controlling and preserving the structures that remain is a prime objective in treating the partially edentulous patient. This concept, as presented by DeVan, is a basic objective of treatment with the removable partial prosthesis. Replacement of structures or mastication surfaces by themselves may not be proper treatment if it jeopardizes the health or survival of the remaining structures.

The occlusion that is developed provides the force factor, which directly affects the remaining structures. Improperly organized or traumatic occlusion on the removable partial denture could institute or accelerate damage to the remaining structures.

Organize Occlusion

Basic factors to be considered in developing occlusion in removable partial denture treatment are

1. The occlusal plane.
2. Anterior guidance.
3. Condylar guidance.
4. The occlusal scheme.

THE OCCLUSAL PLANE

The first consideration in developing occlusion is the evaluation and establishment of the correct position of the occlusal plane. Without this controlling base line, it is impossible to develop organized and compatible interarch contacts. This condition is most obvious when a posterior tooth is elongated beyond the occlusal plane and extends into a depression in the opposing arch—the elongated tooth can create interference in opening and closing jaw movements. The greatest difficulty, however, develops when there is horizontal jaw movement that results in immediate contact and interference. Elongation of anterior teeth can cause interference and difficulties of occlusion in excursions and can be an esthetic liability.

The ideal occlusal plane is an imaginary line that starts from a posterior position located in the middle third of the retromolar pad (Fig. 17–1), when the jaws are at the correct vertical dimension of occlusion. The anterior location of the line is on the incisal edge of the maxillary central anterior teeth, which are at the proper position as determined by phonetics and esthetics at the correct vertical dimension of occlusion (Fig. 17–2).

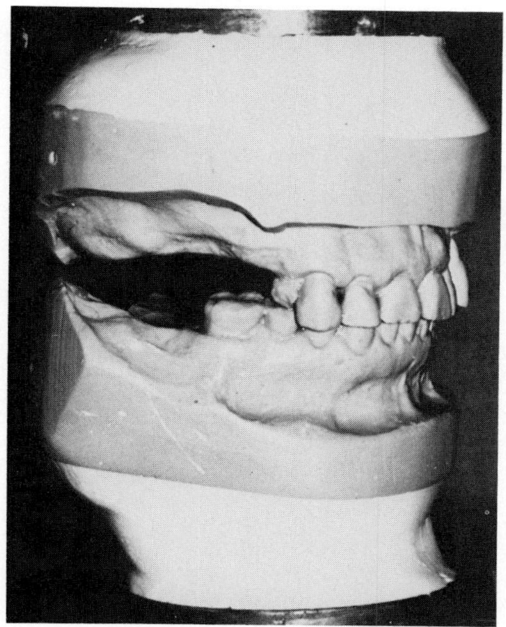

Figure 17–1 ■ The *posterior location* of the occlusal plane lies within the middle third of the retromolar pad. The cast must include this area for occlusal plane orientation.

Once the occlusal plane is established, the occlusal surfaces of the remaining teeth are assessed or positioned in relation to it and modified or restored to develop the occlusal scheme that the operator has selected (Fig. 17–3).

ANTERIOR GUIDANCE

When anterior maxillary and mandibular teeth remain, their positions often determine the path of movement of the jaw in protrusive and lateral excursions. In some situations, excursions may result in immediate and steep opening or vertical movement of the jaw (Fig. 17–4), and in other instances there can be considerable horizontal movement of the jaw before the anterior teeth induce an opening movement.

The significance of anterior guidance is the influence it exerts on the posterior occlusal surfaces. If there is immediate vertical opening, there is less possibility of posterior occlusal interference. If the anterior guidance allows considerable lateral movement, posterior interference can result and requires coordination in placement and adjustment of the occlusal surfaces to remove these interferences.

It is *desirable* to have remaining *anterior teeth in both jaws to provide guidance* (Fig. 17–5). In many situations there is anterior guidance with remaining anterior teeth, but, owing to wear or tooth movement, it is necessary to restore anterior guidance in excursions and the vertical dimension of occlusal contact. Where anterior restoration will be provided with fixed partial dentures, these principles can be used in the fabrication and restoration of the crown anatomy (Fig. 17–6). If the restoration of anterior guidance will be done entirely with a removable partial denture, the principles are incorporated into the restorations in the anterior design of the casting (Fig. 17–7).

When natural anterior tooth guidance is present in conjunction with posterior removable partial dentures, it is desirable to have a separation of the posterior occlusion in excursions.

A most common clinical situation is a *maxil-*

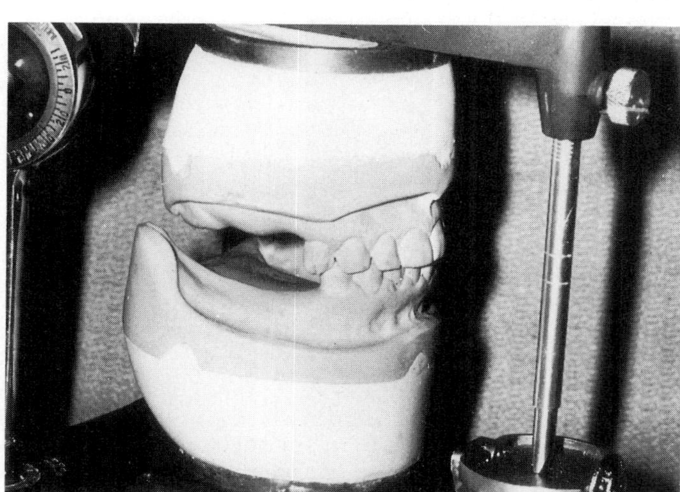

Figure 17–2 ■ The *anterior location* of the ideal occlusal plane is the incisal edge of properly positioned maxillary central incisors, with the casts positioned at the correct vertical dimension.

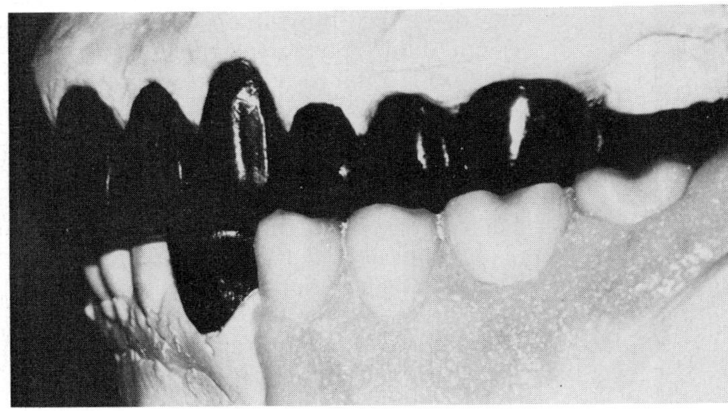

Figure 17–3 ■ A diagnostic wax-up prior to treatment helps to identify occlusal problems and assists in developing ideal occlusion in the finished prosthesis.

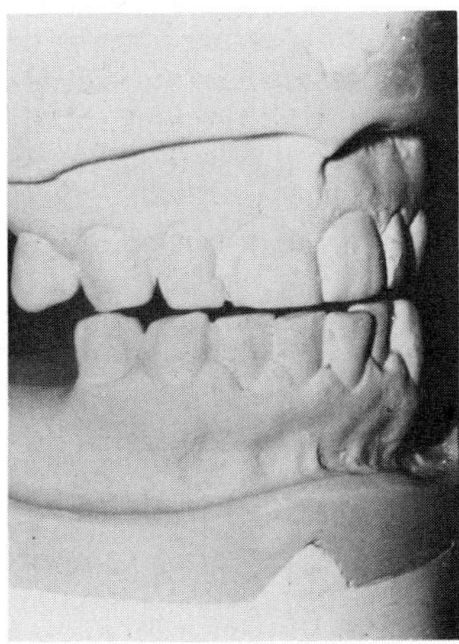

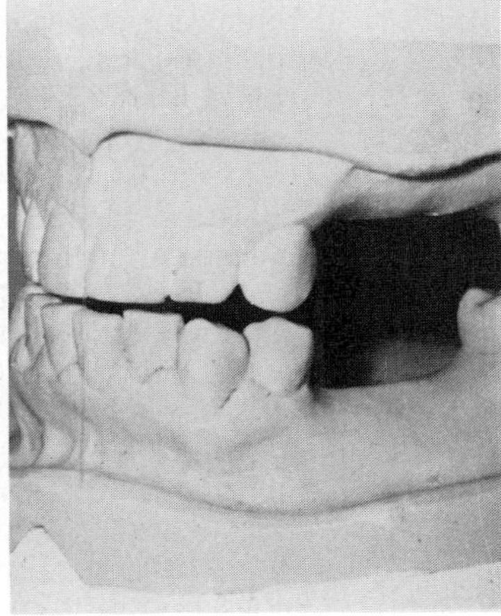

Figure 17–4 ■ The location and number of remaining natural anterior teeth determine anterior guidance. In some movement situations, there is immediate separation of the posterior teeth.

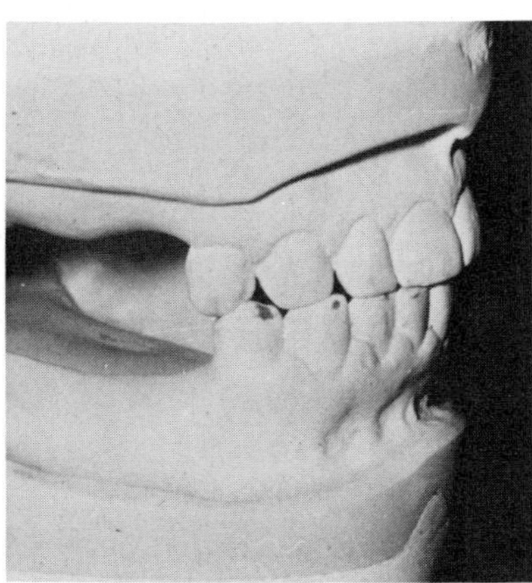

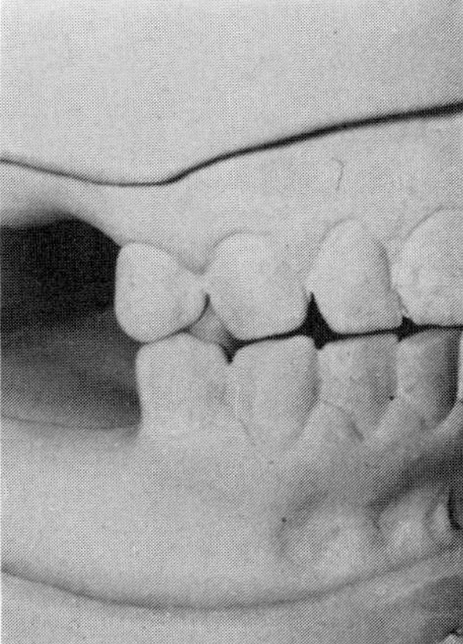

Figure 17–5 ■ Remaining natural anterior teeth contacting in group function in *all* excursions provide ideal anterior guidance.

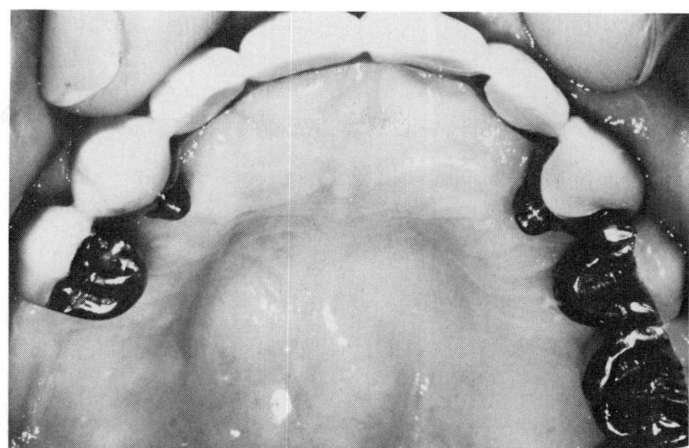

Figure 17–6 ■ Fixed anterior treatment coordinated with a removable posterior prosthesis provides the opportunity to establish ideal anterior guidance.

lary complete denture with a *mandibular removable partial* denture (Fig. 17–8). This condition requires entirely different treatment with respect to anterior guidance. Occlusion is developed, which provides occlusal contacts in centric relation; occlusal contact and balance are also provided for the complete denture in eccentric positions. This anterior and posterior occlusion is necessary to provide stability for the maxillary complete denture as the patient moves through the complete range of motion.

This type of balanced occlusion in all excursions is not necessary for a removable partial denture when remaining anterior natural teeth provide anterior guidance.

CONDYLAR GUIDANCE

The contour of the glenoid fossa is unique in each person. Its measurements can be recorded and transferred to an instrument and have a profound influence in developing occlusion in protrusive and lateral positions.

The measurements of the positions of the patient's glenoid fossae are transferred to the laboratory articulator so that the prosthetic occlusion

1. Will be harmonious and will not interfere with natural tooth guidance.
2. Will provide for development of a balanced occlusal contact in all excursions when a removable partial denture is occluding with a maxillary complete denture.

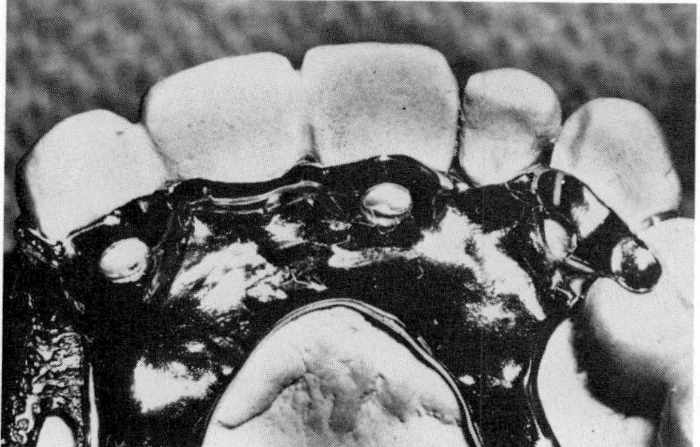

Figure 17–7 ■ In some situations, anterior guidance and occlusal control is developed with the anterior component of the removable partial denture casting.

THE OCCLUSAL SCHEME

Development of the occlusal scheme involves the placement of the prosthetic teeth and the occlusal portions of the metal casting so as to produce proper occlusal contact patterns. A common error is placing the posterior denture teeth to fill in the edentulous spaces (Fig. 17–9). They appear to do so quite well from an occlusal view, but occlusal contact on closure places the tooth and opposing occlusal contacts in an abnormal cusp-to-cusp situation that compromises centric occlusion (Fig. 17–10) and produces interference in excursions. Removal of the excursive interferences changes tooth contours and results in esthetic and occlusal compromise.

The approach to the arrangement of posterior denture teeth that oppose natural teeth is to place the prosthetic teeth in the most advantageous occlusal position for centric and excursive occlusion (Fig. 17–11). This approach develops the best possible control of occlusion and occlu-

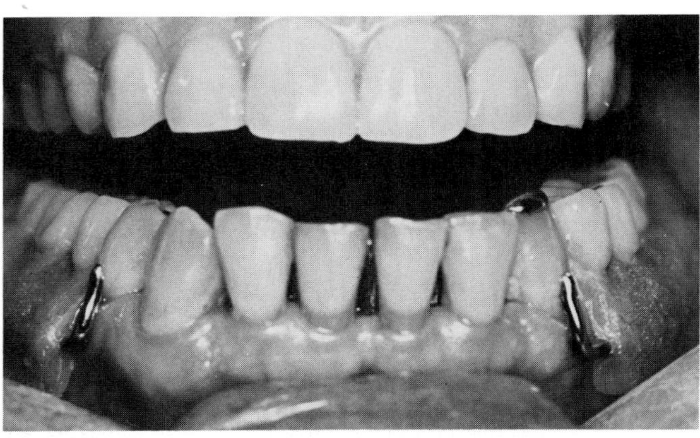

Figure 17–8 ■ When a complete maxillary denture is opposed by a removable partial prosthesis, it is necessary to develop occlusal contacts and balance in all excursive positions in order to stabilize the complete denture.

sal forces. Esthetic difficulties that may result from this approach are located in one small area and can easily be rectified by altering the prosthetic tooth, by recontouring, by adding tooth-colored acrylic to the tooth, or by leaving a slight space.

Since the prosthetic occlusion is now *started* in its proper relationship to existing occlusion, the best possible occlusal scheme for the arch will result (Fig. 17–12), and the entire occlusion will not be jeopardized by improper placement of the first tooth (Figs. 17–13 and 17–14).

Provide Masticating Surfaces

The development of occlusion in posterior extension removable partial dentures against natural teeth requires special consideration. Two factors influence *placement* and *occlusal form* of the denture teeth:

1. The relationship of the remaining natural teeth to the opposing residual ridge.

2. Consideration of the tooth periodontal ligament support opposing the mucosal support of the extension prosthesis.

NATURAL TEETH VS THE RESIDUAL RIDGE

When opposing ridges position the lingual cusp of the maxillary natural tooth over the mandibular ridge (Fig. 17–15), the only contact will be the maxillary lingual cusp against the mandibular denture tooth (Fig. 17–16). The occlusal contact is small and is developed to touch

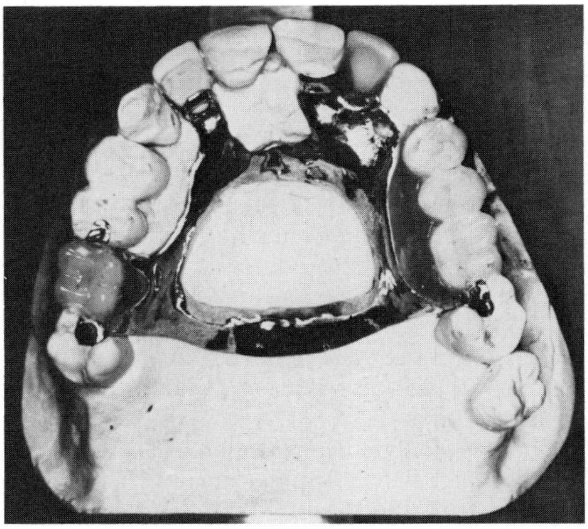

Figure 17–9 ■ Placing the prosthetic teeth to fill existing space may satisfy esthetics but may not satisfy the occusal requirements.

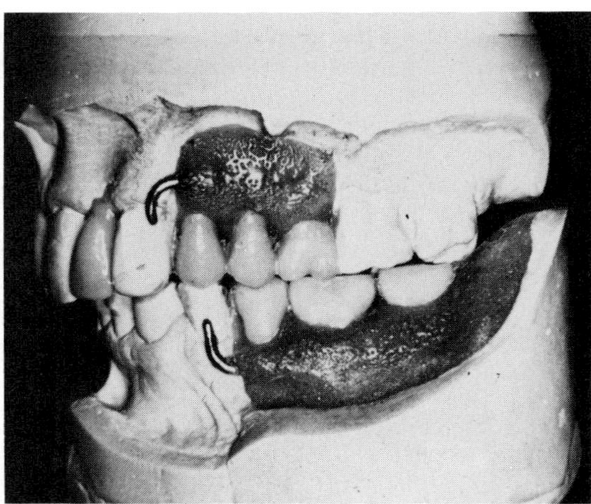

Figure 17–10 ■ Prosthetic teeth placed simply to fill the space can jeopardize the occlusion for proper intercuspation and result in interference in excursions with a cusp-tip-to-cusp-tip contact.

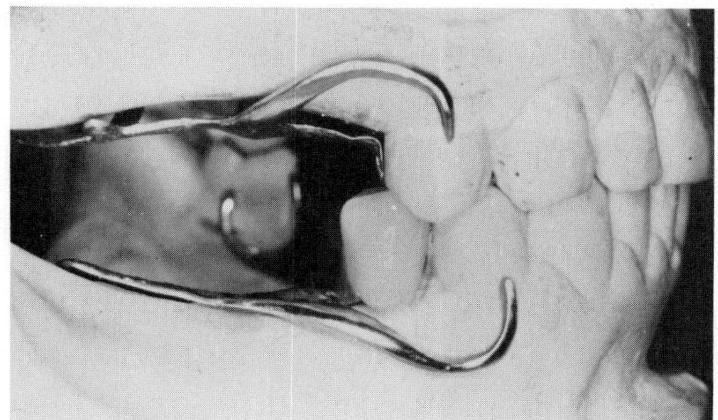

Figure 17-11 ■ Locate the first prosthetic tooth in an ideal position opposite remaining natural teeth in centric and eccentric positions. This may require altering *all* parts of the prosthetic tooth.

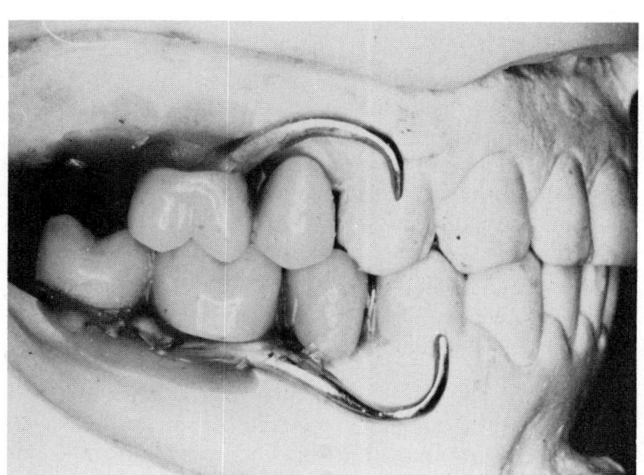

Figure 17-12 ■ If the occlusion is started properly, the remaining prosthetic teeth can be organized into their ideal positions.

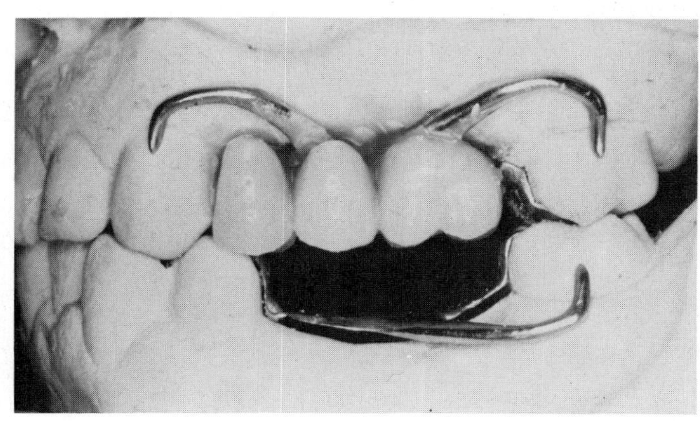

Figure 17-13 ■ Establish the ideal occlusal plane in one arch and fix it in position with a small amount of sticky wax on the tooth and the prosthesis. This insures good attachment with minimal tooth movement.

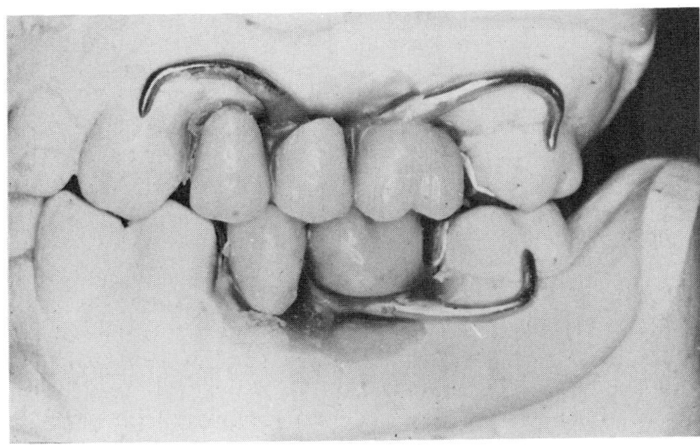

Figure 17–14 ■ The opposing prosthetic teeth are positioned and adjusted for centric and eccentric movements.

in centric relation and for 2 to 3 mm in excursions. When anterior guidance of natural teeth is present, it is advantageous to have the posterior occlusion *disengage* after 2 or 3 mm of eccentric movement (Fig. 17–17).

This type of occlusion (lingualized occlusion) is designed to have only the *lingual cusp* of the *maxillary* tooth in function against the mandibular denture tooth. This design minimizes the size of opposing occlusal surfaces during mastication, reduces and simplifies development and adjustment of occlusion, but still provides the necessary jaw support and mastication requirements. The occlusal width of the mandibular denture tooth is lessened considerably to reduce the surface area, and the central fossa is recontoured into a shallow curve that provides occlusal contact in and around centric relation.

When discrepancies of opposing arches place the residual mandibular ridge opposite the central fossa of the maxillary natural tooth (Fig. 17–18), the same principles of occlusion described above are achieved through recontouring the mandibular denture tooth by removing the lingual cusp and contouring and adjusting the buccal cusp into the central fossa of the natural tooth (Fig. 17–19).

Adjustment of the Occlusal Surface of Prosthetic Teeth

Mixed occlusions requiring coordination of prosthetic teeth to natural teeth rarely have ideal positions and occlusal surfaces. Natural tooth surfaces require recontouring to obtain needed cusps and fossae, to correct positions,

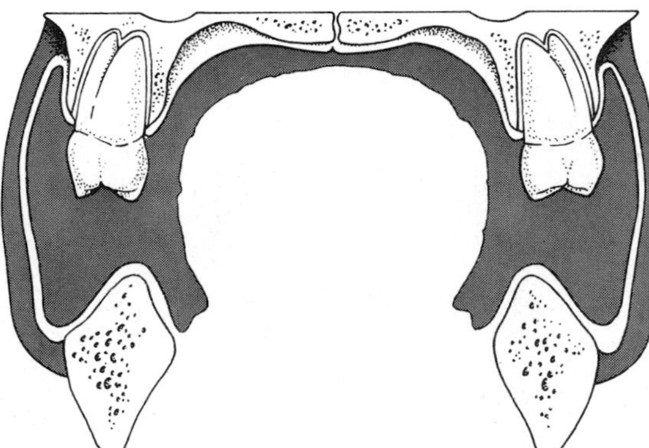

Figure 17–15 ■ The lingual cusp of remaining natural teeth is often positioned directly over the opposing edentulous ridge, which is weaker from a support standpoint.

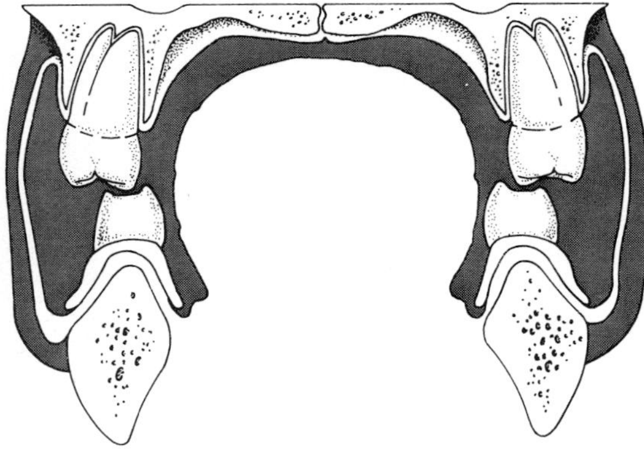

Figure 17–16 ■ The mandibular prosthetic tooth is modified to reduce occlusal size, and the centric contact area is a flat surface. This occlusal scheme is called *lingualized occlusion.*

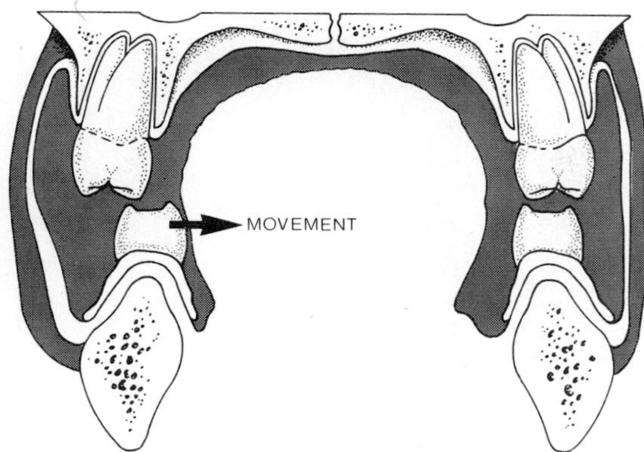

Figure 17–17 ■ When natural anterior tooth guidance is present, it is desirable to have the posterior extension occlusion disengage after 2 or 3 mm of eccentric jaw movement.

and to improve the occlusal plane. The prosthetic tooth is positioned and *adjusted* (Fig. 17–20) to provide the proper occlusal scheme.

Posterior teeth provide the majority of vertical dimension control and require a material that is resistant to wear or abrasion and compatible with natural tooth structure or other materials used on the opposing occlusion of remaining teeth and prosthesis. Materials that provide most of these requirements are quality porcelain and metals. The metals commonly used are gold (Fig. 17–21) and chrome, and when porcelain is used, it is highly polished or glazed and not occluded against gold restorations. Plastic denture teeth are used for posterior occlusion where there is a space problem that requires extensive prosthetic tooth modification or where it opposes a gold restoration. When the plastic posterior tooth is used, an amalgam restoration is placed on the occlusal surface in and around the centric relation area that will be contacted, for control of vertical dimension and to provide mastication surfaces more resistant to wear (Fig. 17–22).

A MAXILLARY COMPLETE DENTURE OPPOSING A MANDIBULAR RPD

When a maxillary complete denture opposes a mandibular removable partial denture, a com-

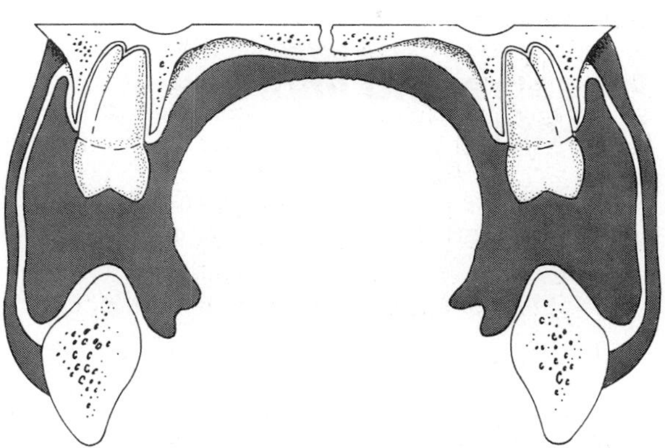

Figure 17–18 ■ In some situations, the edentulous ridge is opposite the central fossa of opposing natural teeth.

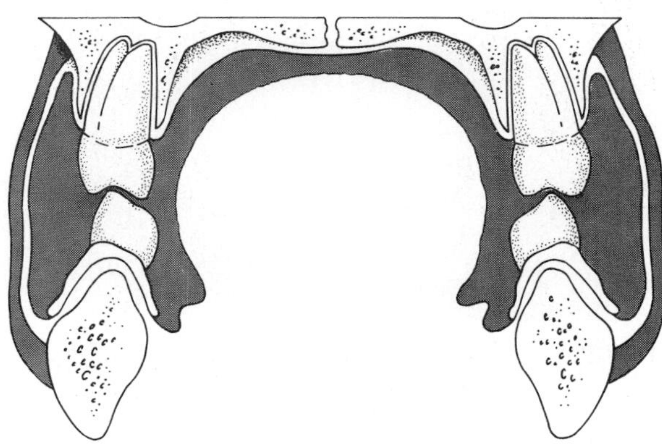

Figure 17–19 ■ The lingual cusp of the mandibular prosthetic tooth is modified to minimize the contact area and still provide sufficient support and function.

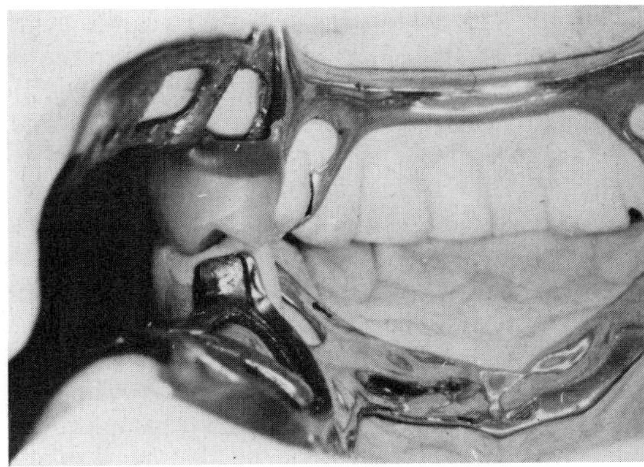

Figure 17–20 ■ Occlusion of remaining natural teeth and metal RPD casting is equilibrated *first*. The prosthetic tooth is then positioned in hyperocclusion and adjusted for ideal contact against the natural tooth and made compatible with all other occlusal contacts.

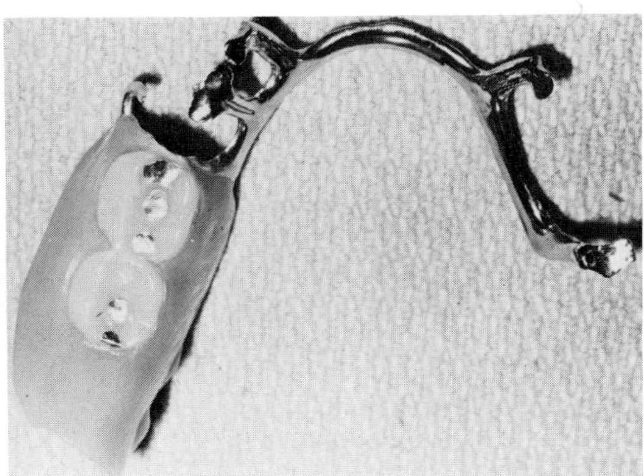

Figure 17–22 ■ Plastic teeth may be necessary for space or esthetic reasons. When they are used, the centric contacts should be protected with casting or silver restorations to reduce the wear factor.

pletely different situation regarding the occlusal scheme exists. It is necessary to provide contacts in *both* centric and excursive movements. The occlusion and posterior balance contacts are developed to provide even occlusal contacts in all excursions.

Preserve and Improve Esthetics

Appearance in removable partial denture treatment is often complicated by difficulty of harmonizing prosthetic replacements with remaining natural teeth (Fig. 17–23). The remaining teeth often present a variety of sizes, colors, and shapes within the same arch. Producing a compatible replacement often requires reshaping, contouring, and characterizing the prosthetic replacement to produce a blending with existing natural features that cannot be altered, owing to a variety of patient or professional reasons.

For anterior teeth, the replacement plastic tooth is the optimal choice. The plastic tooth can be readily altered, contoured, and added to for harmony and blending with remaining structures (Fig. 17–24). The plastic tooth can be individually characterized with colors, stains, and restorations before completion of the pros-

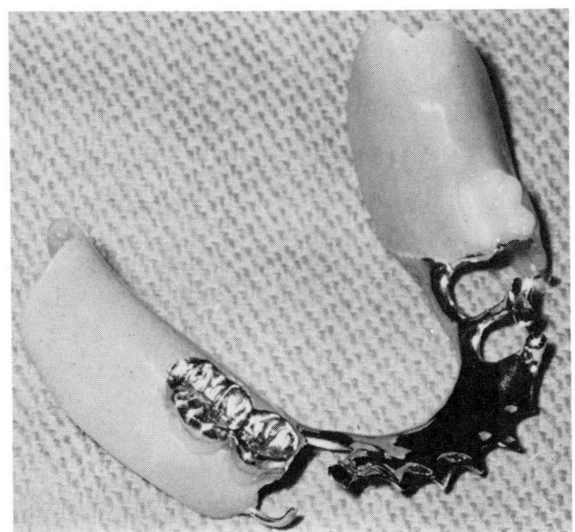

Figure 17–21 ■ For compatibility of wear, metal or porcelain surfaces may be required. Compatible, stable, opposing occlusal surfaces are necessary to maintain the vertical dimension and to control wear.

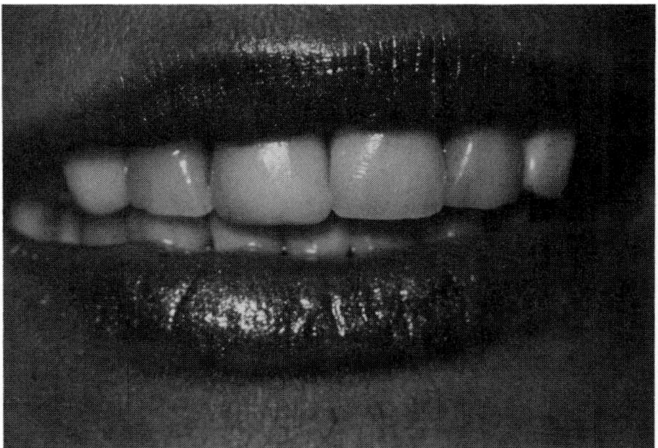

Figure 17–23 ■ Harmonizing the shade and shape of prosthetic teeth with remaining natural teeth can be quite difficult because of variations in the teeth to either side, the metal casting support, and the width of the available space. (See also Color Plate 4, p XX.)

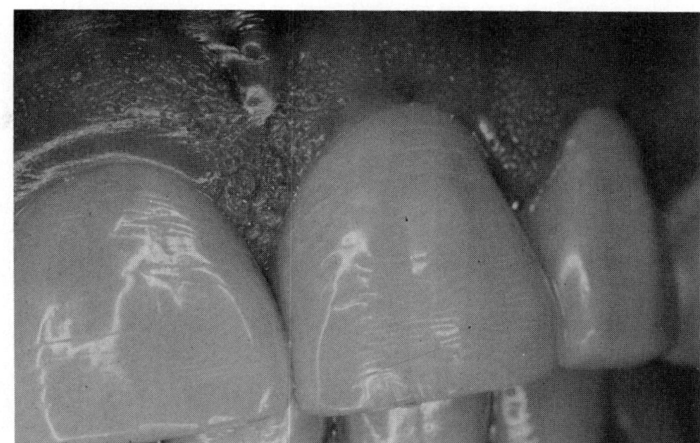

Figure 17–24 ■ Plastic anterior teeth are easy to contour and adjust, are not as abrasive to opposing occlusion, and can be modified easily for shade, hue, and individual character, as shown on the left central incisor. (See also Color Plate 4, p XX.)

thesis and after completion if necessary (Fig. 17–25). Anterior function and guidance can be incorporated in the partial denture casting and remaining natural teeth to minimize the wear factor on the plastic tooth.

Posterior plastic teeth are often used in premolar positions for esthetic reasons. When they are used, it is essential that a metal occlusal surface be provided to reduce wear and to help preserve the vertical dimension of occlusion (Fig. 17–26).

Portions of the *metal casting* of the partial denture that are in the area of tooth replacement are evaluated for appearance. Guiding surfaces and the denture base retention area may need to be recontoured and reshaped to reduce their size if they are visible or if they affect the color of the denture teeth.

At the try-in appointment for evaluation of appearance and esthetics, the final contour, size, and shape of the finished denture base must be reproduced in wax for patient and doctor consideration. Necessary changes such as repositioning of teeth and contouring of the denture base continue to be made until there is mutual agreement between doctor and patient that the appearance is acceptable (Fig. 17–27).

Contour and color of the denture base are quite critical in removable partial denture treatment when the mucosa is visible (Fig. 17–28). Contours and colors that are not compatible with existing structures are quite obvious, and a blending of topography and color is necessary. Color guides for denture bases are used to select a suitable color.

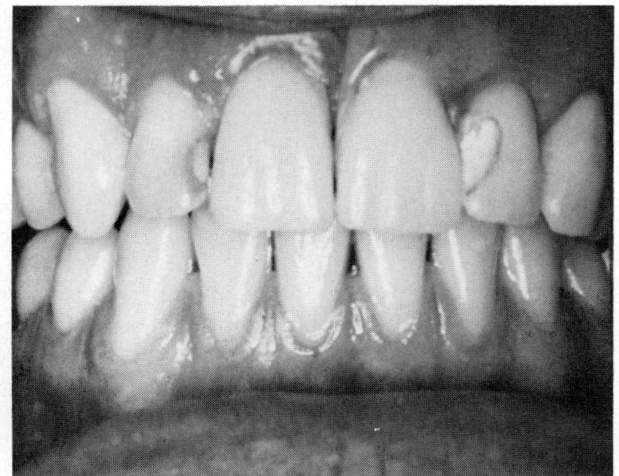

Figure 17–25 ■ After fabrication and insertion, the plastic tooth can be modified and changed if necessary. (See also Color Plate 4, p XX.)

Abnormal Arch Positions

Occasionally, unusual occlusal conditions are present for which orthodontic or surgical treatment is not possible. However, if the occlusal situation is not controlled, there can be extensive destruction of existing structures; an example is the teeth of the mandibular arch being positioned completely lingual to the teeth of the maxillary arch (Fig. 17–29). Continued occlusal activity in this relationship forces the teeth lingually and facially with resultant periodontal difficulties and diminished function. The *objectives of treatment* are

1. *Control of tooth positions.*
2. *Stabilization of the arches.*
3. *Provision of occlusal support* at the proper vertical dimension of occlusion.
4. Provision of mastication surfaces.

The metal casting of the maxillary removable partial denture is designed with fossae on the

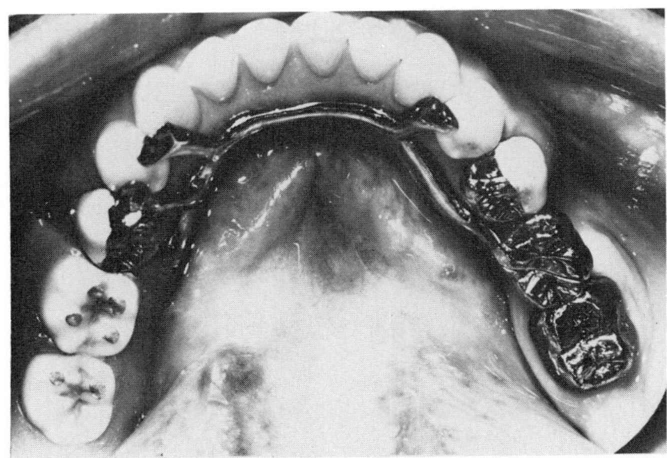

Figure 17–26 ■ Amalgam restorations can be used on posterior plastic teeth to replace or preserve occlusal contacts.

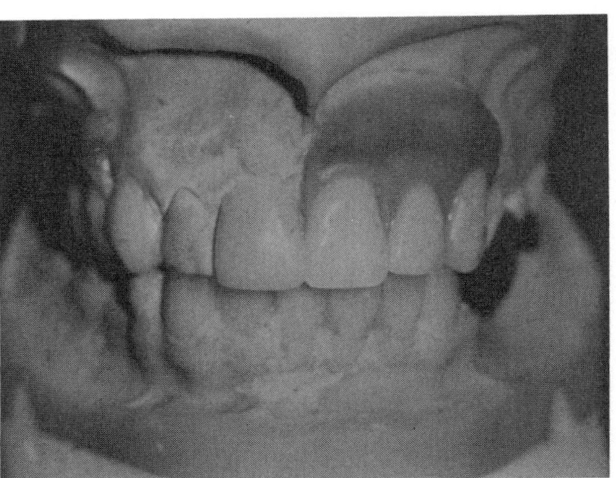

Figure 17–27 ■ The shape and contour of the denture base had a great influence on mold and appearance of teeth and on lip contour. The wax denture base contours are completely formed and shaped at the try-in stage. (See also Color Plate 4, p XX.)

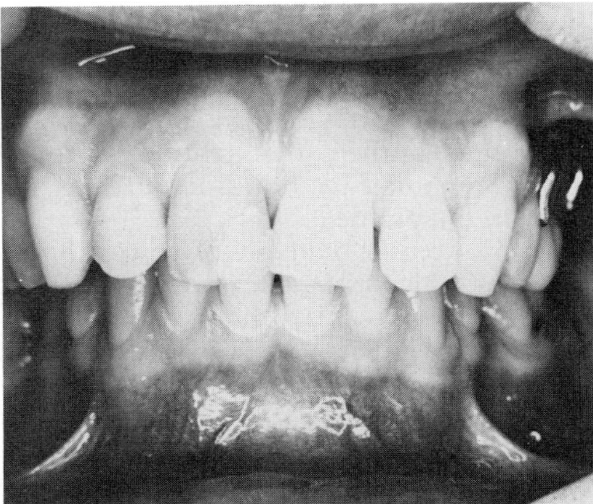

Figure 17–29 ■ Mandibular teeth in complete lingual relationship to the opposing maxillary teeth. When orthodontic treatment is not possible, a removable partial prosthesis can provide arch and occlusion control.

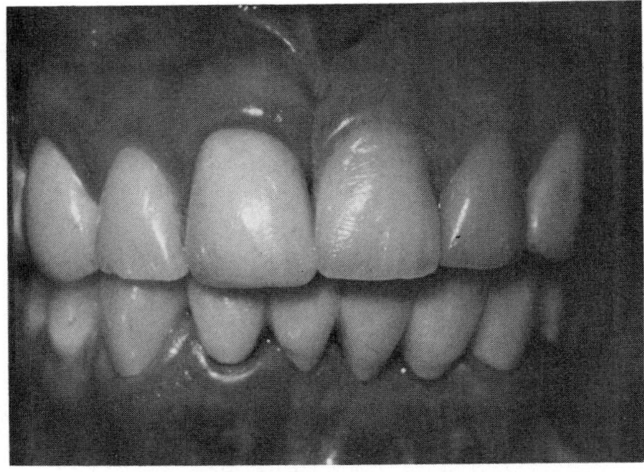

Figure 17–28 ■ The junction of the denture base and mucosa is a smooth, compatible continuation of the existing natural contours. (See also Color Plate 4, p XX.)

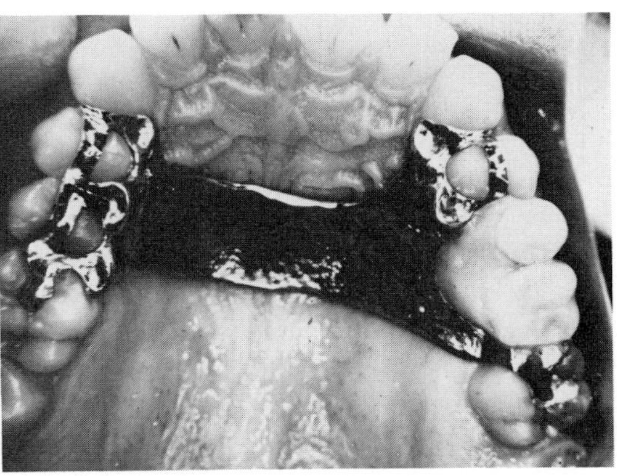

Figure 17–30 ■ A modified lingual design provides positive centric occlusion for the buccal cusps of the opposing teeth and prevents further lateral tooth movement.

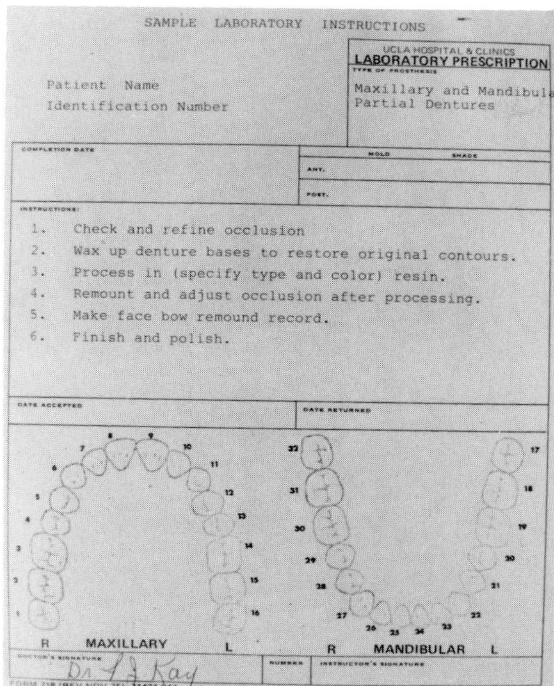

SAMPLE LABORATORY INSTRUCTIONS

UCLA HOSPITAL & CLINICS
LABORATORY PRESCRIPTION

TYPE OF PROSTHESIS

Patient Name
Identification Number

Maxillary and Mandibular Partial Dentures

COMPLETION DATE

MOLD | SHADE

ANT.

POST.

INSTRUCTIONS:

1. Check and refine occlusion
2. Wax up denture bases to restore original contours.
3. Process in (specify type and color) resin.
4. Remount and adjust occlusion after processing.
5. Make face bow remound record.
6. Finish and polish.

DATE ACCEPTED

DATE RETURNED

R MAXILLARY L

R MANDIBULAR L

DOCTOR'S SIGNATURE

NUMBER

INSTRUCTOR'S SIGNATURE

Figure 17–31 ■ Laboratory instructions are complete and include all necessary information.

lingual side of the teeth (Fig. 17–30) to provide the occlusal contacts for the facial cusps of the mandibular teeth; this controls the vertical relationship and restores some mastication function. Placing continuous rests in the central fossae of the maxillary teeth ensures unity and stabilization of the arch and directs the forces in the long axis of the teeth. While the treatment is not ideal, it will help fulfill the concept of saving the remaining structures.

Laboratory Instruction

Upon completion of the occlusal development and the esthetic procedures, the prosthesis is returned to the laboratory for processing in the finished form.

Complete and detailed instructions are required for the technician to understand and fulfill the desires of the doctor and the patient (Fig. 17–31). These instructions include

1. The necessary refinements of occlusion—centric and eccentric.
2. Orders for tooth modifications, changes, staining, or restorations.
3. Specific details of denture base contour and color.
4. Orders for postprocessing occlusal adjustments.
5. The date for completion.
6. A copy of articulator information (face bow record—articulator setting).

REFERENCES

Occlusion

Cohn R: The relationship of anterior guidance to condylar guidance in mandibular movement. J Prosthet Dent 6:758–767, 1956.

Colman AJ: Occlusal requirements for removable partial dentures. J Prosthet Dent 17:155–162, 1967.

Craddock FW: The accuracy and practical value of records of condyle path inclination. J Am Dent Assoc 38:697–710, 1949.

Henderson D: Occlusion in removable partial prosthesis. J Prosthet Dent 27:151–159, 1971.

Jeffreys FE and Platner RL: Occlusion in removable partial dentures. J Prosthet Dent 10:912–920, 1960.

McCracken WL: Occlusion in partial denture prosthesis. Dent Clin North Am March:109–119, 1962.

Reitz PV: Technique for mounting removable partial dentures on an articulator. J Prosthet Dent 22:490–494, 1969.

Wallace DH: The use of gold occlusal surfaces in complete and partial dentures. J Prosthet Dent 14:326–333, 1964.

Esthetics

DeVan MM: The appearance phase of denture construction. Dent Clin North Am March:255–268, 1957.

Frush JP and Fisher RD: Introduction to dentogenic restorations. J Prosthet Dent 5:586–595, 1955.

Tilman EJ: Molding and staining acrylic resin anterior teeth. J Prosthet Dent 5:497–507, 1955.

Wolfson E: Staining and characterization of acrylic teeth. Dent Abstr 1:41, 1958.

chapter 18

Insertion principles and procedures

The objectives at insertion are

Intraarch control: the best possible adaptation of the finished prosthesis to the remaining teeth and soft tissues to restore the arch.

Interarch control: (1) final maxillomandibular registrations, and (2) refinement of occlusion.

Patient instructions (see Chapter 19).

Intraarch Control

The objective of this procedure is to obtain the ultimate prosthesis adaptation and support from the remaining teeth and mucosa. There should be maximum compatibility of the casting and the tissue surface of the denture base. The impression and fabrication procedures are subject to technical and procedural errors during fabrication. These errors could be in impressions, registrations, casts, or processing. There is also the possibility of tissue changes since the impressions were made. With the finished prosthesis, these factors can be identified and corrected to provide the best possible adaptation and support at completion.

TISSUE SURFACE REFINEMENT

1. A complete visual and digital examination is made of the finished prosthesis (Fig. 18–1) for spicules, rough or sharp areas, or processing irregularities (Fig. 18–2). The patient is informed of the insertion steps.

2. Pressure indicator paste (Fig. 18–3) (PIP) is placed in liberal amounts on the tissue surface and spread with a stiff bristle brush to form deep grooves in the paste (Fig. 18–4).

3. The prosthesis is placed in the mouth (Fig. 18–5) and removed and examined for pressure areas where the paste is displaced (Fig. 18–6) or for lack of adaptation demonstrated by little or no compression of the PIP ridges.

4. The pressure areas are relieved with an acrylic bur, and the PIP process is repeated until there is even flattening of the PIP ridges (Fig. 18–7).

PERIPHERY REFINEMENT

1. Disclosing wax is placed on the peripheral surface of the denture base to identify overextension of the denture base onto the tissues of the mouth, when in function (Fig. 18–8).

2. A roll of the wax (which is more resistant to pressure than PIP) is evenly adapted to both inner and outer periphery surfaces (Fig. 18–9).

3. The prosthesis is placed in the patient's mouth, held firmly in place on the teeth, and the patient is instructed to move the jaw, cheeks, and tongue through the normal movements.

4. The prosthesis is removed and pressure areas, located where the denture shows through the wax, are relieved (Figs. 18–10 through 18–12).

5. The disclosing wax process is repeated

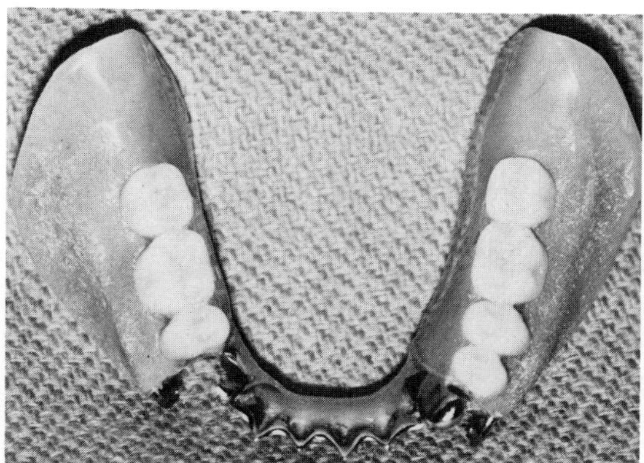

Figure 18–1 ■ The finished prosthesis is inspected for contour, completeness, and smoothness.

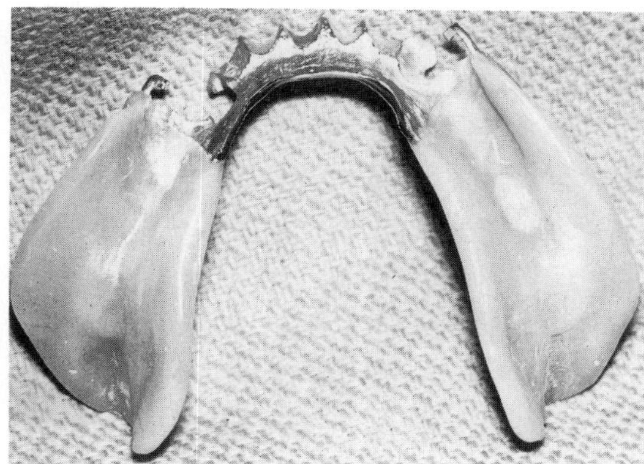

Figure 18–2 ■ The tissue surface is checked for sharp and rough areas, especially at the plastic-metal junctions.

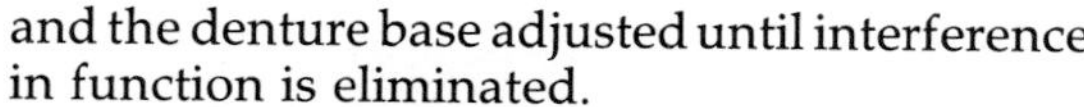

and the denture base adjusted until interference in function is eliminated.

The prosthesis has now been adapted and fitted as closely as possible to the structures of the arch for maximum support (Fig. 18–5).

Interarch Control

A careful assessment of clinical and laboratory procedures reveals the potential for errors derived from the following:

1. Tissues not completely recovered from irritation or displacement.
2. Errors in the surface of the impression.
3. Changes or damage to the cast.
4. Record bases that were not adapted to the tissues properly.
5. Dimensional changes of waxes and registration materials.
6. Errors in the patient's jaw position and records.
7. Changes in the patient's temporomandibular joint (TMJ) tissues.
8. Articulator mounting errors.
9. Investing, packing, processing, and dimensional errors.

This potential for error during fabrication of the prosthesis requires that all steps be accepted as *tentative* until the finished prosthesis is available for the final and most accurate checks. This in no way suggests that all procedures up to the insertion steps should be less than as ideal as possible, but there should be a series of ongoing checks, evaluations, and corrections of previous procedures to reduce the potential for error in the finished prosthesis.

Interarch control is determined by the occlusal surface contacts between the maxillary and mandibular arches. Adjustment and refine-

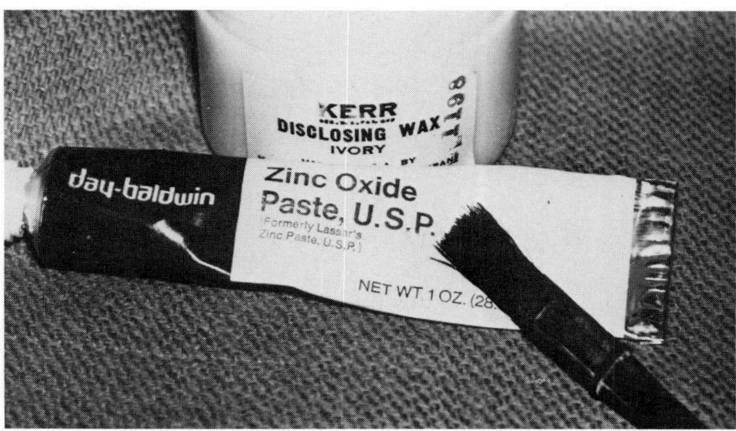

Figure 18–3 ■ Pressure indicator paste is used to evaluate the adaptation of the plastic denture base to the mucosa.

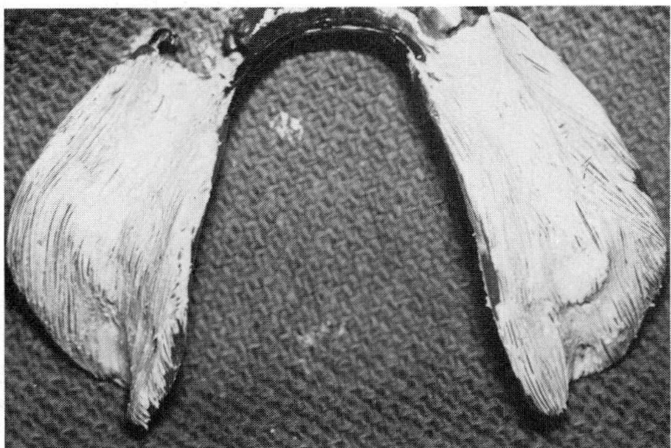

Figure 18–4 ■ A sharp bristle brush is used to liberally apply the PIP and produces deep, definite grooves in the paste.

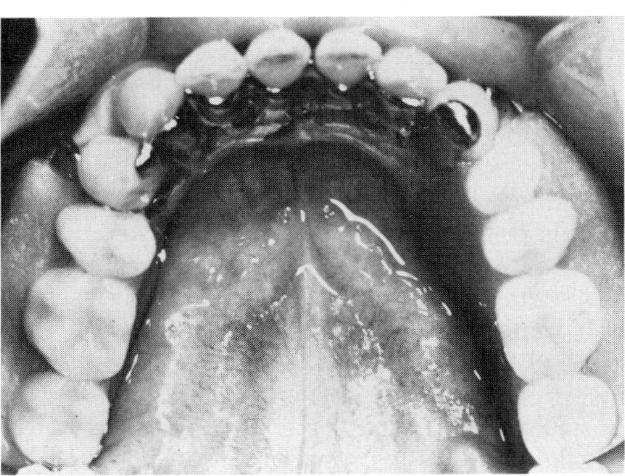

Figure 18–5 ■ The prosthesis is placed in the mouth and seated with gentle finger pressure.

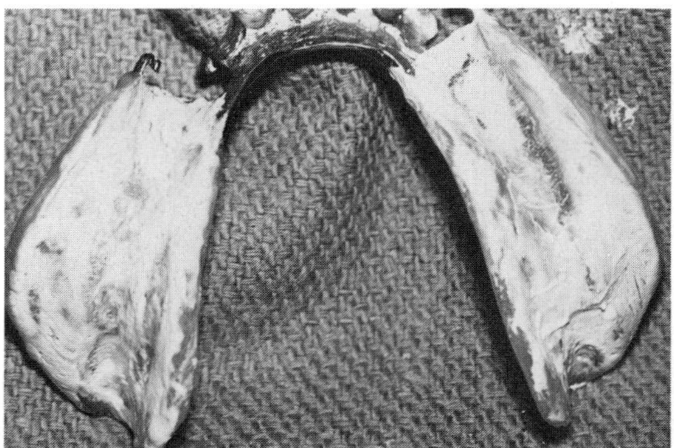

Figure 18–6 ■ Inspection of the tissue surface reveals areas of excessive contact where the paste is removed and areas of no contact where the brush marks are undisturbed.

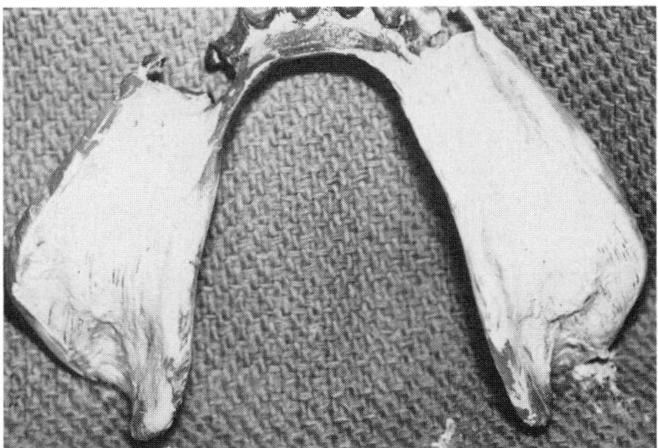

Figure 18–7 ■ Areas of pressure are relieved with a plastic bur until the PIP try-in demonstrates even contact in all areas.

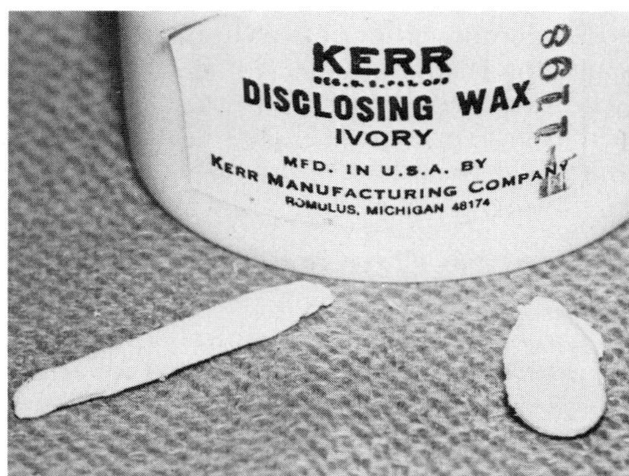

Figure 18–8 ■ The extension and contours of the peripheries are evaluated by using disclosing wax formed in a roll or applied by syringe.

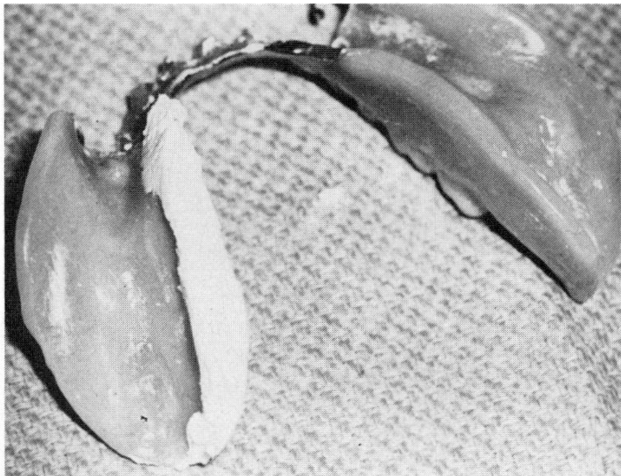

Figure 18–9 ■ The disclosing wax is placed on the inner and outer surfaces of the denture base, which is then placed in the patient's mouth, with instructions given to move the tongue and the cheeks in normal action.

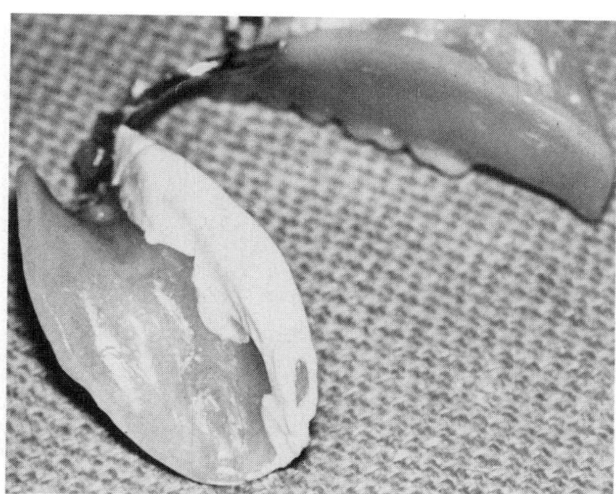

Figure 18–10 ■ The areas of interference with muscle activity show through the wax. These areas are reduced.

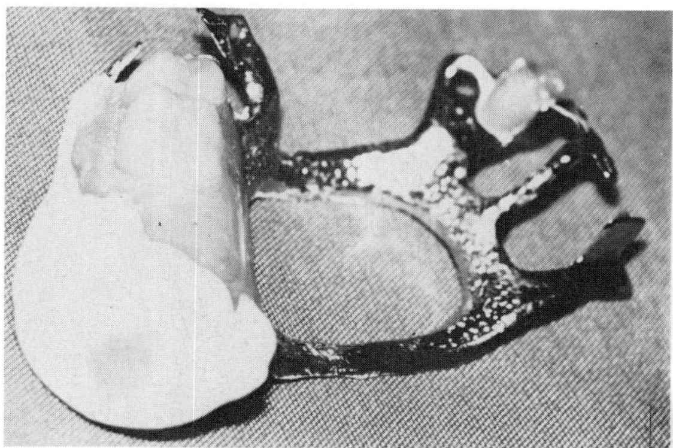

Figure 18–12 ■ When evaluating a maxillary prosthesis, wax is placed over the tuberosity area to identify contact with the ramus of the jaw in lateral movement.

ment of these surfaces must be coordinated and compatible with the anatomy and jaw motions of each individual patient *at the time of insertion* of the prosthesis.

The most positive and precise method of refining interarch occlusion is to transfer a record of the occlusal surfaces of each arch to a laboratory situation, where the final adjustments can be accomplished (Fig. 18–13). In the partially edentulous mouth, this procedure requires transfer to the articulator of the finished prosthesis and a replica of the occlusal surfaces of remaining natural teeth. These teeth must retain their position in relation to the prosthesis, as established at the fitting of the finished denture to the individual arch.

The production of individual arch occlusion and the relationship of remaining natural teeth to the prosthesis are accomplished as follows:

1. The fitted prosthesis is placed in the patient's mouth.
2. An alginate impression (occlusal surfaces *only*) is made of the prosthesis and of the remaining teeth (Fig. 18–14).
3. The impression is removed with the prosthesis in place.
4. Low fusing metal (Fig. 18–15) is poured into the alginate impression to reproduce the natural teeth (Fig. 18–16). (Note: *Only occlusal surfaces are reproduced.*)
5. The prosthesis and the metal occlusal surfaces are removed from the impression (Fig. 18–17).

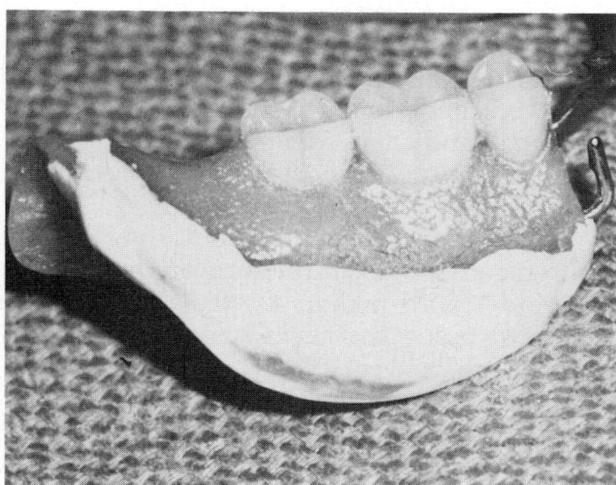

Figure 18–11 ■ In some muscle activities, the interference is in the width of the denture base and not in the length.

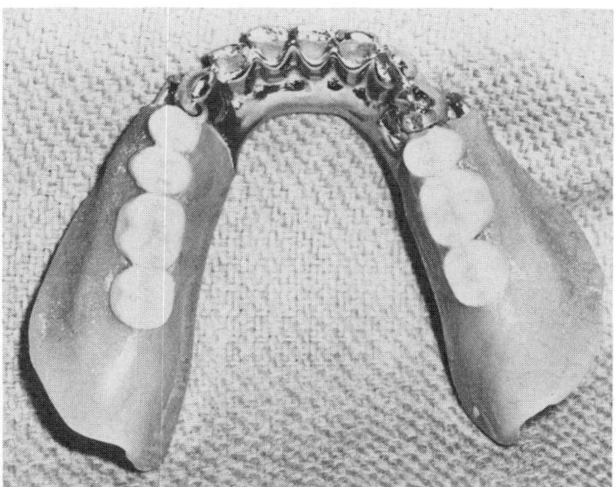

Figure 18–13 ■ For final occlusal equilibration on the articulator, the natural teeth are reproduced in low fusing metal and placed in position in the prosthesis; this will duplicate all occlusal surfaces as they present in the mouth.

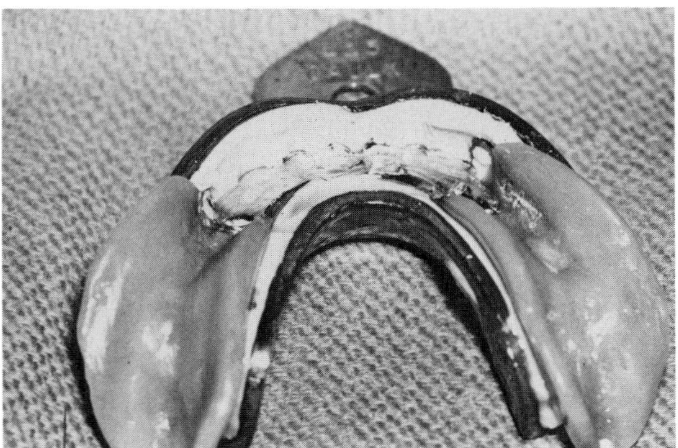

Figure 18–14 ■ To produce the metal replica of the natural teeth, an impression is made with the prosthesis in place in the mouth and removed with the prosthesis embedded in the impression.

This procedure reproduces the occlusal surfaces of the entire arch, including the prosthesis itself, with the natural teeth in metal. This is a quick, effective, and durable reproduction of the relationship developed at the fitting of the prosthesis.

The low-fusing metal is melted *only* to the flowing point and *not* overheated, which would increase the dimensional change. All water and moisture are removed from the alginate impression before pouring. Only occlusal surfaces of the teeth are poured in metal. Do not pour excessive material into retainer undercuts or other casting or denture undercuts.

When the metal has solidified, cool it under water, remove it from the partial denture and set it aside for later mounting.

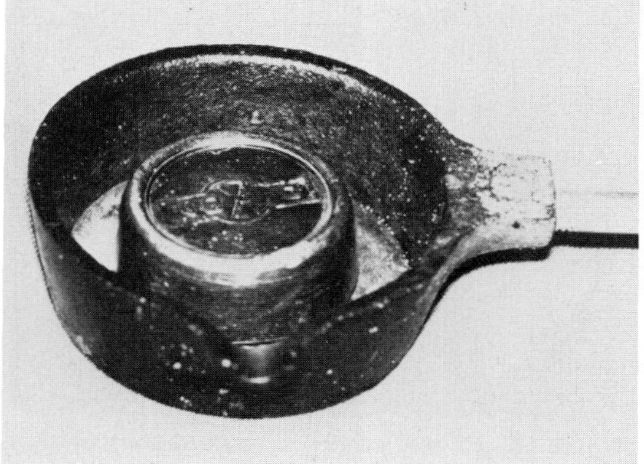

Figure 18–15 ■ The low-fusing metal is melted in a ladle until it just reaches pouring viscosity in order to minimize distortion.

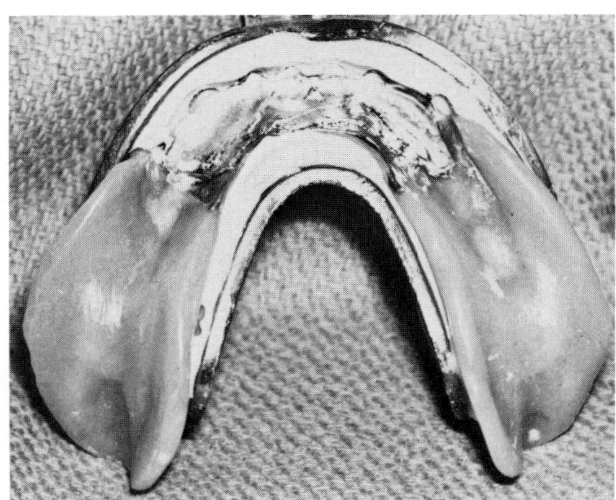

Figure 18–16 ■ Only the occlusal surfaces of the teeth are poured; *do not* pour metal into the retainer or other undercuts.

FACE BOW RECORD

A face bow record may be requested and produced by the laboratory at the time of the processing procedure. If the laboratory face bow index is not available, a face bow measurement is recorded on the patient *with the prosthesis in place.* The reproduction in metal of the natural teeth is placed in the prosthesis and secured with sticky wax. The maxillary prosthesis and metal teeth are mounted on the articulator using the face bow registration. The plaster mounting involves *only* the peripheries of the prosthesis and the base surface of the metal teeth, which can be easily removed and then returned to an exact-keyed position.

CENTRIC RECORD

The final maxillomandibular registrations are now recorded, transferred to the articulator, mounted, and checked with a second set of interarch records for accuracy of transfer in mounting on the articulator.

1. The patient must *not* touch the denture teeth together or exert pressure on the dentures prior to record-taking. Occlusal inaccuracies can cause tissue displacement or change patient jaw closure pattern.
2. The prosthesis with complete palatal coverage and with a posterior palatal seal requires closure on cotton rolls for 5 minutes in order to properly seat the post-dam.
3. A centric relation record is made with the material of choice (Fig. 18–18).

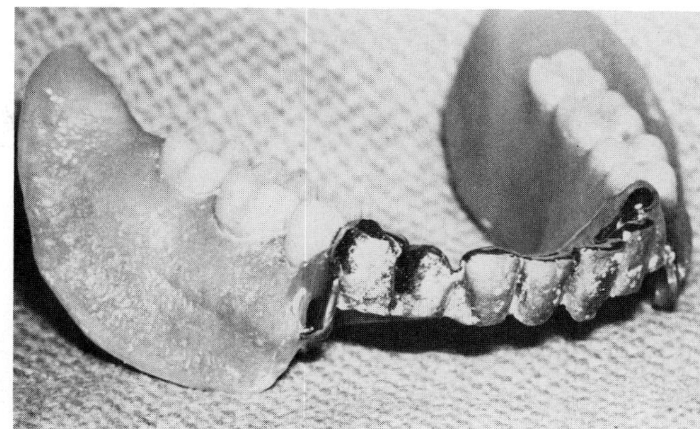

Figure 18–17 ■ The occlusal reproduction is identical to the occlusion in the mouth. The metal occlusal surfaces are removed from the prosthesis to ensure ease of separation.

4. The metal teeth are placed in the prosthesis and secured with sticky wax (Fig. 18–19).
5. The mandibular arch is positioned against the maxillary arch, using the interocclusal record, and secured together and mounted on the articulator (Figs. 18–20 through 18–22).
6. The centric relation record is taken again in the patient's mouth (Fig. 18–23) and placed on the mounted casts, and the accuracy of the first articulator mounting is confirmed (Fig. 18–24). If the two centric mountings do not coincide, the mounting procedure is repeated until two compatible records are obtained.

Materials used for interocclusal records are modeling composition, plaster, acrylic, elastic impression materials, registration paste, and wax. A registration material that sets to a hard, unchanging form is the most accurate. The material should have minimal resistance to closure of the jaws and have a reasonably quick setting time.

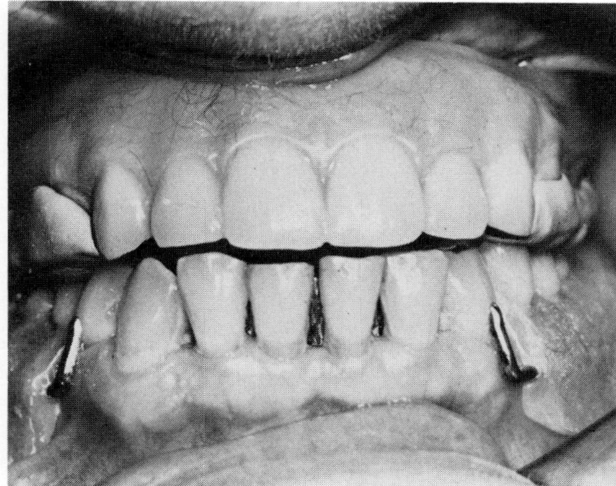

Figure 18–18 ■ A centric relation record is made in the patient's mouth with low heat modeling composition uniformly softened in a water bath at 140° F.

One of the most ideal materials is a low-fusing modeling composition (Fig. 18–25). The material can be quickly softened in a water bath at 140°F and adapts securely to the prosthesis, which, with the composition attached, can be immersed in a water bath for uniform softening. This modeling composition sets quickly, is easily trimmed to shallow cusp indentations (Fig. 18–26), is unchanging when set, and can be quickly softened to retake a record.

PROTRUSIVE RECORD

A protrusive record is made in the patient's mouth with the jaw positioned a minimum of 6 mm forward. This interarch position is recorded with one of the occlusal record materials used for the centric relation record.

The condyle inclinations of the articulator are adjusted to coincide with the protrusive record (Fig. 18–27).

Protrusive recordings made with the finished prosthesis in the mouth are the most accurate and repeatable because of the stability of the dentures.

EQUILIBRATION AND OCCLUSAL REFINEMENT

The rationale for doing a patient articulator remount and equilibration is to obtain a definite, repeatable, proven relationship of the maxillary and mandibular arches prior to final adjustments of opposing occlusal surfaces. The occlusion developed at this time affects the freedom of mandibular movement and influ-

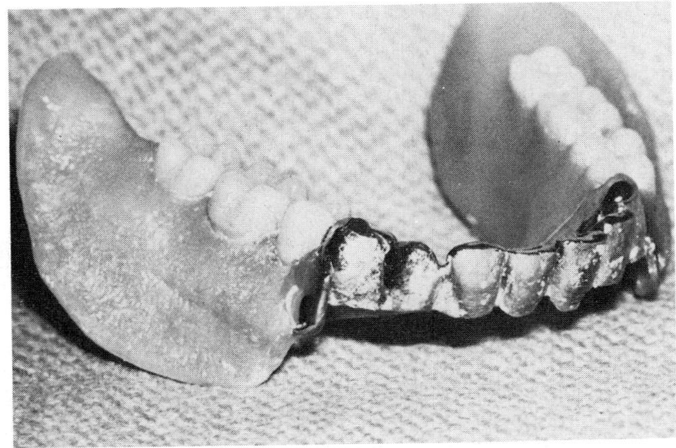

Figure 18–19 ■ The prosthesis is removed from the mouth; the metal teeth are positioned and fixed in place with sticky wax.

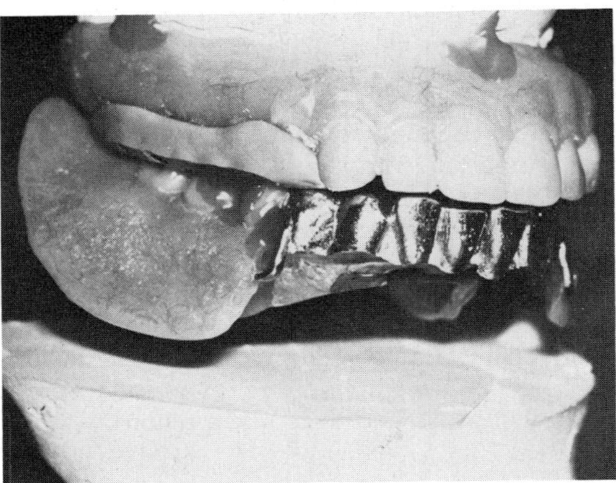

Figure 18–20 ■ The maxillary prosthesis is positioned on the articulator in the face bow record mounting cast, and the mandibular prosthesis with metal teeth in place is secured in the interocclusal record with sticky wax. (Note the mandibular plaster platform.)

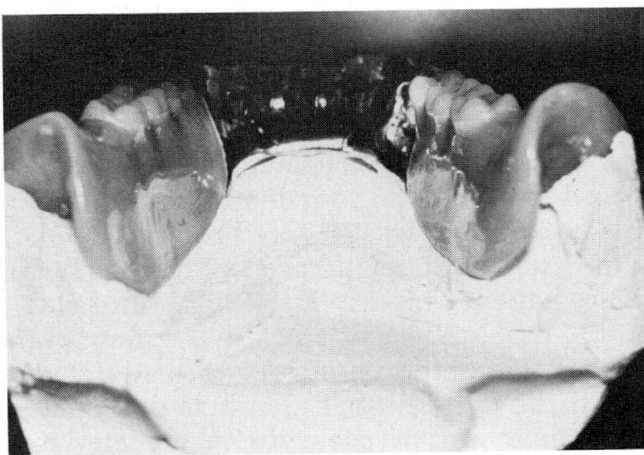

Figure 18–22 ■ The plaster mounting covers *only* the peripheral borders of the prosthesis and metal teeth. *Do not* extend it into the prosthesis undercuts; this would interfere with separation.

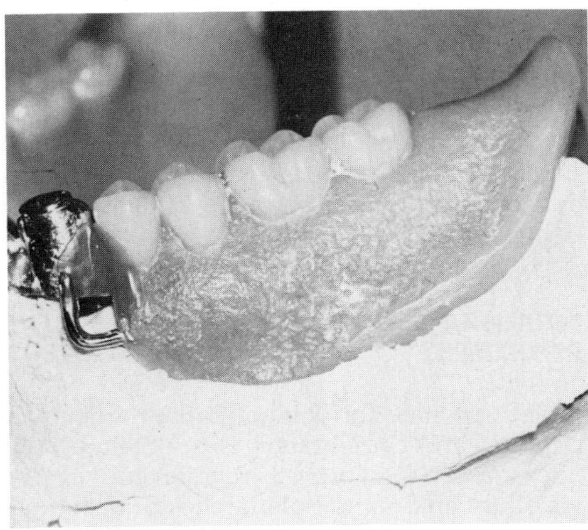

Figure 18–21 ■ The mandibular prosthesis and teeth are mounted onto the articulator with quick-setting plaster.

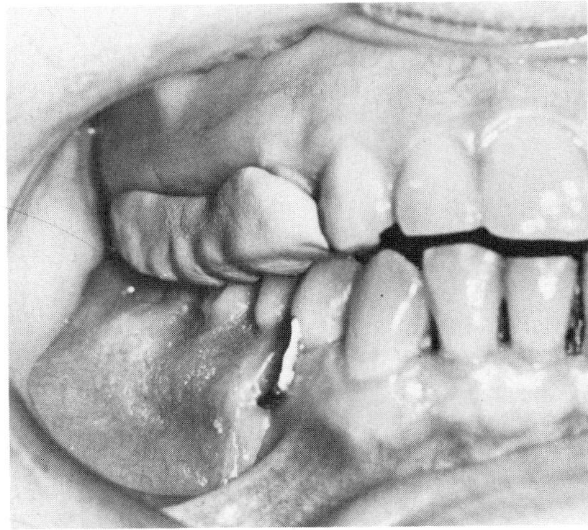

Figure 18–23 ■ A second centric relation record is made in the mouth to check the accuracy of the first record and of the articulator mounting. The same modeling composition is used by resoftening it in the water bath.

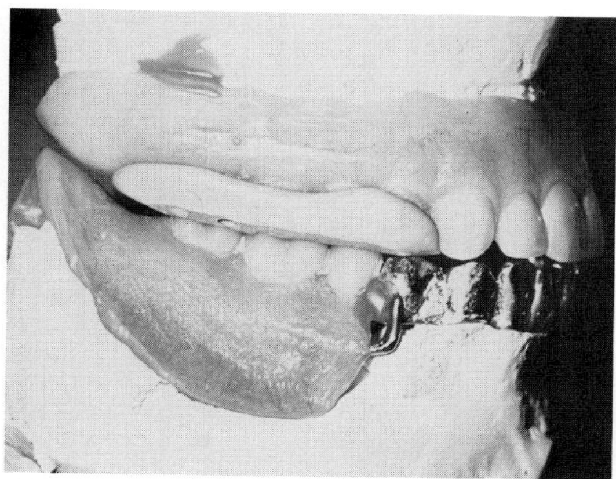

Figure 18–24 ■ The second record is tested on the articulator to see if the teeth fit in the occlusal record. If both records are identical, you are assured of an exact transfer from the patient's mouth to the articulator.

ences the forces delivered to teeth and support tissues. Adjustments on the articulator are easily observed, the movements are repeatable, and refinement can be precise and quick.

The Basic Rules of Equilibration

1. Adjust for *centric relation* first (Fig. 18–28). Place the maxillary lingual cusp in the mandibular fossa. Contour the fossa for positive centric stops.
2. Adjust the mandibular tooth surfaces for *eccentric movements* (Figs. 18–29 and 18–30).

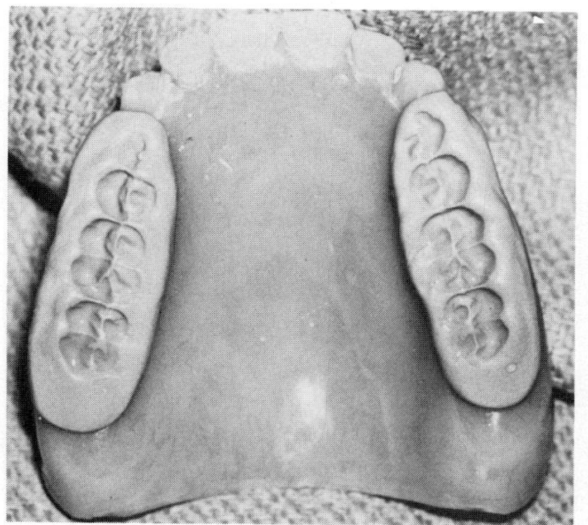

Figure 18–25 ■ Low-fusing modeling composition is a quick, accurate, reusable, and stable material for interocclusal records.

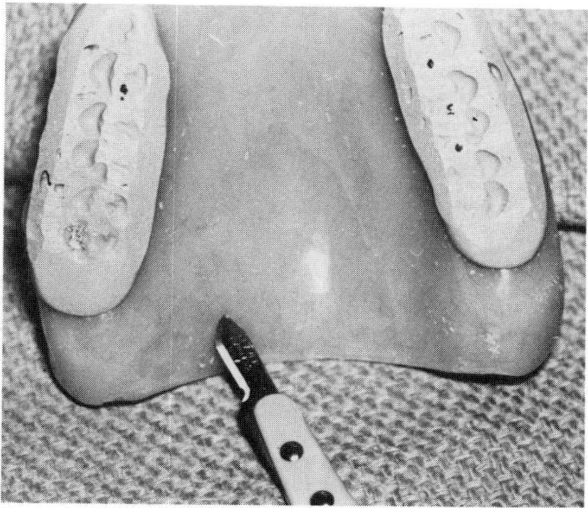

Figure 18–26 ■ When the registration is being tested for accuracy in the mouth or on the articulator, the indentations in the composition are reduced to shallow cusps with a sharp knife to ensure complete setting of the cusp tips.

Natural Teeth Opposing Denture Teeth

1. Make adjustments on denture teeth opposing the natural teeth.
2. When it is necessary to alter natural teeth, perform the alteration on the cast, mark the cast, and reproduce the alteration in the patient's mouth.

Finish and Polish

1. Check for smooth movement of opposing occlusal surfaces in all articulator positions. Eliminate rough or bumpy movements.

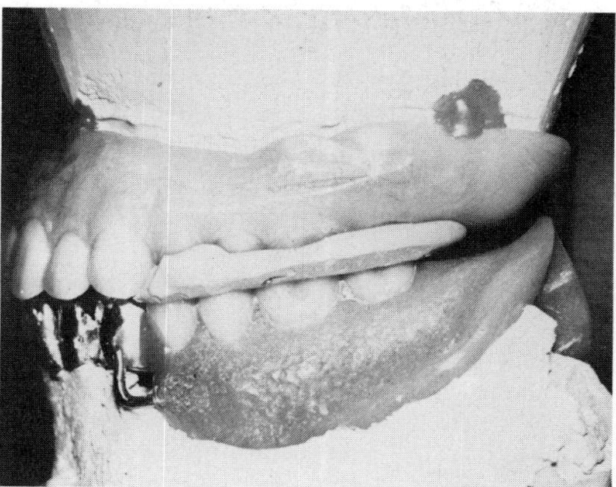

Figure 18–27 ■ A protrusive record is made in the mouth, and the articulator condyle settings are adjusted.

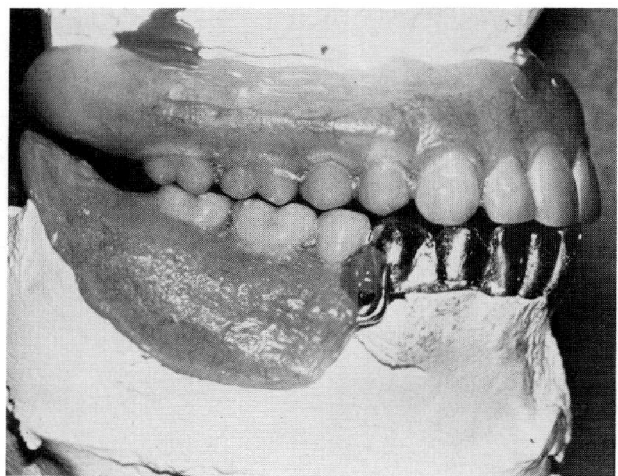

Figure 18–28 ■ Interferences in centric relation closure are removed.

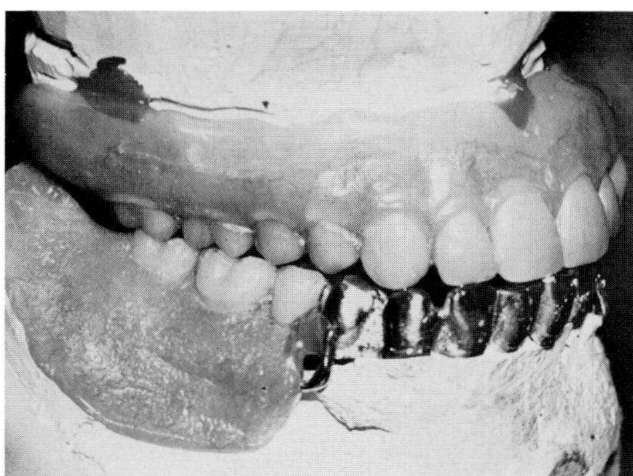

Figure 18–29 ■ Occlusion is harmonized in lateral excursions.

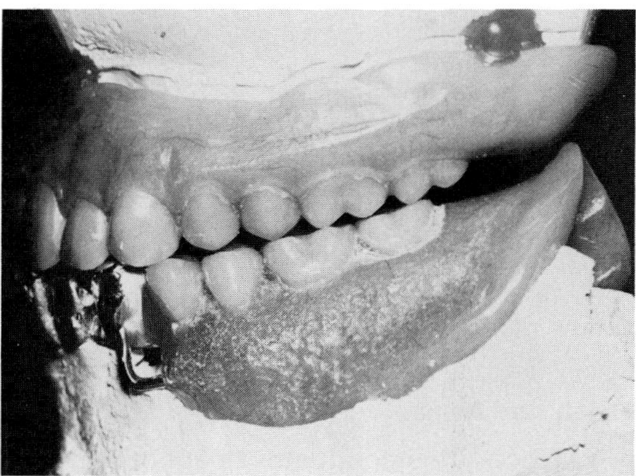

Figure 18–30 ■ Equalized occlusal contacts are provided in protrusive movements.

2. Inspect and smooth all surfaces; restore anatomy as much as possible.
3. Highly polish porcelain teeth.
4. Smooth and round all metal edges.
5. Highly polish peripheral edges that will contact tissues.

Intraoral Evaluation

The adjusted and polished prosthesis is placed in the patient's mouth and the following final checks are made:

1. A centric relation check for simultaneous, even contact of denture and natural teeth (Fig. 18–31).

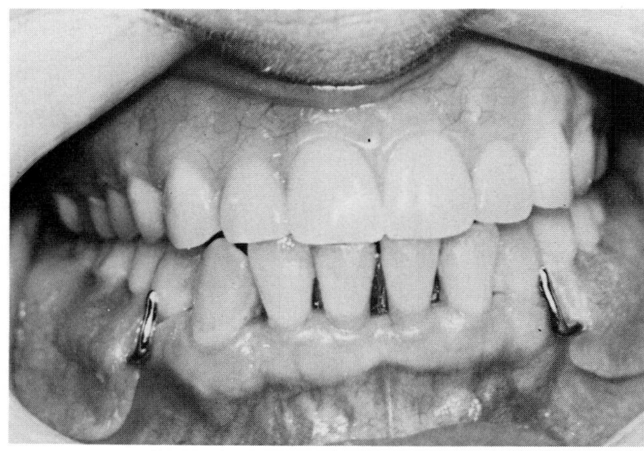

Figure 18–31 ■ The prosthesis is inserted in the mouth and intraoral examination is made for equalized contacts in all excursions.

2. Check for planned anterior guidance of natural teeth in excursions. Ensure that there is no interference of posterior teeth in lateral and protrusive movements.

3. Ask the patient if there is pressure discomfort or sharp areas.

REFERENCES

McCracken WL: Occlusion in partial denture prosthesis. Dent Clin North Am March: 109–119, 1962.

Schuyler CH: Fundamental principles in the correction of occlusal disharmony—natural and artificial. J Am Dent Assoc 22:1193–1202, 1935.

chapter 19

Patient preparation and postinsertion instruction and care

Patient preparation and instruction are continuing, ongoing communications that are a part of every appointment and procedure. The patient will retain more information for a longer period if it is written and repeated several times. It is important that patients be informed and conditioned as to what to expect with use of a removable partial denture, such as the feeling of fullness or of a foreign object in the mouth. They must be reassured that adjustment to function and use takes time, but that perseverance will result in acceptance and adaptation. The importance of cleanliness of remaining teeth, tissues, and prosthesis must be emphasized many times. Explicit instructions for maintenance are essential. Patient education is not a single procedure; it is ongoing.

WHEN TO INSTRUCT PATIENTS IN DENTURE CARE

Patients are instructed, educated, and conditioned during the entire period of treatment.

Little of what you say will be retained if the instructions are given while you are actually treating a patient. He or she is more interested in what you are doing than in listening to instructions. This is especially true when a prosthesis or other material has just been placed in the mouth.

WHY PATIENT INSTRUCTION IS NECESSARY

Younger patients are not always willing to accept an artificial replacement as readily as are more mature individuals; this is especially true with removable prostheses.

If irritation develops on a tissue or tongue surface, the patient is likely to remove the partial denture, place it in a drawer, and not remember it until a much later date, when he or she becomes "dentally conscious" again, usually because of pain or discomfort.

Patients have no way of knowing how to care for their dentures. *It is your responsibility to instruct them as part of their treatment.*

SPECIFIC REMOVABLE PARTIAL DENTURE INSTRUCTIONS

Instruct the patient in the following procedures:

Placement of Dentures

Place the denture by using the fingers—never "bite" it into place. This could bend or break the denture or harm the remaining teeth. Dentures have a definite direction or path of insertion. Practice placement with a mirror. If the denture seems to bend or does not slide smoothly into place, check the direction of insertion.

Removal of Dentures

Always remove partial dentures during the night unless specifically instructed to do otherwise. Store them in water.

To avoid bending a denture or causing tooth damage, remove the denture in the same direction or path as that in which it was inserted.

Cleaning of Dentures

1. Clean the dentures and the natural teeth after every meal or snack (Fig. 19–1).
2. Keep a brush at work as well as home.
3. Use care when cleaning the dentures to avoid dropping them. Scrub over a basin filled with water.
4. Regular soap is the best cleaning agent.
5. Hold the denture so as to avoid squeezing and bending flexible parts.

Denture Compatibility

It will be several days or weeks before denture no longer feels like a foreign object.

Do not expect immediate masticating effectiveness. It takes practice to learn to "use" the dentures.

Phonetic difficulties are usually resolved by reading aloud or practicing words which are giving trouble.

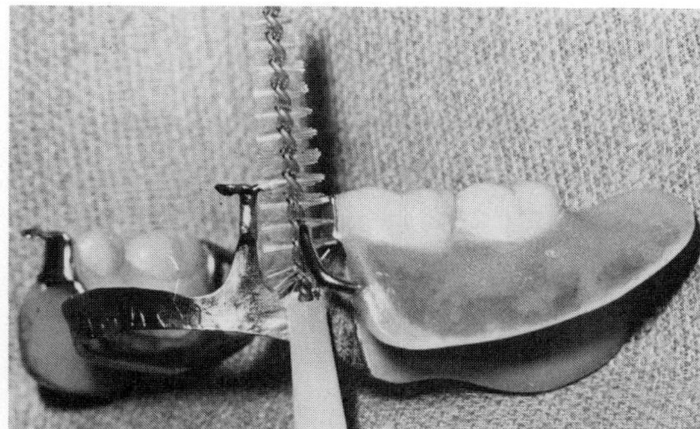

Figure 19–1 ■ The prosthesis must be cleaned after each meal or after snacking. A tapered brush is best to clean guiding surfaces and denture base areas, using regular hand soap. Cleaning or denture liquids are satisfactory *after* scrubbing, but soaking does not remove plaque.

ROUTINE DENTURE EXAMINATIONS

The Newly Inserted Denture

The patient is given a 24-hr postinsertion appointment. Areas causing irritation or discomfort should be removed and relieved immediately. Pressure indicator paste is used to identify pressure areas. Question the patient concerning areas of discomfort.

If further difficulties are anticipated, give the patient a second 24-hr appointment.

Always give an appointment 1 week following insertion. This ensures that the patient will get through the accommodation stage with minimum difficulty.

Stannous fluoride gel 0.4% (Fig. 19–2) is prescribed for daily application to all parts of the prosthesis that contact a tooth surface. The gel is applied in a thin layer with a cotton swab after cleaning of remaining teeth and prosthesis (Fig. 19–3).

Always give an appointment slip to ensure that the patient remembers the correct time and date.

Periodic Examination

1. Impress removable partial denture patients with the necessity for routine 6-month

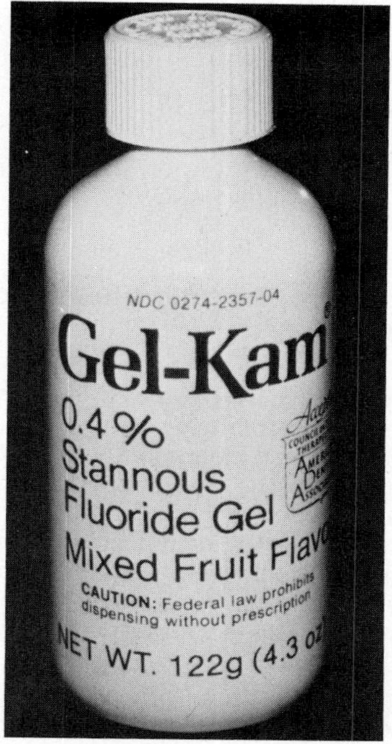

Figure 19–2 ■ Stannous fluoride gel (0.4 percent solution) will help prevent the development of caries in places where the prosthesis is in contact with the tooth structure.

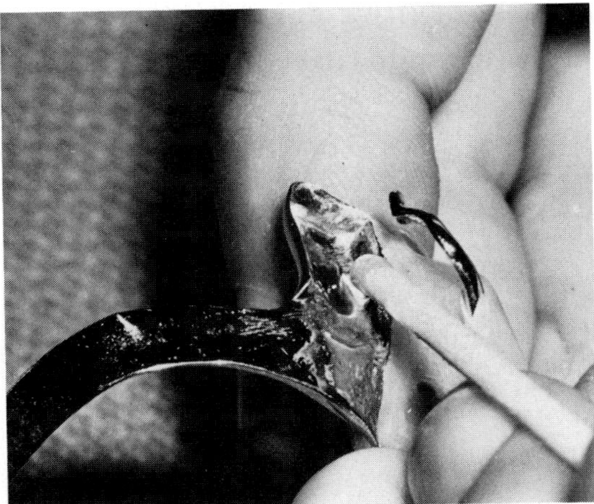

Figure 19–3 ■ Stannous fluoride (0.4 percent solution) is applied once a day at all tooth contact surfaces with a cotton swab.

examinations, and place their names on recall file; the dental record is most useful for this purpose. Place a note on the face of the chart with the recall date plainly visible.

2. For a complete recall examination and evaluation, the denture must be removed for 24 hours prior to the appointment. This allows for tissue and occlusion examination without displacement by the prosthesis.

WRITTEN INSTRUCTIONS

The following are written instructions given to the patient to take home.

Instructions for Removable Partial Denture Patients

The denture you have received is meant to be a replacement for your missing teeth and to assist you in keeping your oral cavity in good health. It will restore support to the jaw, increase your chewing ability, and improve your appearance.

If your mouth is to remain healthy, there are certain points that should be called to your attention to assist you in adjusting to your new denture and in taking care of it. This is your responsibility.

LEARNING TO USE YOUR DENTURE

1. Please be patient and expect that it will take a week or ten days before your denture will really feel as if it is a part of your body.

2. Speech: If you have difficulty pronouncing certain words, practice reading them aloud, and you will soon master the correct pronunciation.

3. Do not expect to chew easily and effectively immediately. You must learn to use the new denture; this will take time. Take small amounts of food cut into small pieces with your knife and fork, and start with softer types of food. Learning to use the denture effectively is your part of the treatment. Take the time to eat meals slowly during this "learning" period.

PLACING AND REMOVING DENTURES

1. Place and remove the denture with your fingers—never "bite" it into place.

2. There is one definite path of insertion and removal. If the denture tends to "bind" or is difficult to place or remove, stop and make sure you are using the correct path of insertion. Do not force the denture when placing or removing it.

CLEANING DENTURES

Your mouth and your denture must be kept as clean as possible all the time. Failure to do so may result in damage to your natural teeth and to your gums.

1. Remove and clean your dentures and natural teeth after each meal and snack. (At very minimum, rinse your mouth and denture clean of food debris.)

2. Regular soap or toothpaste can be used for cleaning. Keep a brush at home and at your place of work.

3. Dentures are slippery when wet. Scrub them over a basin filled with water, or over a towel. If you should drop the denture and bend any of the metal parts, *do not* attempt to straighten it yourself. See your dentist.

4. Apply stannous fluoride gel 0.4% each day to all parts of the denture that touch your remaining teeth *after* cleaning the denture and brushing your remaining teeth.

OVERNIGHT CARE

Always leave the denture out of your mouth at night. Your mouth, like the rest of your body, requires a period of rest.

Always keep the denture in water when it is not in your mouth. This prevents the plastic parts from drying out and warping.

Denture cleaners placed in the overnight water bath are good for use *after* the dentures have been *scrubbed.*

Develop the habit of examining your mouth in the mirror. This is the best insurance against disease and damage to your tissues. *Examine* cheeks, tongue, and gums carefully. Look for food debris or accumulation around teeth and gums, especially at the gum line and behind teeth; clean the mouth until debris and accumulations are gone. Examine your teeth for decay, stains, or brown deposits, especially at the gum line. Test your remaining teeth for excessive movement or looseness.

DIFFICULTIES

Be sure to return 24 hours after receiving your denture. Sore or irritated teeth and soft tissues must be treated immediately.

Dentures are not a permanent treatment. The remaining natural teeth decay and gums change or resorb, just as they did when you had all your natural teeth. Periodic examination and treatment by the dentist is *most necessary.*

See your dentist for examination and prophylaxis treatment every 6 months. Have an examination whenever there is

a. Soreness or irritation of teeth or gums.
b. Evidence of decay.
c. Excessive movement of the denture.
d. Calculus or stain on dentures or on natural teeth.

Home remedies for ill-fitting dentures aggravate a bad situation and cause greater bone and tissue loss. See your dentist if you have a problem.

Partial Denture Reline

Examination and evaluation of the removable partial denture patient is scheduled every 6 months. Determining if there are tissue and bone changes of the edentulous support area under the extension portion of the prosthesis is a primary concern. Proper evaluation requires removal of the prosthesis for a 24-hr period prior to examination to allow the support tissues to return to their natural contours. The adaptation of the prosthesis to the mucosa can then be checked for even contact with pressure indicator paste and the ridge can be observed for possible changes or resorption.

Further evaluation of changes in ridge support are made by observing the amount of movement that occurs when force is placed on the extension portion of the prosthesis. Extensive denture movement is evidenced by the lifting of the indirect retainer rests off their rest seats (Fig. 19–4).

Another method of evaluating changes requiring relining is the use of articulating ribbon or celluloid strips between the occlusal surfaces.

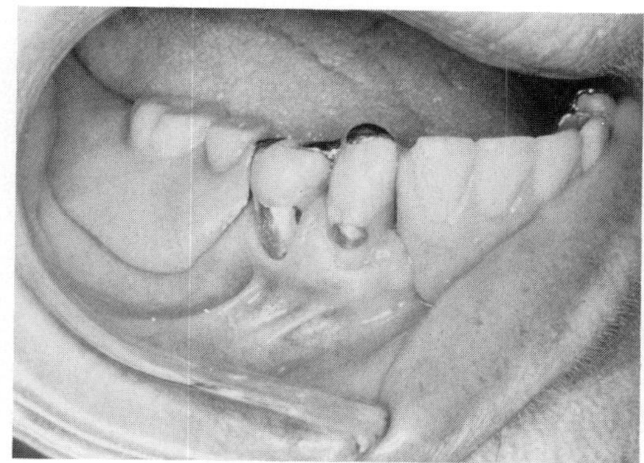

Figure 19–4 ■ The need for partial denture reline is determined by excessive displacement of the denture base when pressure is placed on the prosthetic teeth over the edentulous area. The indirect retainer or metal rest on the canine lifts off the tooth when excessive ridge change or resorption has occurred.

If there has been bone resorption or ridge support changes, the occlusal surfaces will not record or hold the strips (Fig. 19–5).

RELINE PROCEDURE

The reline procedure is basically the same as the altered cast procedure.

1. Remove the denture for 24 hr or until the edentulous areas are healthy.
2. Remove enough acrylic resin from the tissue surface of the denture base to allow at least

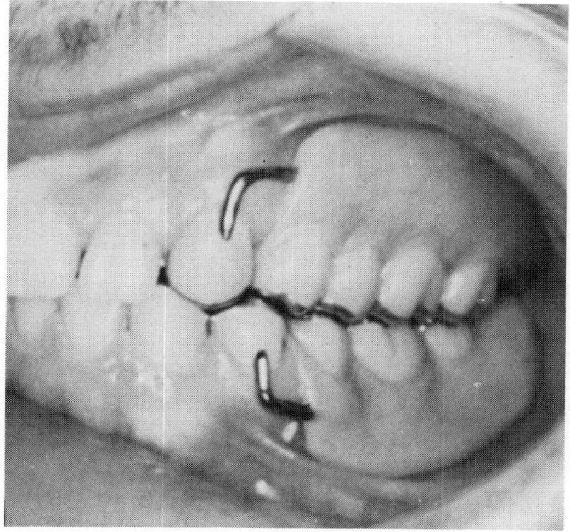

Figure 19–5 ■ The need for reline is demonstrated when the occlusal surfaces of the prosthesis will not grip and hold articulating ribbon or plastic strips.

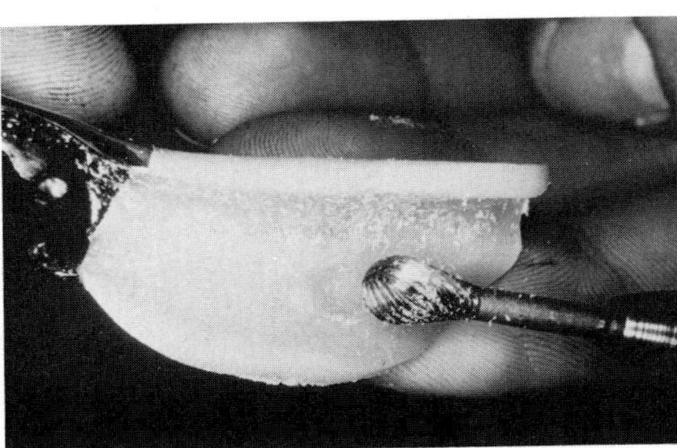

Figure 19–6 ■ Before a reline impression is made, 1 mm of the denture base is removed from the tissue side to provide space for the impression material.

1 mm of space between base and tissue (Fig. 19–6).

3. Mold the periphery with gray stick modeling composition warmed in a water bath at 140°F.

4. Remove all modeling composition that has flowed onto the tissue side of the denture base.

5. Make a final impression with ZnOE paste, while holding the metal framework in place on the teeth (Fig. 19–7).

6. Flask the denture and replace the impression material with acrylic resin (Fig. 19–8).

7. Insert the denture, following the *same procedure as that described for insertion of a new denture.*

8. Postinsertion instructions and follow-up appointments are *identical* to those described for a new denture.

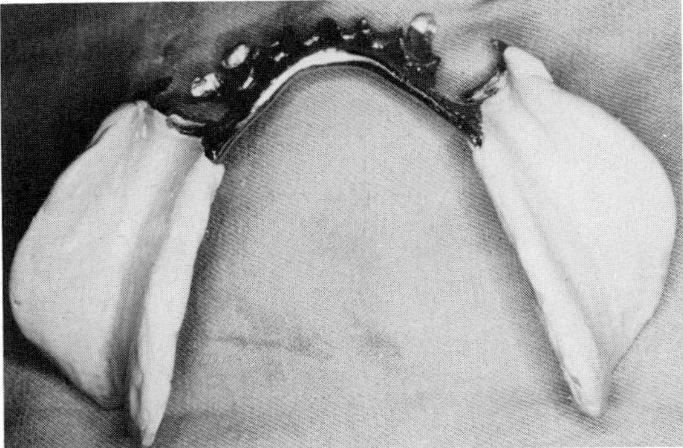

Figure 19–7 ■ An impression of the edentulous area is made with ZnOE impression paste while the metal casting is held firmly in place on the remaining natural teeth. (This procedure is identical to the altered cast impression procedure.)

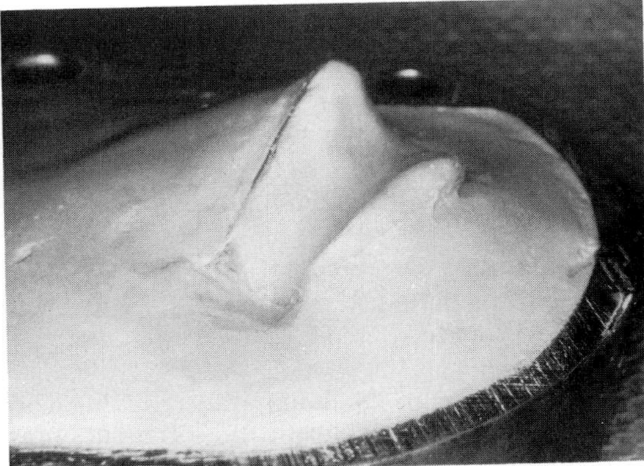

Figure 19–8 ■ The prosthesis with the new impression is flasked, packed, processed, and inserted with the same procedures used in making a new partial denture.

Periodontal-Involved Patients

Patients with extensive periodontal involvement, including loss of many teeth and much of the supporting structures around remaining teeth, present difficult treatment planning problems. The basic tooth positions and occlusal plane are often in disarray (Fig. 19–9). Anterior-posterior contacts between remaining teeth are gone (Fig. 19–10), and the teeth stand alone. The teeth are often twisted or tipped and forced into abnormal facial or lingual positions. The arch is further compromised by extensive periodontal involvement and loss of teeth.

A basic premise of diagnosis, evaluation, and treatment is to stabilize the arch during the evaluation and periodontal treatment, while

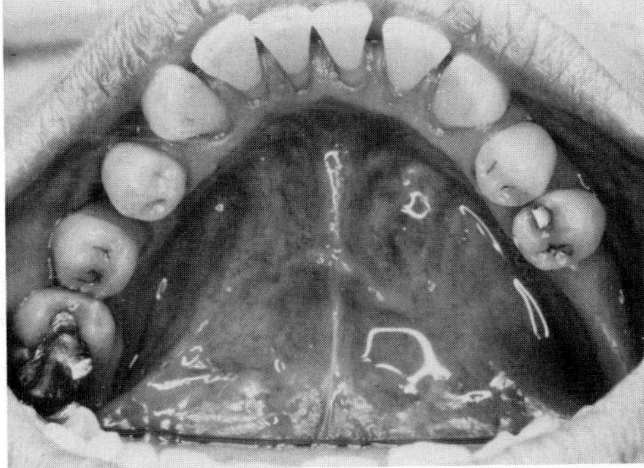

Figure 19–9 ■ Periodontally involved teeth usually present disorganized occlusions, with teeth mobile and turned in abnormal positions.

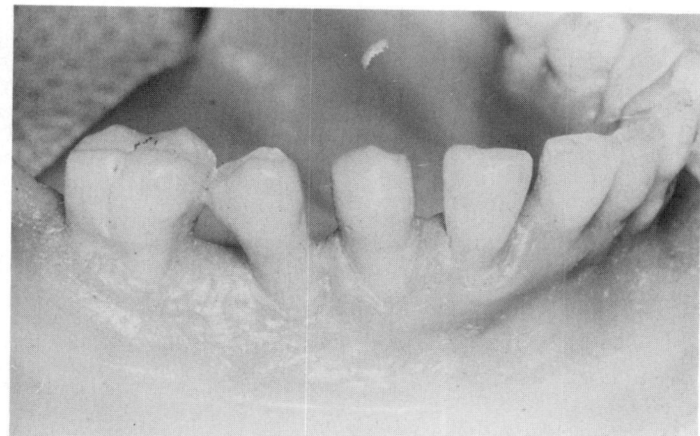

Figure 19–10 ■ A common complication of periodontally involved conditions is loss of anterior-posterior tooth contact, resulting in loss of arch stability.

deciding which teeth or areas will respond to treatment and which teeth can be retained.

Stabilization of the arch can quickly and effectively be accomplished through the use of a removable casting (Fig. 19–11). This type of casting could be considered a splint or treatment casting (Fig. 19–12).

The advantages of a removable stabilizing casting are that it

1. Immediately stabilizes each tooth.
2. Unites the entire remaining arch.
3. Is removable for periodontal and restorative treatments.
4. Organizes and restores the occlusal plane.

The advantageous effects of stabilizing and reducing tooth movement during treatment are well appreciated and utilized by the periodontist. The removable casting does not interfere with surgical procedures and placement of packs, since the casting can be coated with petroleum jelly and placed and removed while the pack material is soft. This allows removal of the splint for optimal cleaning access. The casting controls tooth movement during the healing period, promoting maximum healing results.

All remaining teeth are united to act as an organized unit against opposing occlusal forces.

The splint is usually restricted to the remaining teeth, unless esthetics require replacement of teeth in edentulous areas. Attempts to restore extension areas at this time complicate and jeopardize the remaining teeth.

If periodontally involved teeth do not respond to treatment and a tooth must be removed, it can be added to the treatment prosthesis without redoing the casting.

In many instances the removable cast splint may be a long-term treatment because of compromised periodontal conditions, the need for flexibility of treatment, geriatric considerations,

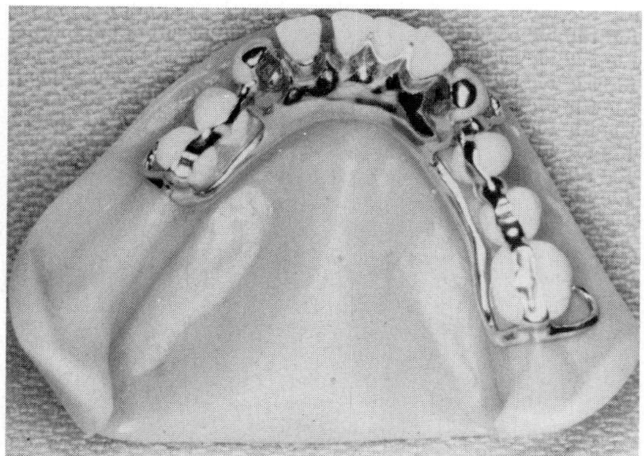

Figure 19–11 ■ A removable casting immediately unites and stabilizes the remaining teeth, controlling movement and position.

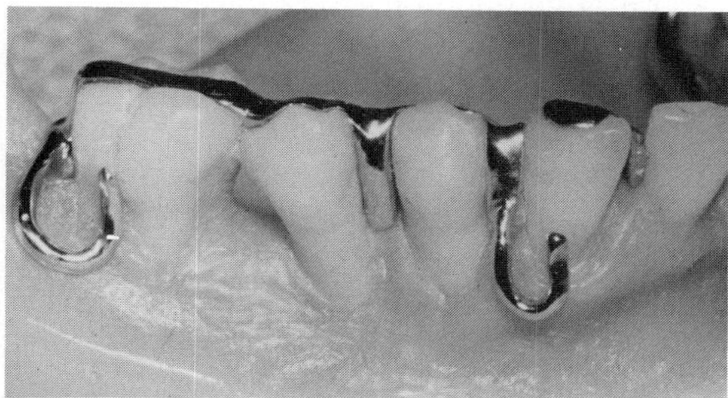

Figure 19–12 ■ The removable casting provides anterior-posterior bracing and helps to restore the proper occlusal plane during and after periodontal treatment.

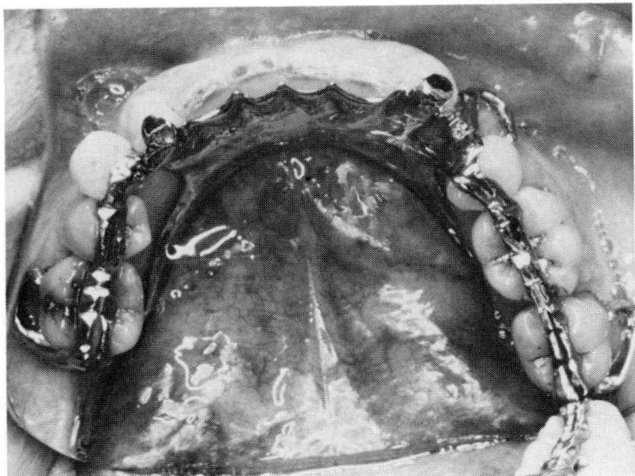

Figure 19–13 ■ Metal removable casting can provide long-term treatment for advanced periodontally involved situations in which prognosis is guarded or uncertain. Teeth that do not respond to treatment can readily be added to the prosthesis.

health problems, and financial considerations (Fig. 19–13).

REFERENCES

Patient Instruction

Hickey JC: Responsibility of the dentist in removable partial dentures. J Ky Dent Assoc 17:70–87, 1965.

Maison WG: Instructions to denture patients. J Prosthet Dent 9:825–831, 1959.

Plainfield S: Communication distortion. The language of patients and practitioners of dentistry. J Prosthet Dent 22:11–19, 1969.

Ramsey WO: The relation of emotional factors to prosthodontic service. J Prosthet Dent 23:4–10, 1970.

Savage RD and MacGregor AR: Behavior therapy in prosthodontics. J Prosthet Dent 24:126–132, 1970.

Schabel RW: Dentist-patient communication. A major factor in treatment prognosis. J Prosthet Dent 21:3–5, 1969.

Reline

Blatterfein L: Rebasing procedures for removable partial dentures. J Prosthet Dent 8:441–467, 1958.

Steffel VL: Relining removable partial dentures for fit and function. J Prosthet Dent 4:496–509, 1954.

Wilson JH: Partial dentures—relining the saddle supported by the mucosa and alveolar bone. J Prosthet Dent 3:807–813, 1953.

Periodontal Involvement

Applegate OC: The interdependence of periodontics and removable partial denture prosthesis. J Prosthet Dent 8:269–281, 1958.

Kratochvil FJ: Maintaining supporting structures with a removable partial prosthesis. J Prosthet Dent 25:167–174, 1971.

McKenzie JS: Mutual problems of the periodontist and prosthodontist. J Prosthet Dent 5:37–42, 1955.

Nevin RB: Periodontal aspects of partial denture prosthesis. J Prosthet Dent 5:215–219, 1955.

Rudd KD and O'Leary TJ: Stabilizing periodontally weakened teeth by using guide plane removable partial dentures. A preliminary report. J Prosthet Dent 16:721–727, 1966.

Schuyler CH:The partial denture as a means of stabilizing abutment teeth. J Am Dent Assoc 28:1121–1125, 1941.

chapter 20

Laboratory and clinical procedures

LABORATORY PROCEDURES

Impressions and Casts

Laboratory procedures associated with impressions and the production of accurate casts are dependent on *materials, technique, and preciseness.*

Impression materials vary in their properties and require individual consideration. Alginates are poured *as quickly as possible* because of their inherent characteristic of absorbing or losing water easily and quickly, causing distortion of the impression material. Because of this property, it is important that alginate impressions be kept in a humidor (Fig. 20–1) but *not* submerged in water, even during the short time before they are poured.

Other impression materials for removable partial dentures do not have as critical a time-moisture factor. The rubber impression materials do not require immediate pouring but should be placed in a humidor to prevent drying or distortion, especially if a custom acrylic tray was used.

HANDLING CONSIDERATIONS

Special care must be taken with all impressions to prevent distortion in the posterior or molar portion. A common cause of distortion in this area is setting the finished impression on the bench surface, with the impression material extending over the end of the tray and becoming the support area (Fig. 20–2). This can result in separation of the impression material from the tray, especially when the additional weight of the stone or plaster is added, resulting in distortion of the impression and cast. A simple, effective method of preventing this distortion is to support the tray containing the impression by the tray handle, using a support jig or a metal strip added to the bench or shelf (Fig. 20–3).

MIXING AND POURING STONES

The dental stones are primarily used during the fabrication of removable partial dentures in the production of diagnostic and working casts.

A basic laboratory procedure when pouring the impression is to obtain the proper water:powder ratio by weight and measure (Fig. 20–4). Since there are many types and brands of dental stones available, it is most important that individual manufacturers' information be followed because changes in ratios affect the expansion of each material. A second basic characteristic that must be considered is the different expansion changes that occur if the material is allowed to set in air or in water: Allowing the cast to set with the base in water increases expansion.

Mixing of the powder and water must be thorough and complete in order to provide a consistent, smooth, finished product.

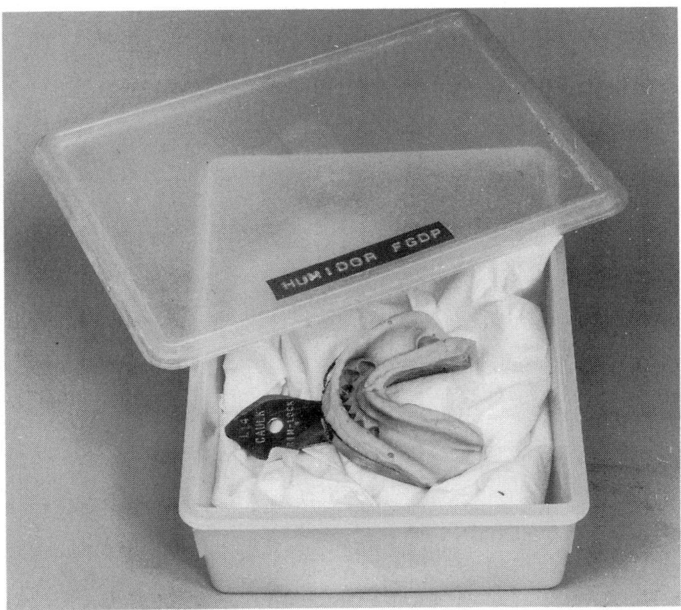

Figure 20–1 ■ Storage in a simple humidor minimizes changes in impression materials until they are poured.

PRODUCTION OF THE CAST

There are two methods of pouring the stone into the impression:

The Double-Pour Method

This procedure, as indicated by its name, requires the initial pour of stone to fill in all tooth and tissue surfaces up to the peripheral border of the impression material (Fig. 20–5). The first pour is allowed to achieve the *initial set,* and then the base portion of the cast is formed by a second mix of stone. The impression with the first pour of stone is inverted onto the second pour, and the base is shaped to the proper dimensions (Fig. 20–6).

The rationale for the two-pour technique is that the impression is in an upright position during the pour and set of the stone, when the tooth and tissue surfaces are being formed. Atmospheric pressure and the weight of the stone tends to force the stone onto the impression surfaces, producing better contact and duplication.

The Single-Pour Method

This method requires one mix of stone, which will be used to produce the entire cast. The

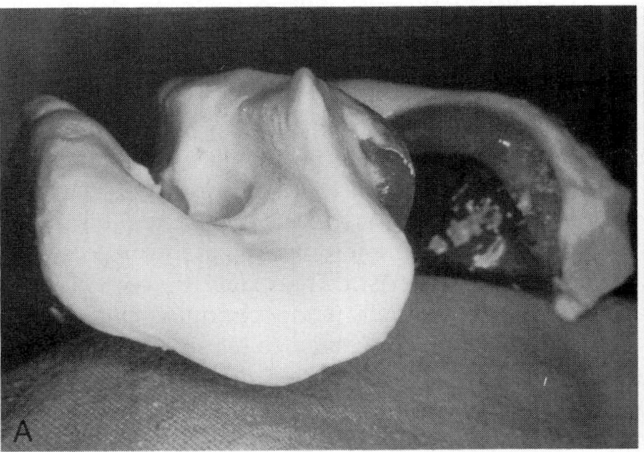

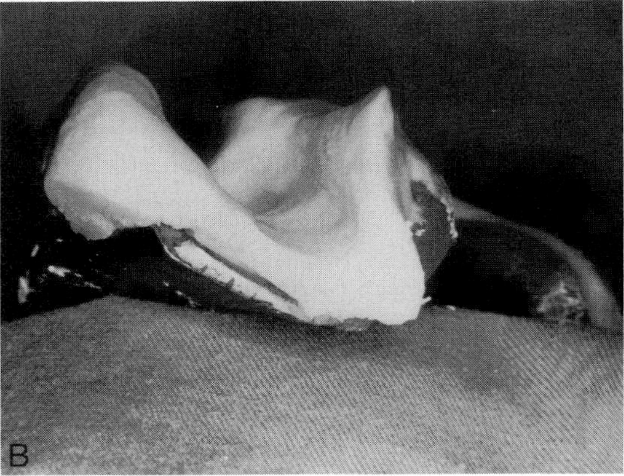

Figure 20–2 ■ *A,* If a part of the impression material touches the bench top, it can distort the impression. *B,* Check the posterior portion of the impression for possible separation of the impression material from the tray.

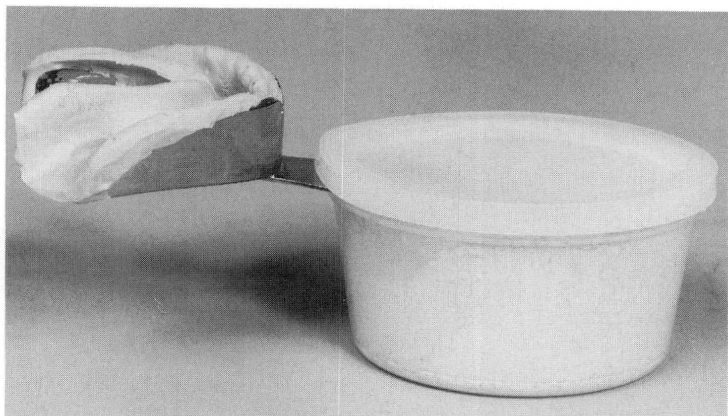

Figure 20–3 ■ To prevent distortion of the impression, the tray should be suspended by the tray handle.

stone is prepared and poured into the impression to cover all surfaces. The impression tray with the stone in a fluid state is inverted onto stone to form the cast base. The base portion is shaped to the desired form, and the stone is allowed to set.

The single-pour or inverted method requires special consideration and care to prevent the stone mix from losing contact with the surface of the impression material during inversion and as a result of atmospheric pressure.

Whenever stone is being poured into an impression, it is most important that the stone be applied in small amounts and *vibrated* into all areas. It is necessary to *observe* the flow of the stone onto each area of the impression, which ensures accurate reproduction of the surfaces and eliminates air that can be trapped between the impression material and the stone.

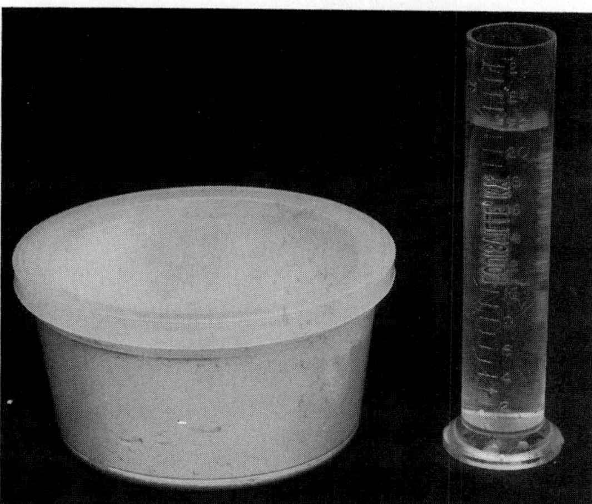

Figure 20–4 ■ To provide a cast that will correctly reproduce the dimensions of the mouth, the powder must be weighed and the water measured according to the manufacturer's directions. Failure to do so will produce less accurate casts.

Record Bases

It is often necessary to fabricate record bases for the registration of maxillary-mandibular jaw positions and to transfer these positions to a laboratory situation on the articulator.

The record bases are needed where insufficient natural teeth remain to properly orient the casts. The bases must

1. Accurately fit the tissues of the mouth and cast.
2. Be rigid and stable.
3. Retain a precise position in the mouth and on the cast.
4. Not interfere with closure and contact of remaining teeth.

Laboratory preparation of the cast for the record base requires a wax-out of undercut areas of the teeth and soft tissues (Fig. 20–7). The stone surface of the cast is protected with two coats of separating medium. The auto-curing acrylic material used to form the record base can be applied by the "sprinkle-on" method or by adaptation of the acrylic in the plastic stage. It is important that the base be *well adapted* to the *edentulous area* and have definite *occlusal stops* and *position contacts* with remaining teeth (Fig. 20–8).

Care must be taken when removing the record base after polymerization to prevent damage to the cast. Immersion of the cast and acrylic in water at 140°F for 2 minutes prior to separation greatly facilitates removal.

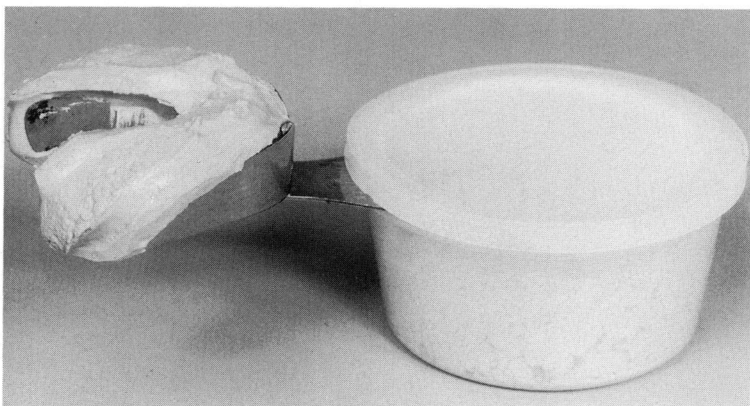

Figure 20–5 ■ The most accurate method to produce a cast is the double-pour method, in which the tooth-tissue surfaces are poured with the tray held in a suspended position, and the stone is allowed to achieve its initial set.

The record base is shaped and polished for the best possible acceptance by the patient and with the least possible interference with jaw movements and occlusion.

It is often possible to place small, thin plastic occlusion rims on the record base. This provides a stable rim, reducing the possibility of dimensional errors. The registration material can be placed directly on the plastic record base.

Articulator Mountings

The two articulator mountings are the face bow mounting record for the maxillary cast and the maxillomandibular record for the mandibular cast.

MAXILLARY CAST MOUNTING

The objective is to place the cast of the maxillary arch on the articulator in an exact reproduction of its position in the patient's head. The face bow apparatus is a holder or jig that measures and records the location of anatomic landmarks from the patient and transfers the recorded measurements of these locations to an instrument — the articulator.

In the laboratory procedure, it is necessary to be sure that the anatomic location points are in the correct positions on the articulator before attaching the cast with stone or plaster.

Laboratory Articulator Considerations

1. The hinge axis position.
2. The cast position in the bite fork record.

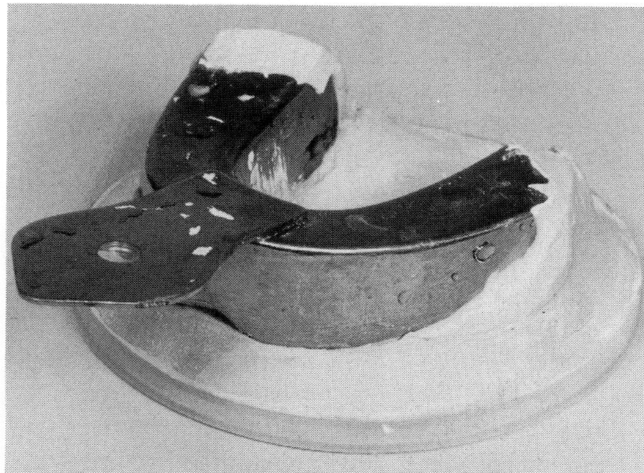

Figure 20–6 ■ The base of the cast is produced by a second mix of stone, after the initial setting of the first pour.

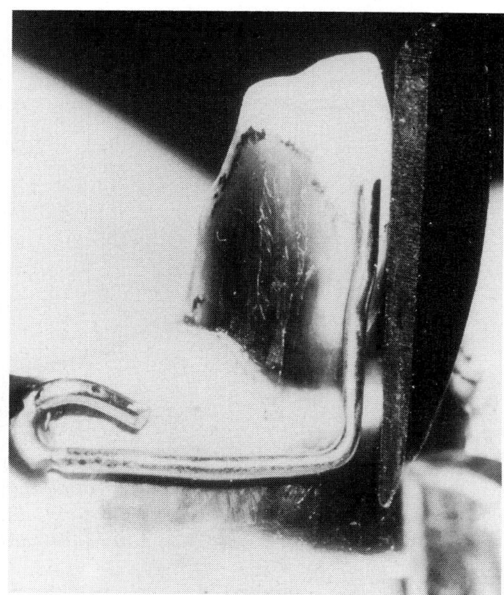

Figure 20–7 ■ Tooth and tissue undercuts are filled with wax prior to fabrication of a record base to mount casts for diagnostic or laboratory purposes.

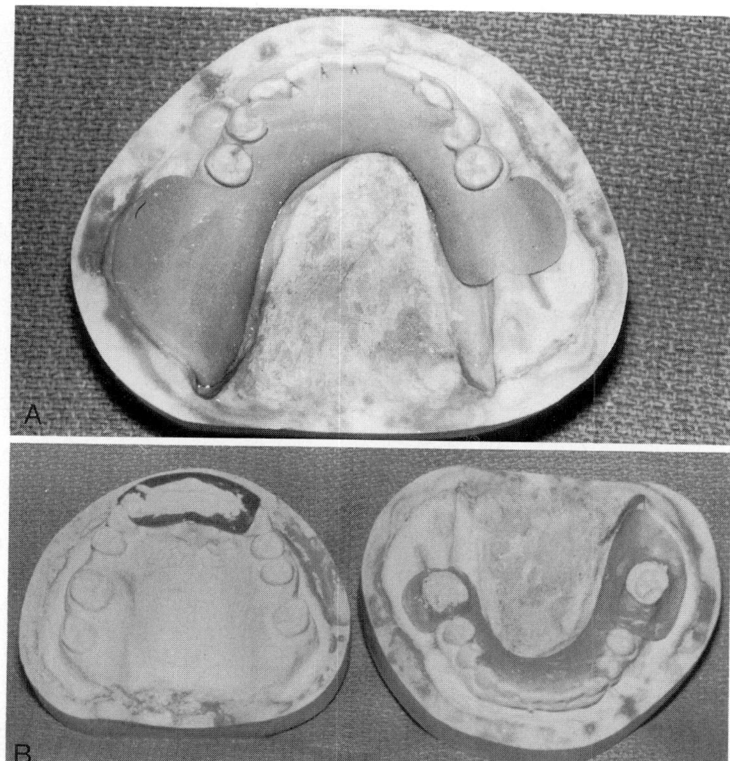

Figure 20–8 ■ *A*, Record bases must be well adapted to the edentulous areas and have positive occlusal stops for exact position in the mouth and on the casts. *B*, Occlusal registration material is placed on the record base to record the interocclusal position of the arches.

3. The attachment of the cast to the instrument without distortion of the location points.

The *hinge axis* location of the face bow record on the articulator depends on the ability to adjust the hinge axis of the articulator (inward and outward) to adapt to the face bow record. If the axis of the instrument is adjustable, the face bow record is *not moved*, and the articulator hinge axis is moved in *equal* measure on *both* sides outward to the face bow (Fig. 20–9).

If the hinge axis location of the articulator is *not* adjustable, the face bow is adjusted with *equal* movement on *both sides* to fit the articulator (Fig. 20–10).

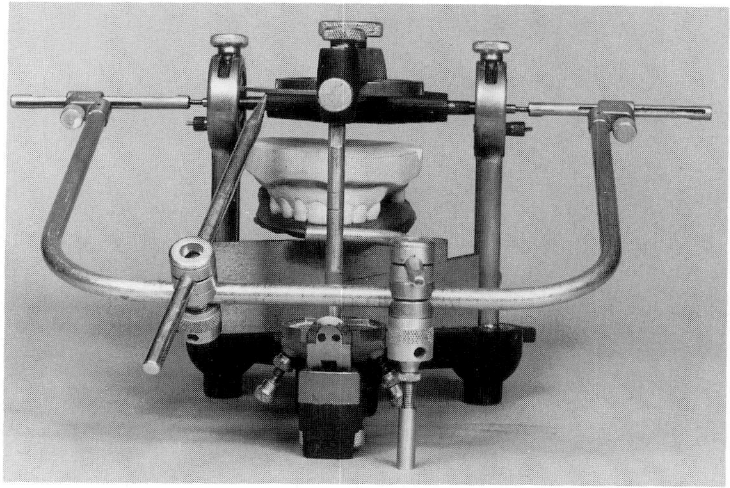

Figure 20–9 ■ Articulators with an *adjustable intercondyle axis* are moved *equally* outward on each side to engage the face bow. The face bow settings are *not moved.*

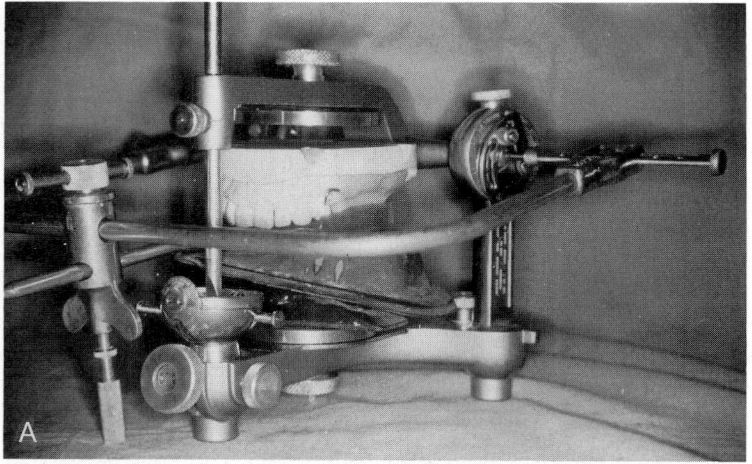

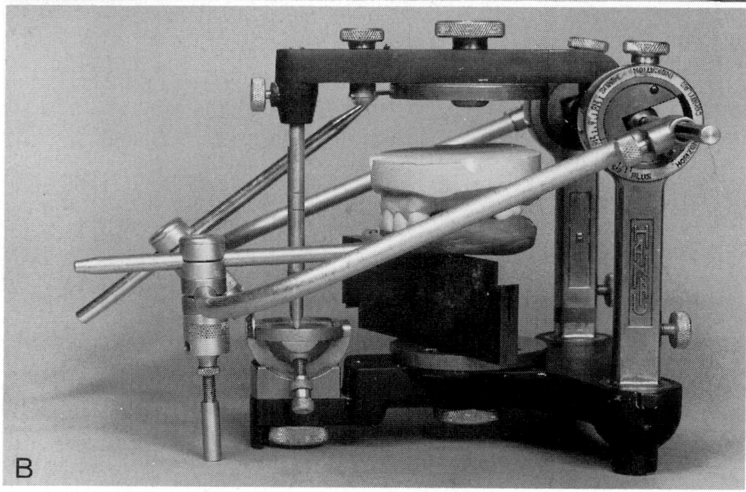

Figure 20–10 ■ *A*, For articulation with a *nonadjustable* intercondyle axis, the face bow is adjusted *equally* on *both* sides to establish contact. *B*, The maxillary cast is securely fixed to the bite fork with wax. Index notches have been cut into the base of the cast for positive positioning.

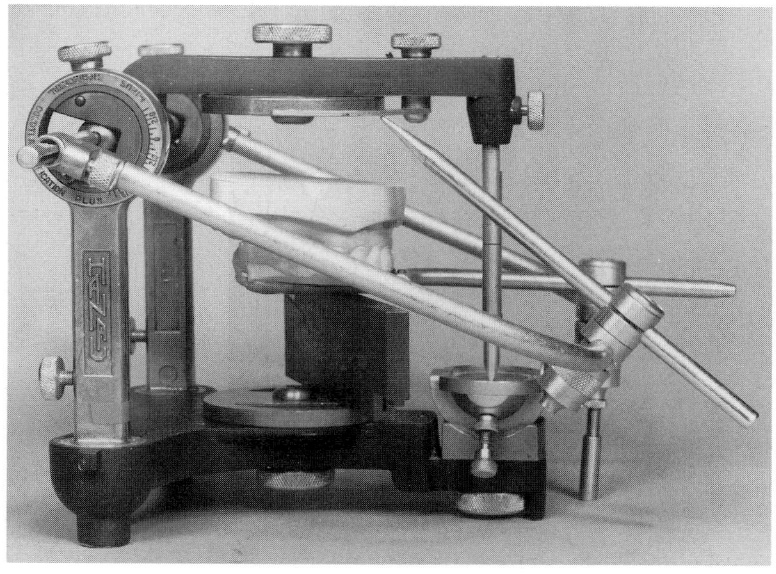

Figure 20–11 ■ To reproduce an upright patient head position on the articulator, move the face bow until the orbital pointer touches the orbital plane attached to the upper member of the articulator.

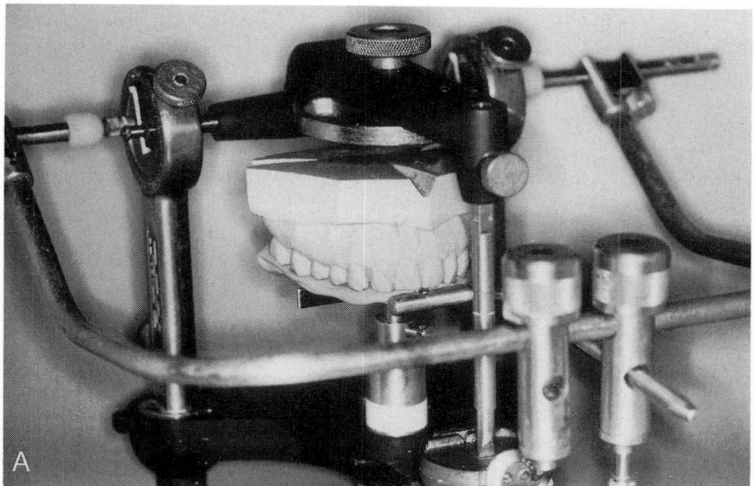

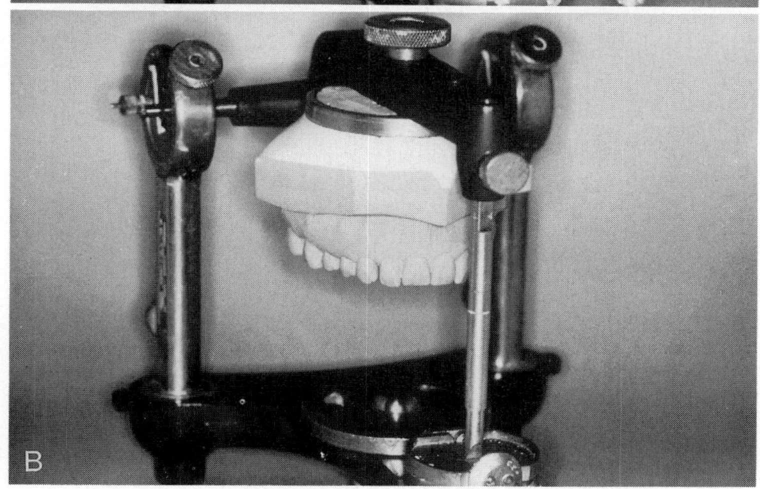

Figure 20–12 ■ *A*, Support the cast and bite fork with a prop to prevent the weight of the mounting plaster from moving the cast. Adjustable devices are available to support the cast and bite fork in the correct position. *B*, The finished mounting of the maxillary cast.

The *maxillary cast*, with index notches cut into the base, is carefully positioned in the occlusal index of the bite fork, which is attached to the face bow and secured with sticky wax (Fig. 10B). If the maxillary arch is to be presented on the articulator in a position duplicating the patient's standing with the head in an upright position, the intraorbital pointer is positioned to the infraorbital plane attachment on the articulator (Fig. 20–11). The maxillary arch is now located in the same position on the instrument as that which it occupies in the patient's head.

Attachment of the maxillary cast to the articulator is accomplished with stone or plaster. Two possibilities of changes that can cause errors are

1. Dimensional change of the mounting material.
2. Change in position of the face bow apparatus.

The dimensional change of the stone or plaster is affected by the water : powder ratio and by the amount of material being used. Care in measurement of materials can control the first factor, and reduction in the amount of space between cast and articulator can reduce the second.

The weight of the maxillary cast and the attachment stone, together with placement and manipulation changes, can cause distortion of the face bow record. It is necessary to provide additional support to the cast for stability prior to attaching the cast to the articulator (Fig. 20–12).

MANDIBULAR CAST MOUNTING

Attachment of the mandibular cast to reproduce centric relation position is dependent upon the same accurate *placement* of the inter-

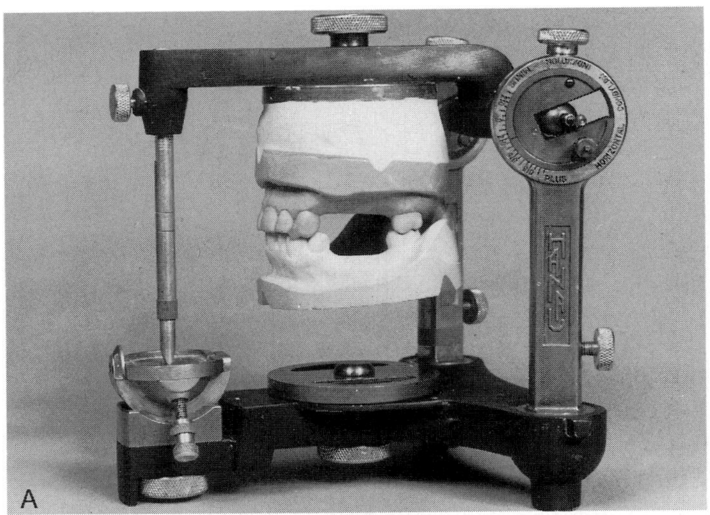

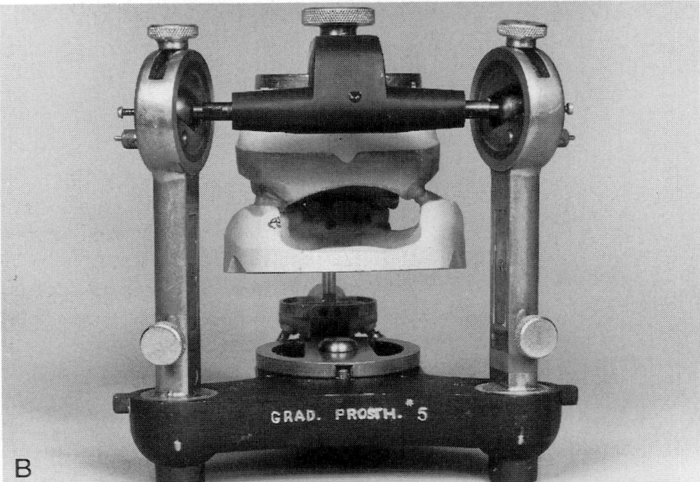

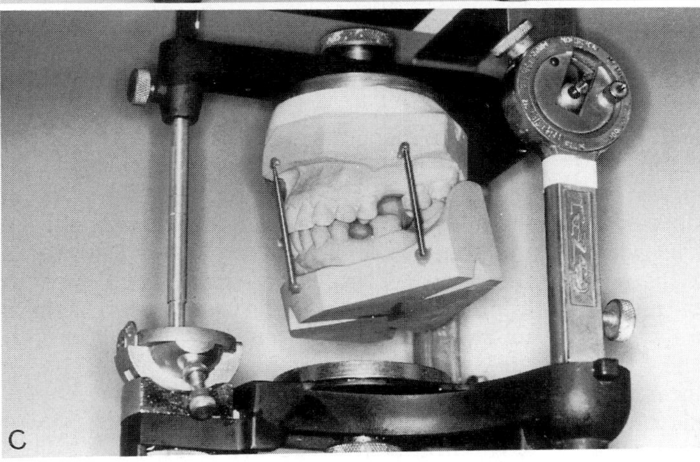

Figure 20–13 ■ *A*, The lower cast must be securely attached in proper position with sticky wax prior to mounting. *B*, Where possible, attach the cast bases directly to each other to ensure a secure relationship for interocclusal position. *C*, Metal extensions such as burs may be necessary to ensure the position of one cast in relation to the other.

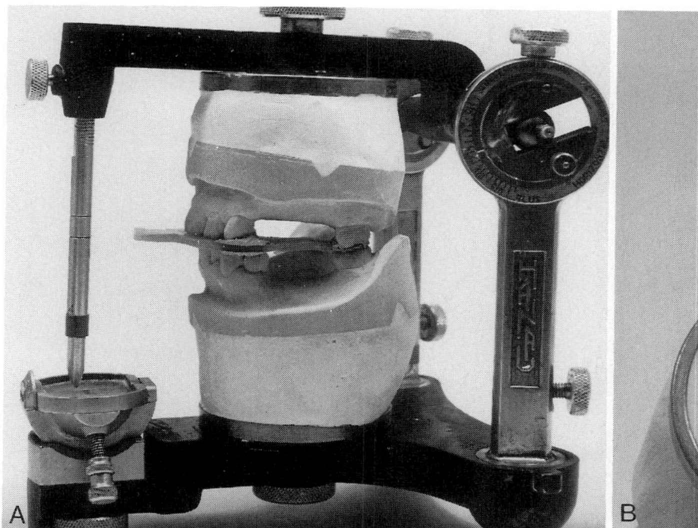

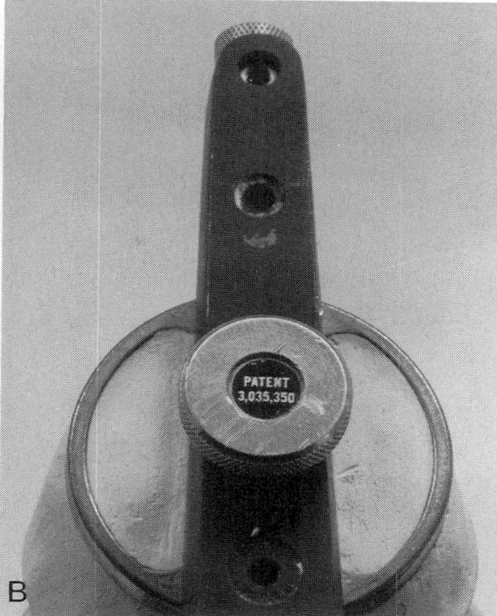

Figure 20 – 14 ■ *A*, An interocclusal record between the teeth causes a separation of the occlusal contacts of the teeth. *B*, When the teeth are separated by an interocclusal record, the incisal pin is opened to the amount equal to the thickness of the record.

occlusal registration against the occlusal surfaces and on avoidance of dimensional changes of the stone or plaster attachment materials.

The casts must be *securely* attached to each other to prevent positional changes during the mounting or attachment procedure. Sticky wax applied directly between the casts provides a firm, unchanging method of maintaining position (Fig. 20 – 13).

If the interocclusal record requires an increase in the vertical dimension of occlusion in the patient's mouth, the vertical dimension setting of the articulator is increased by that same amount (Fig. 20 – 14).

Removable Partial Denture Casting

MOST ADVANTAGEOUS POSITION (MAP)

Reproduction of the MAP in the laboratory uses the tripod marks that are located on the master cast. The master cast is secured on the survey table and the basic eye survey is repeated, which locates the approximate position (Fig. 20 – 15). The vertical arm of the surveyor is then *fixed* in position at one of the tripod marks, and the survey table is moved to see if the tip of the vertical arm coincides with the other two tripod marks. The angle of the MAP is changed until all three tripod marks contact the tip of the *fixed* vertical arm of the surveyor (Fig. 20 – 16). The cast is now in the identical MAP determined previously, so that the casting can be fabricated to coincide with the planned guide surfaces and retention areas.

On the *maxillary* cast, score the area for the metal-tissue seal, as prescribed, to provide a metal-tissue post-dam for the palate (Fig. 16B).

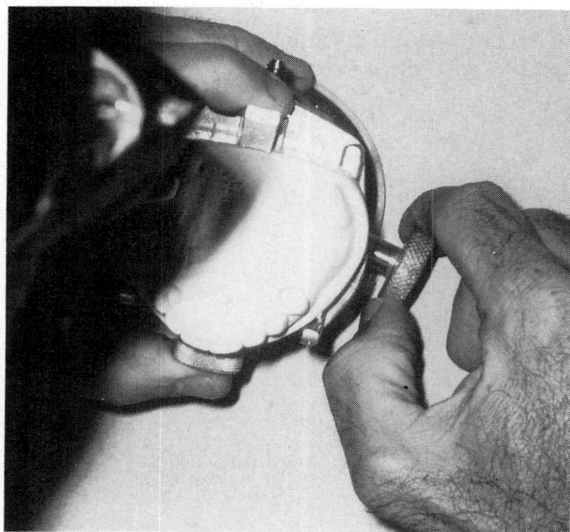

Figure 20 – 15 ■ The master cast used for fabrication of the RPD casting is positioned by eye survey and checked with the surveyor to be sure that the cast is in the original treatment plan position or MAP.

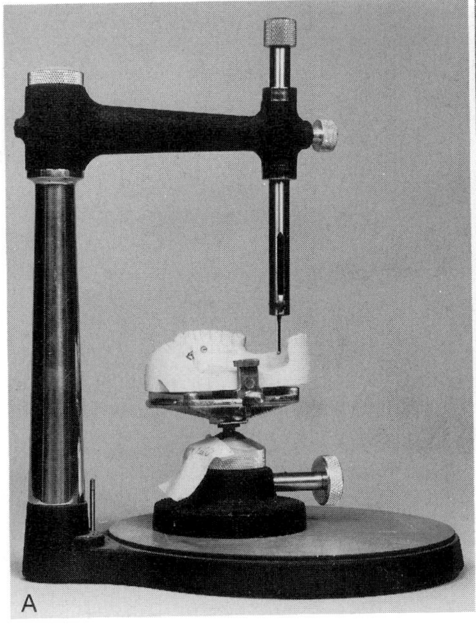

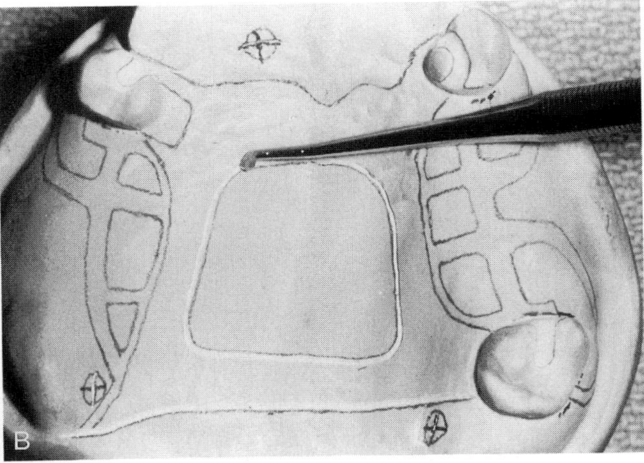

Figure 20–16 ■ *A*, Repositioning the master cast in the MAP at the laboratory is accomplished by contacting the three widely separated marks on the cast with the arm of the surveyor in a fixed position. *B*, A groove is cut into the border area of the prosthesis to provide a palatal seal where the metal will join the tissue.

WAX-OUT OF UNDESIRABLE UNDERCUTS

To fabricate a removable partial casting requires making a second cast of high-heat investment material. This refractory cast is made from an impression or duplication of the master cast. The form for the metal casting is done in wax on this refractory cast and reproduced in metal. Parts of the final casting are in intimate contact with the teeth and soft tissues, and other parts have planned spaces between the casting and tissues. Tissue undercuts can prevent placement (Fig. 20–17); planned spaces provide an area to attach plastic to metal (Fig. 20–18). To reproduce these spaces under the finished casting, they must be created on the master cast with wax, and then duplicated on the refractory cast and eventually under the finished metal casting.

Wax is placed over the area where the denture base retention is located, in order to provide space for the acrylic. One layer of 22-gauge adhesive-coated casting wax provides the necessary thickness. In the edentulous area, where the acrylic will join the metal, the wax is cut to a sharp right angle to form a clean finish line (Figs. 20–19 and 20–20).

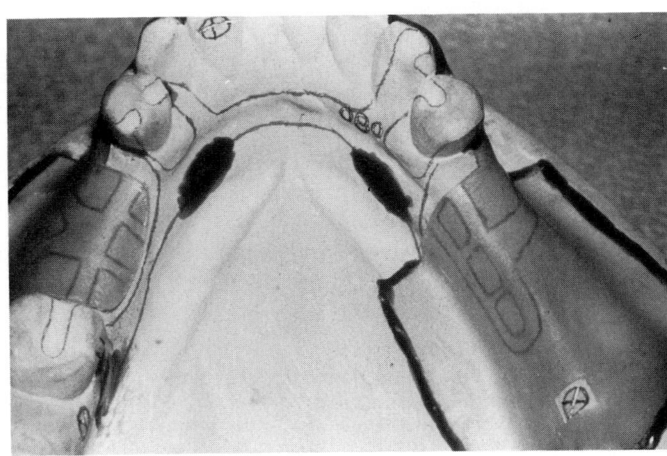

Figure 20–17 ■ Areas where the metal casting should stand away from the mucosa or where undercut areas would prevent seating of the casting are relieved with wax on the master cast.

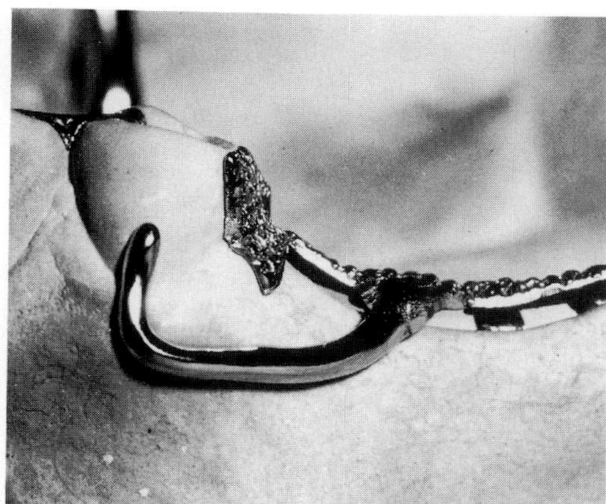

Figure 20–18 ■ It is necessary to provide space between the tissue and the casting in the denture base retention area. The acrylic must attach itself around the metal with sufficient bulk for strength.

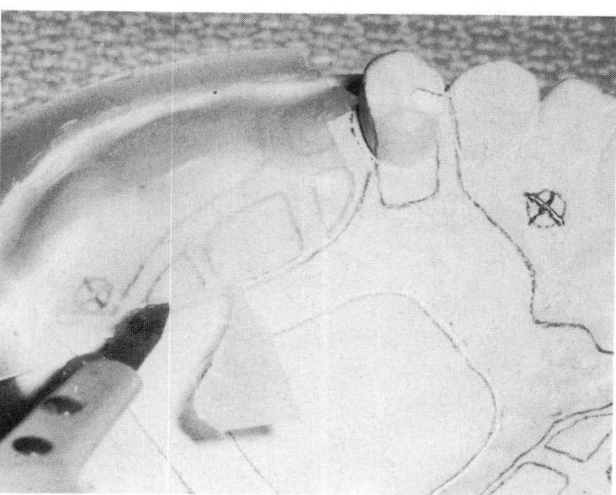

Figure 20–19 ■ The wax relief on the master cast in the denture base retention area is cut to a sharp right angle to produce a sharp finish line in the final casting.

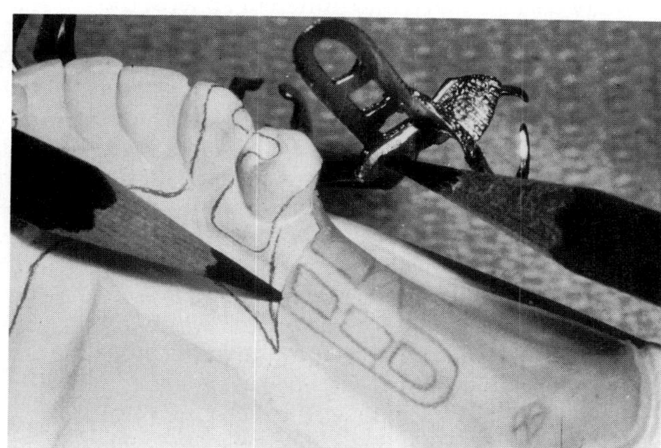

Figure 20–20 ■ For the mandibular prosthesis, the sharp metal-plastic finish margin is curved downward and well distal to the natural tooth.

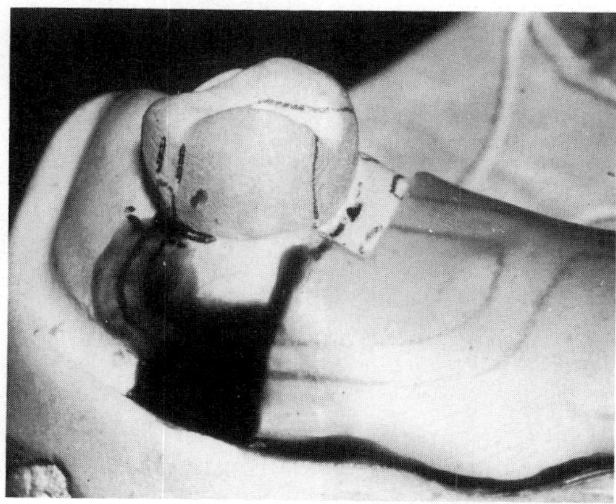

Figure 20–21 ■ Wax is placed on the master cast in tissue undercut areas to prevent interference when the casting is seated over these areas.

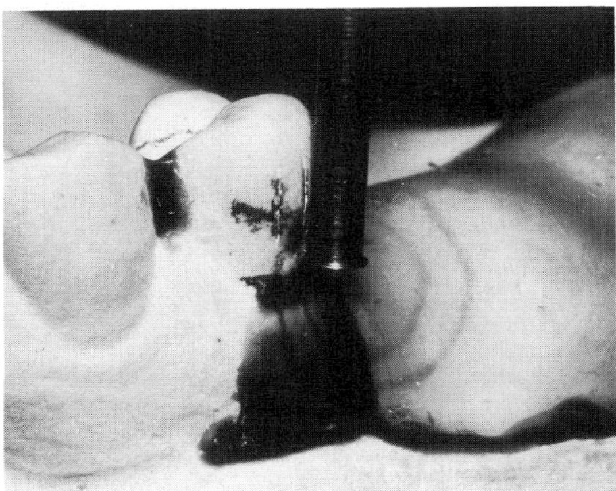

Figure 20–22 ■ *Planned undercut retention* areas on the teeth are *not* waxed out. The casting must touch the tooth at this point. The amount of undercut required is precisely measured and positioned with the undercut gauge.

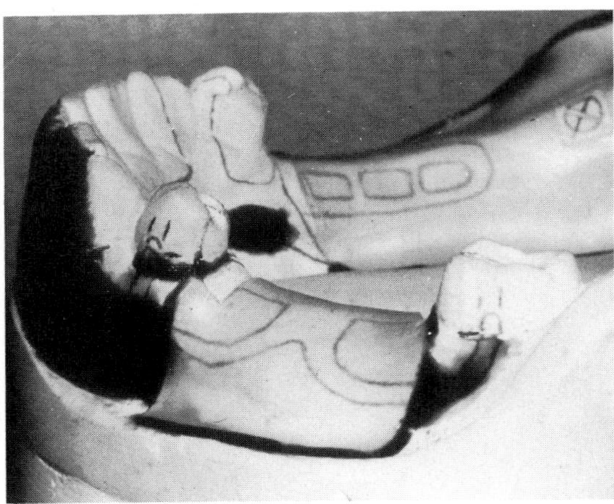

Figure 20–24 ■ Any cast undercuts that are not involved with the metal casting are eliminated by applying wax. This helps to prevent distortion when the master cast is duplicated.

Inlay wax is flowed into undercut areas of the teeth and soft tissues that would interfere with the placement and removal of the casting (Fig. 20–21). An *exception* is the *planned retention* undercut areas on the teeth (Fig. 20–22). Any excess wax in undercut areas is trimmed away with the wax cutting instrument attached to the surveyor, with the cast positioned in the MAP (Fig. 20–23).

Eliminate with wax all other undercuts on the master cast that will not be involved, in order to reduce the potential for distortion when removing the refractory cast from the duplicating material (Fig. 20–24).

REFRACTORY CAST PRODUCTION

The procedure for duplication of the master cast into a refractory cast will vary, depending upon the type and properties of the duplication and refractory cast materials. Basically, the following principles apply to all materials and procedures:

1. Place a metal or plastic sprue-former mold on the master cast to form a cone or funnel for metal entry.
2. Place the waxed-out master cast in warm water at 120°F for 15 min.
3. Center the master cast in the base of the

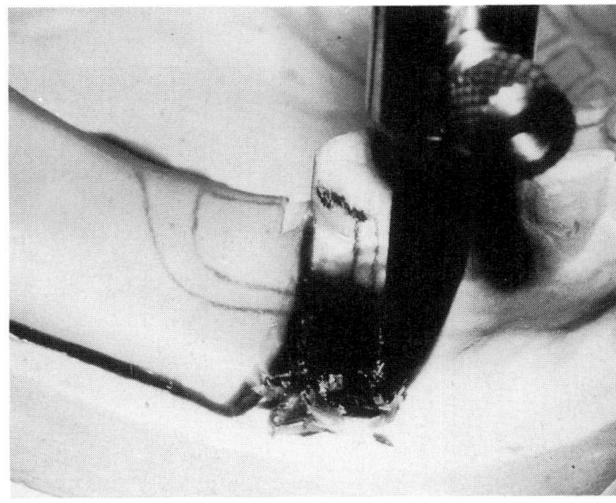

Figure 20–23 ■ Excess wax is cut away with the wax carving blade provided with the surveyor.

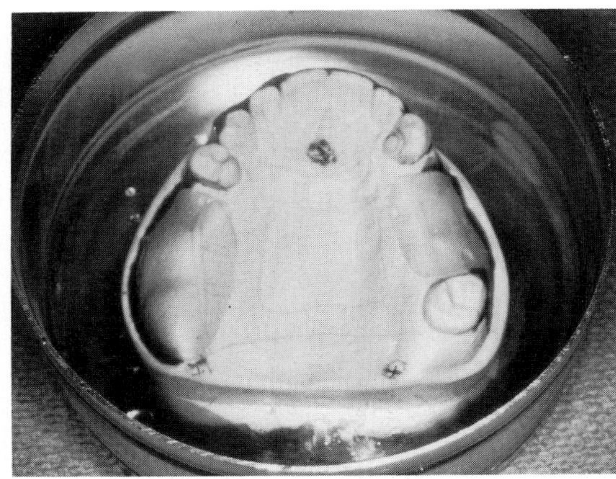

Figure 20–25 ■ The master cast is secured in the duplicating flask ready to receive the impression material.

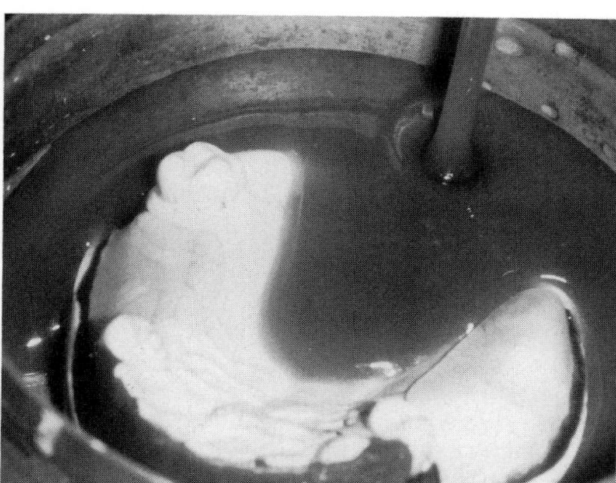

Figure 20–26 ■ The duplication material is flowed slowly over the master cast to prevent bubble formation on the surface of the cast.

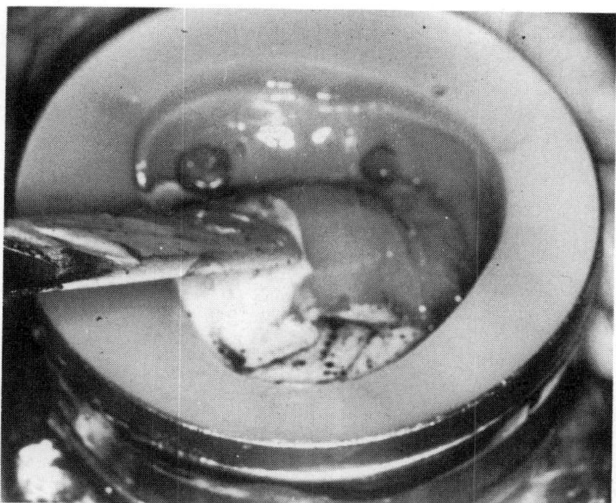

Figure 20–28 ■ After the duplication material is cooled and set, the master cast is removed, and refractory material is poured to produce a high heat refractory cast on which the metal for the RPD casting will be formed.

duplication flash, and secure it with wax to prevent movement (Fig. 20–25).

4. Place and seal the top portion of the flask.

5. Check the duplicating material for correct temperature and smooth consistency.

6. Flow the duplicating material over the cast slowly to prevent surface bubble formation, and fill the reservoir (Fig. 20–26).

7. Place the *base* of the flask in cool running water for 1 hr.

8. Carefully remove the master cast from the duplicating material with air and examine the duplication surface for defects (Fig. 20–27).

The duplication impression is poured with refractory cast investment, which is prepared according to the individual manufacturer's directions (Fig. 20–28). Refractory cast materials vary for different types of metals. Metals that have a high melting temperature require an acid-bound material for accurate reproduction and to support the higher temperatures.

Separation of the refractory model is done with care, as the surface of most refractory materials is quite soft and can be easily mutilated by contact. Do not touch areas that will be used for the partial casting contact (Fig. 20–29).

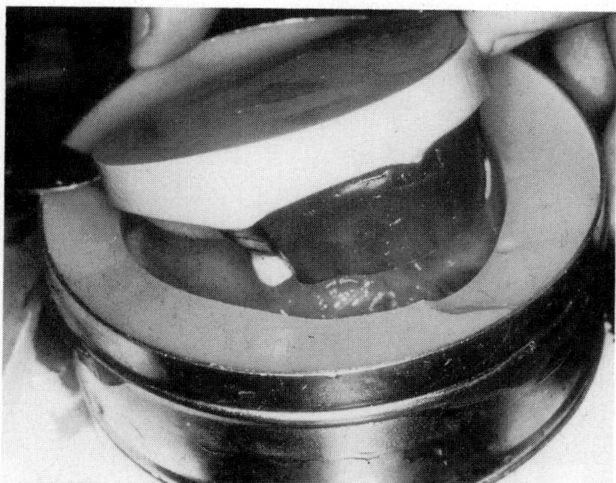

Figure 20–27 ■ The master cast is carefully removed from the duplication material.

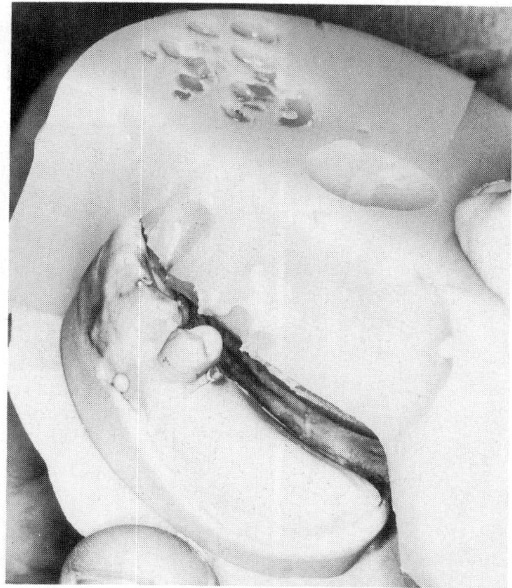

Figure 20–29 ■ Handle the refractory cast by the base to avoid destroying surface detail on the teeth.

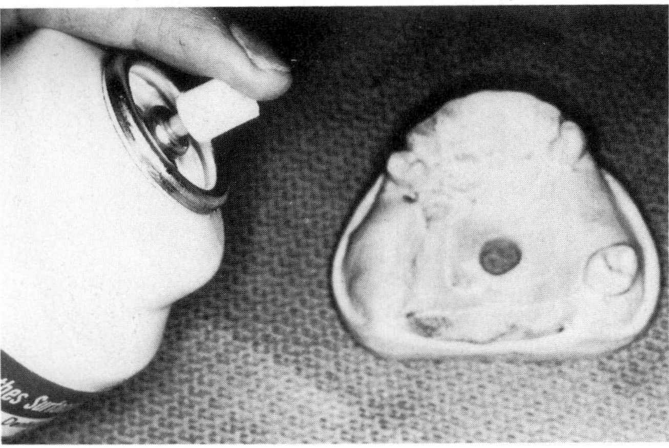

Figure 20–30 ■ The surface of the refractory cast is treated by spraying or dipping in sealer to provide a hard, sticky surface for applying the wax to form the RPD casting.

1. Check the size of the cast and the position of the sprue casting hole within a casting ring to ensure proper placement.
2. The surface of most refractory casts must be treated by dipping or lightly spraying with sealer to form a hard, protective surface and to facilitate the adhesion of the wax (Fig. 20–30).
3. The accuracy of the refractory cast can be checked with the occlusal index that was used for checking the master cast.
4. The outline of the partial denture design can be lightly traced on the refractory cast with a red wax pencil (Fig. 20–31). The design on the diagnostic cast is used as a guide.
5. The refractory cast is ready for the application of a wax pattern that will provide the form and contour for the metal casting.
6. In some cases requiring extensive occlusal restoration and opposing occlusal contacts, it may be necessary to mount the refractory casts on the articulator. When indicated, the face bow and interocclusal registrations, as previously described, are used for articulator mountings. The occlusal contours are then developed in wax and reproduced in metal.

FABRICATING THE WAX PATTERN FOR THE CASTING

1. The framework design is lightly sketched on the treated refractory cast, duplicating the design on the diagnostic cast. Red waxed pencil is used, with care taken not to damage the cast.
2. Hard wax of the inlay type is flowed onto all rest areas to reduce the possibility of chipping or wear (Fig. 20–32). (Avoid flowing wax *beyond* the design, which results in excessive metal in the finished casting.)

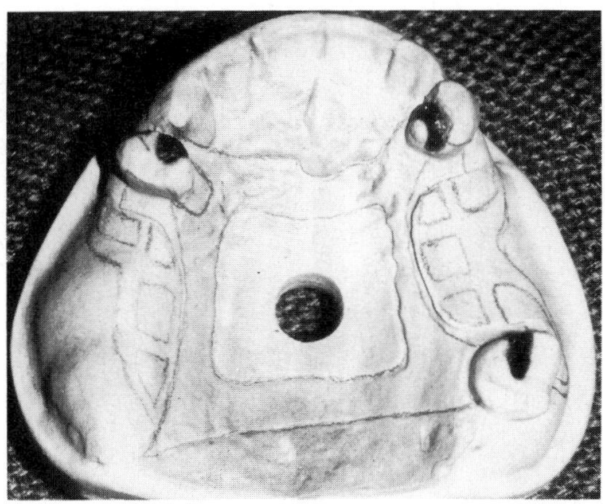

Figure 20–31 ■ The outline of the partial design is lightly drawn on the cast as a guide for applying wax. A sprue hole is positioned in the center of the cast.

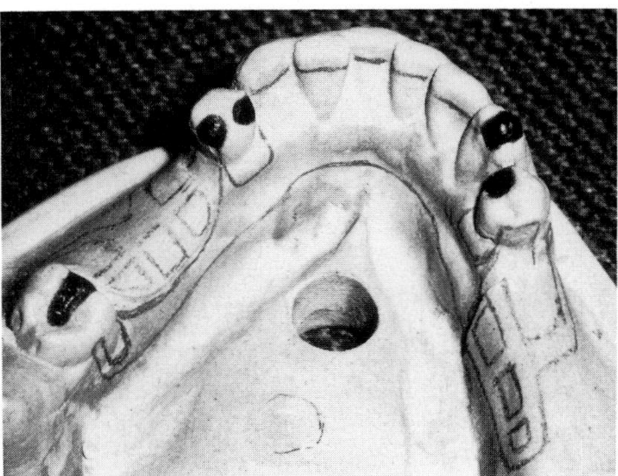

Figure 20–32 ■ Hard inlay type wax is first applied to all rest areas to help prevent damage to the cast in these crucial locations.

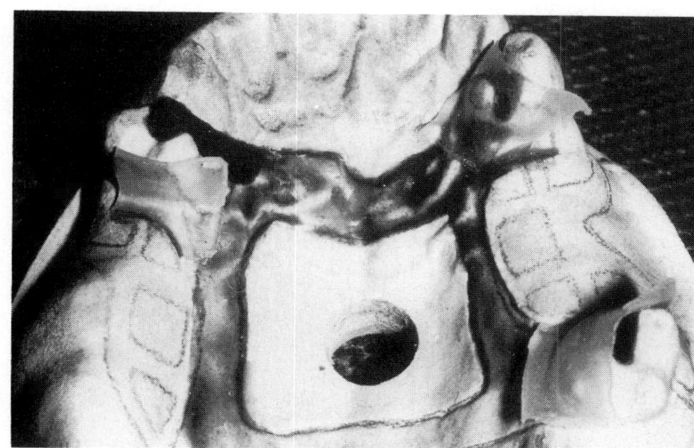

Figure 20–33 ■ Wax is placed in all beaded borders and in areas that will require additional thickness for strength.

3. Flow the wax into beaded areas, finish lines, and over rouge for additional thickness and smoothness (Fig. 20–33).

4. *Mandibular cast*—Place the lingual bar (6-gauge, pear-shaped), with the heavy surface down, in the prescribed position, and lute it in place (Fig. 20–34).

5. *Maxillary cast*—The center of the posterior palatal connector is strengthened by placing an 8-gauge, ½-round wax pattern in the center of the design. Slightly flatten the wax pattern for a smoother finish (Fig. 20–35).

6. *Maxillary cast*—Select a piece of 24-gauge sheet wax, either smooth or pebble-surface (Fig. 20–36), cut a small hole in the center, and make a cut from the hole to the outer surface. This will aid in adaptation. Adapt this sheet over the design for major connectors and guiding surfaces (Fig. 20–37) and onto the area of denture base retention for 1 mm (Fig. 20–38). The wax is adapted with finger pressure and the eraser of a pencil cut to the shape of a V. Trim the wax to the outline with a sharp instrument (Fig. 20–39).

7. The denture base retention is formed with 12-gauge, ½-round wax forms (flat side down) in the edentulous areas (Fig. 20–40). Wax junctions with the connectors are built up to a strong fan-shaped union by adding extra wax.

8. Retainers are positioned, using preformed plastic patterns. *Adhesive liquid is placed on the cast before positioning the patterns* (Figs. 20–41 and 20–42). The taper of the retainer is altered as necessary with wax and is joined with the main body of the partial denture in a strong bond by adding wax (Fig. 20–43).

9. Finish lines are formed with 18-gauge round wax (Fig. 20–44).

10. Additional wax is added where necessary for strength, contour, and smoothness.

11. If necessary, a second layer of sheet wax may be added for bulk or smoothness (Fig. 20–45).

12. All surfaces are smoothed with a light flame or with cotton and water (Fig. 20–46).

13. Finish lines are checked for sharpness, and excessive wax beyond the design is removed (Fig. 20–47).

14. Check the placement of the denture teeth to ensure that there are sufficient space and no interference problems (Fig. 20–48).

WAX FORMS USED

For the Maxillary Arch

8-gauge ½-round (posterior palatal strap)
12-gauge ½-round (base retention)

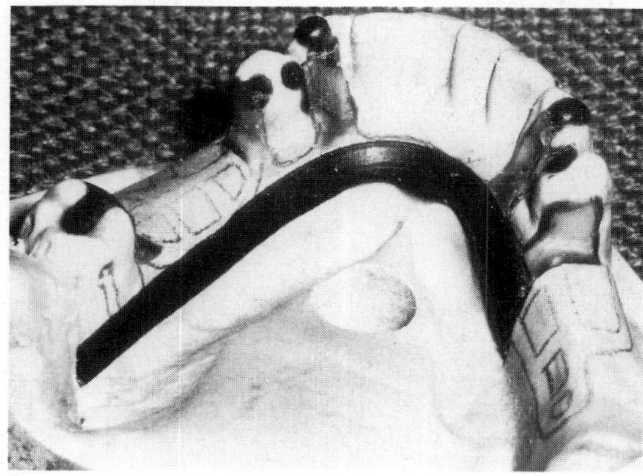

Figure 20–34 ■ The lingual bar of pear-shaped wax is positioned with the bulky side down on the mandibular cast.

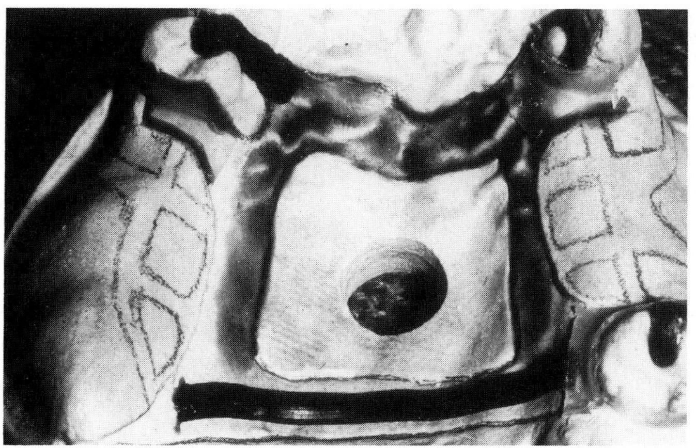

Figure 20–35 ■ A $\frac{1}{2}$-round wax form is placed in the center of the posterior palatal bar for strength.

18-gauge round (finish lines)
Pebbled tan *or* smooth green sheet (palatal connectors)
Clear 22- to 24-gauge with a sticky side (proximal plates)
I bar, plastic preformed

For the Mandibular Arch

6-gauge $\frac{1}{2}$-round pear-shaped (lingual bar, flat side against tissue, thick margin toward the vestibule)
12-gauge $\frac{1}{2}$-round (base retention)
18-gauge round (finish lines)
Clear 22- or 24-gauge with sticky side (proximal plates)
I bar, plastic preformed
($\frac{1}{2}$- and full-round rods, in 4- to 5-in lengths)

Detailed information for the casting design is transmitted to the laboratory and the technician by means of the diagnostic cast. Specific problems of occlusion and contour are known only to the doctor, who has a clinical knowledge of the situation. This information must be communicated to the laboratory. A check at the wax-up stage by the doctor allows for modifications, changes, and additions to the wax pattern prior to casting. A knowledge of wax-up procedures and methods is essential if the doctor is to be able to alter wax patterns and to demonstrate to the laboratory technician exactly what is being requested.

INVESTING, CASTING, AND FINISHING

These procedures are accomplished by the laboratory in most instances. The finished casting is returned to the doctor for approval and evaluation in the patient's mouth.

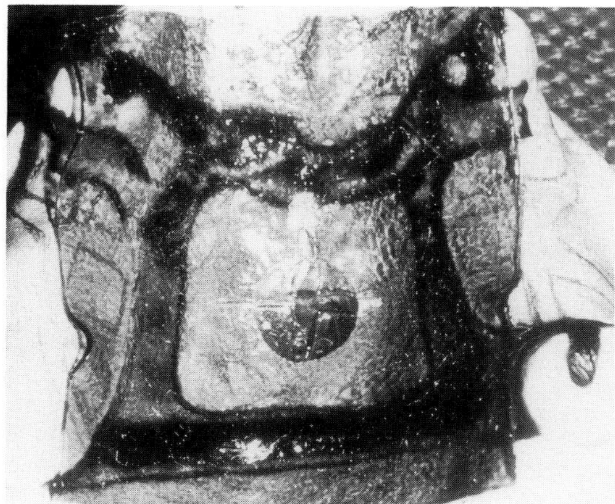

Figure 20–36 ■ A sheet of 24-gauge wax is applied over the entire surface of the cast and trimmed to the outline of the metal casting.

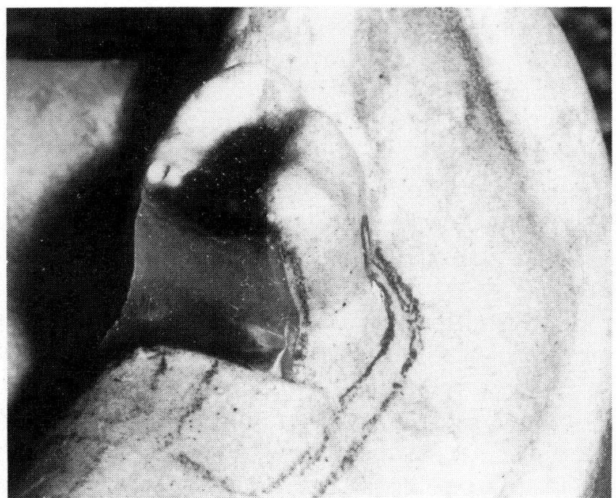

Figure 20–37 ■ The sheet wax is adapted and trimmed to conform to the tooth and tissue area that will be reproduced in metal.

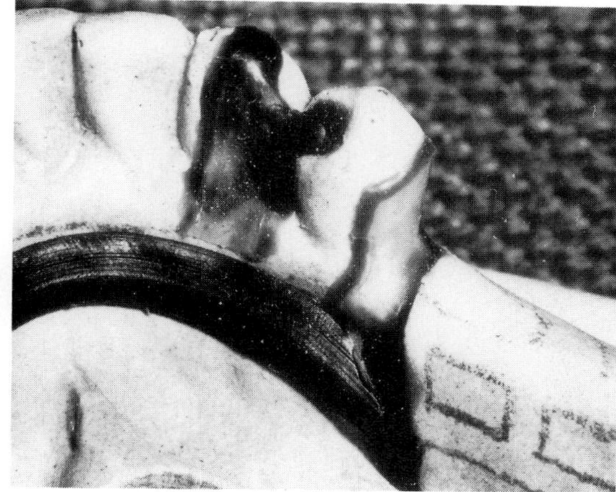

Figure 20-38 ■ The sheet wax extends onto the denture base retention area and is securely waxed to the refractory cast.

EVALUATION OF THE FINISHED CASTING

1. The metal must conform to the design.
2. There must be no excess metal in the rest areas.
3. The guiding surfaces must be in contact with the tooth surface.
4. There must be sharp and definite finish lines.
5. There must be metal-tissue contact where requested.
6. There must be good contours, shape, and smoothness.
7. There must be proper taper, position, and contact of retention areas.

Comparison of the finished casting on the master cast with the submitted diagnostic cast

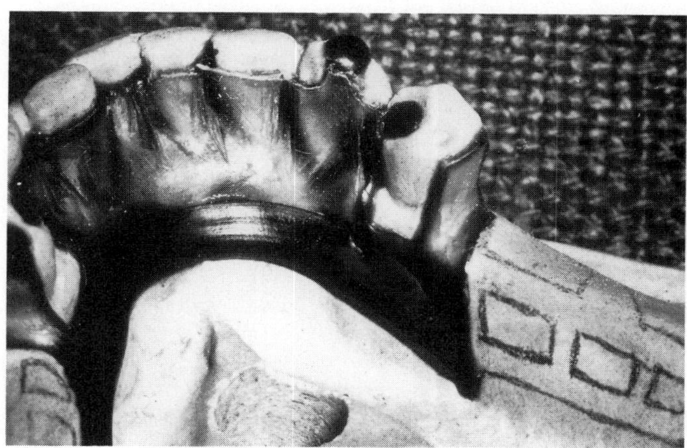

Figure 20-39 ■ The wax is trimmed to the *exact outline* that is required for the finished metal casting.

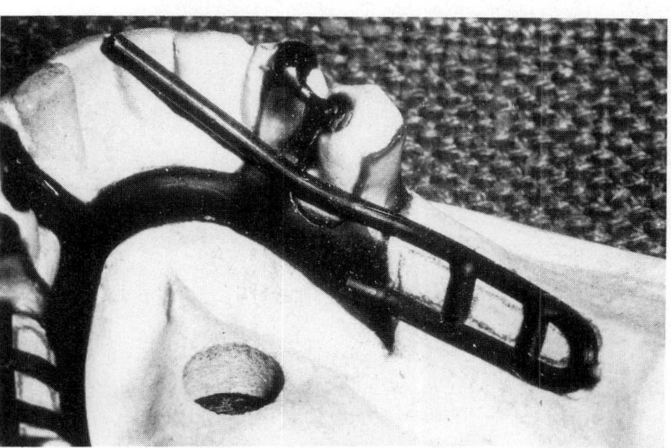

Figure 20-40 ■ Denture base retention is formed with 12-gauge wax firmly attached to the body of the wax pattern, with additional wax for bulk and strength.

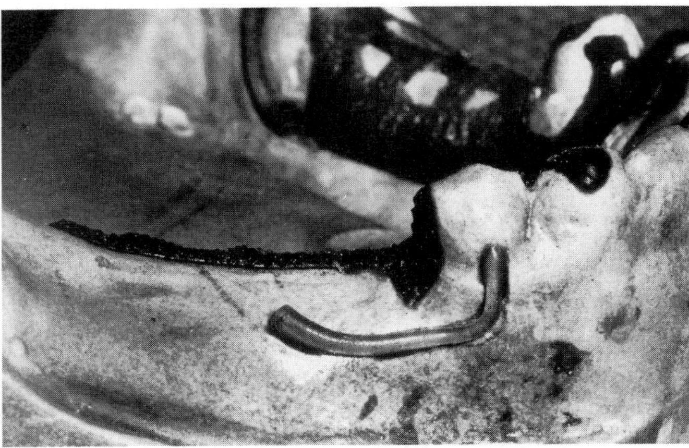

Figure 20–41 ■ Preformed, tapered plastic retainers are positioned over a special adhesive applied to the refractory cast surface.

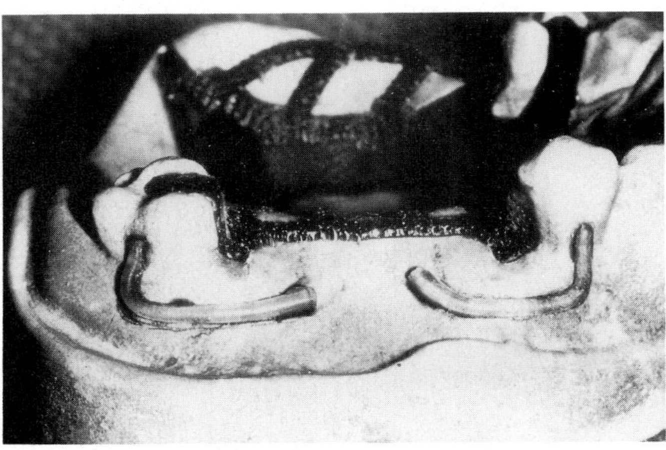

Figure 20–42 ■ The tip of the retainer must be placed in the exact position determined with the surveyor and undercut gauge for correct retention.

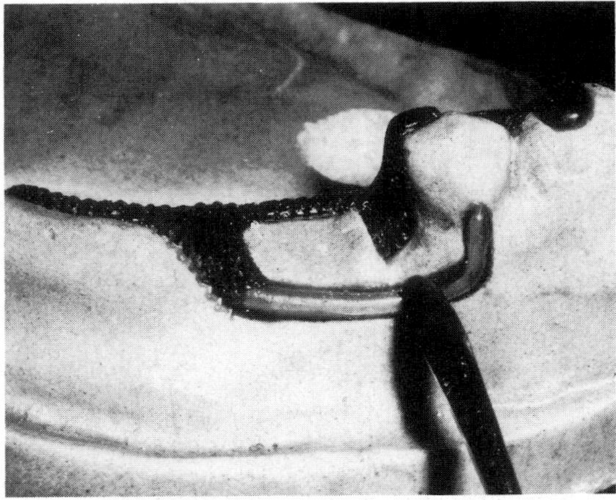

Figure 20–43 ■ The retainer is connected with the denture base retention with extra bulk for strength. The bulk and taper of the retainer can be altered by adding wax.

provides a good basis for communication, evaluation, and production of a completed casting that follows design specifications (Fig. 20–49).

FITTING THE CASTING TO THE MASTER CAST

Precise adaptation of the casting to the master cast ensures good adaptation in the patient's mouth and prevents unnecessary time and adjustment in the operatory. Fitting the casting requires the greatest of care and respect for the stone master cast to prevent damage during the process. If the casting is adjusted on an undistorted stone cast, it will fit in the mouth equally well. The doctor may perform this procedure or request that the laboratory do the final fitting.

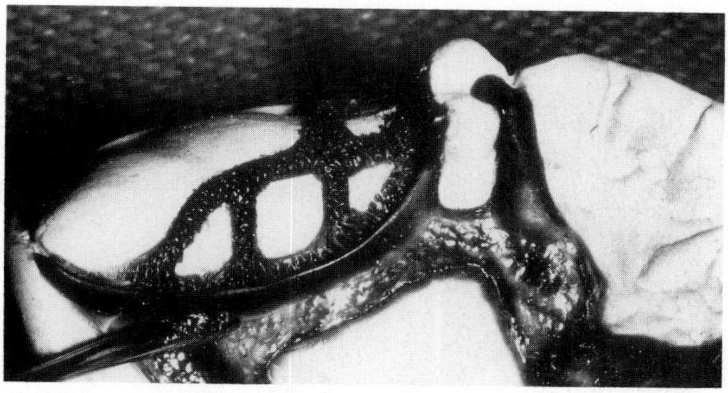

Figure 20–44 ■ External finish lines for the junction of plastic and metal are formed by adding 18-gauge round wax and carving it to a sharp margin.

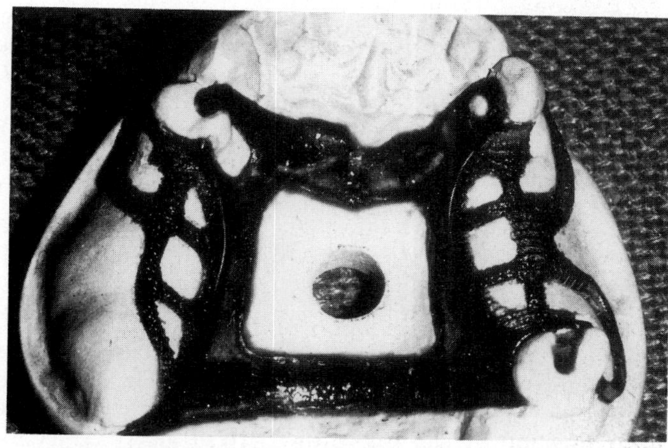

Figure 20–45 ■ When additional bulk for strength is necessary, a second layer of sheet wax is placed and smoothed.

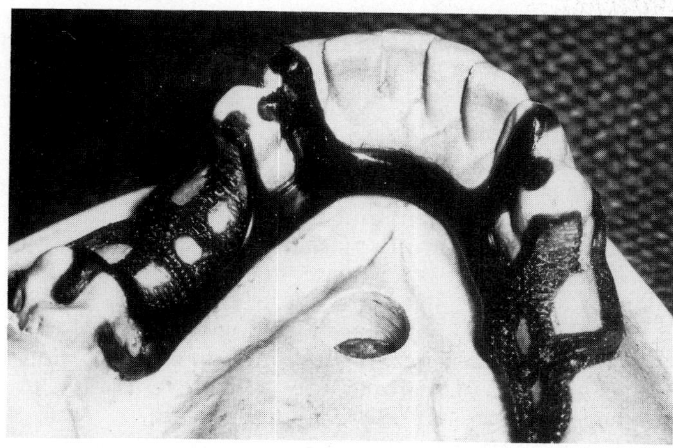

Figure 20–46 ■ The surface of the pattern can be smoothed with a light flame and polished with wet cotton.

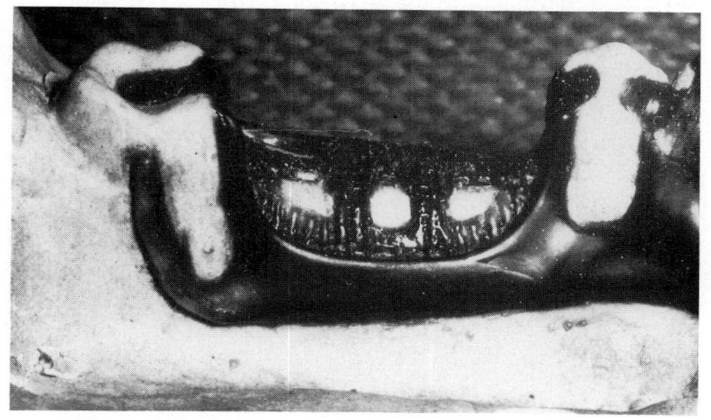

Figure 20–47 ■ Final contouring to the exact duplication required for the finished casting saves finish time on the completed casting.

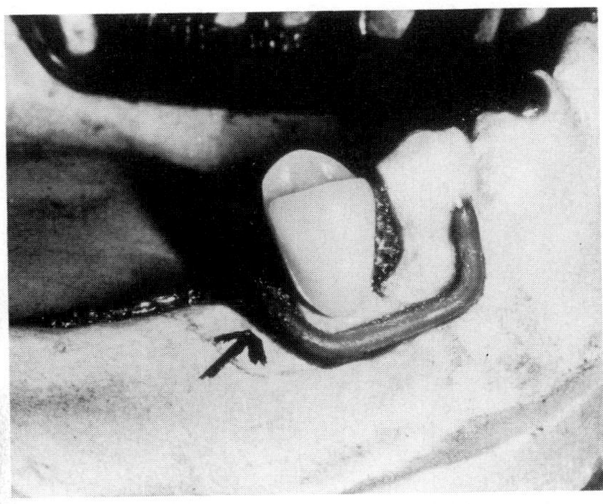

Figure 20–48 ■ Check the placement of the prosthetic denture tooth to ensure that there is sufficient space.

Procedure

1. Remove tooth retention undercuts from the stone cast. These areas are *planned undercut areas* and will offer resistance to seating (Fig. 20–50).
2. Position the casting in the path of insertion on the stone cast until resistance is encountered (Fig. 20–51). Do not use force.
3. Locate points of resistance visually, by the presence of stone particles, or by disclosing material on the casting.
4. Relieve the metal casting at interference points.
5. Repeat the steps until the casting slides smoothly and easily into place (Fig. 20–52).
6. Inspect all areas for proper fit and adaptation.

This laboratory procedure of fitting and adjusting to the master cast saves time and eliminates grinding in the operatory and prevents damage and pressure to the abutment teeth.

DEVELOPING OCCLUSION

The principles of developing occlusion have been discussed in Chapter 17 and are incorporated with the laboratory steps to ensure production of the required final result. Many doctors request that the technician place the denture teeth, while others may prefer to arrange the teeth themselves. Both must know the scheme of occlusion requested and the basic principles of occlusion and articulation.

The occlusion with the metal casting in place on the articulator are evaluated for

1. Correct occlusal contact against opposing teeth and prosthesis.
2. Proper vertical dimension.
3. Correct position of the plane of occlusion.

The necessary adjustments are made if indicated.

Procedure for Placing Teeth

1. Select teeth of mold and size to correspond and harmonize with the remaining natural teeth. The space available will influence selection to a degree. It is usually necessary to *reshape most surfaces* of the denture tooth.
2. Position *the first prosthetic tooth* for proper occlusal functional position *opposite the remaining natural teeth* (Fig. 20–53).
3. Adjust the cervical and interproximal surfaces as necessary to achieve the best occlusal position.
4. The occlusal surface of the tooth is adjusted to all functional positions (i.e., centric and eccentric).
5. The remainder of the teeth are positioned and adjusted to obtain their best possible position in all excursions.
6. When the entire posterior opposing occlusions (both maxillary and mandibular) are re-

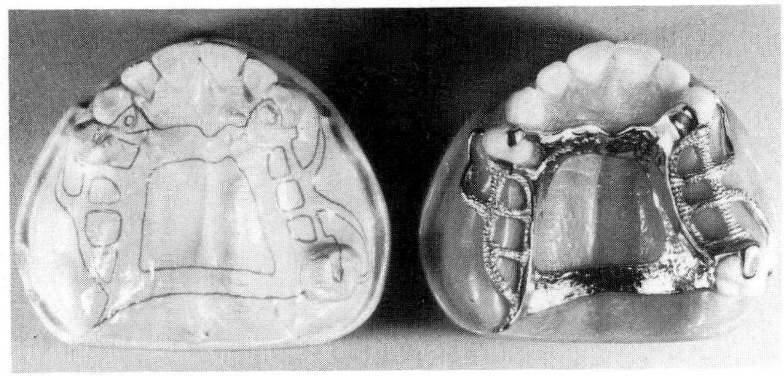

Figure 20–49 ■ The finished casting placed on the master cast can be compared with the design on the diagnostic cast to ensure that the prescribed design has been reproduced.

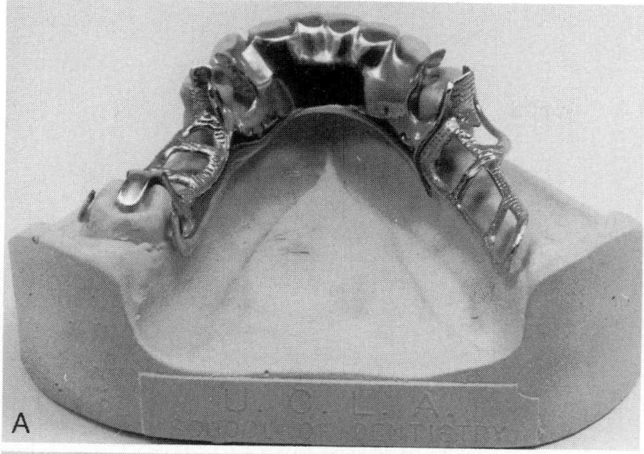

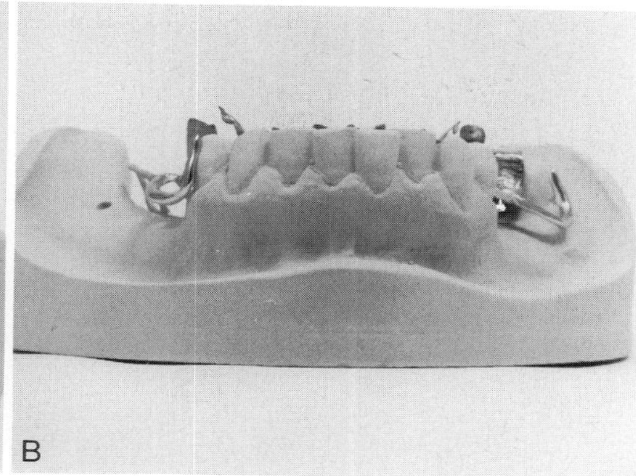

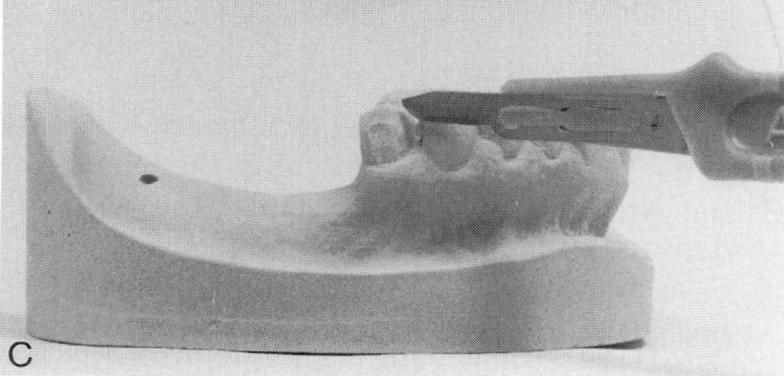

Figure 20–50 ■ *A*, When the finished casting is fitted to the master cast, the retention areas are removed, since they are planned undercuts. *B*, The undercut or retention portion of the stone cast tooth must be removed to allow easy seating of the ridged parts of the casting. *C*, The retention portion of the stone cast is removed with a sharp scalpel.

placed, it is advantageous to position one arch *first* in the most proper location and to then place the opposing teeth (Fig. 20–54).

No matter who develops the occlusion—doctor or technician—they both must evaluate the occlusion and placement of teeth on the articulator before the next step in fabrication is accomplished (Fig. 20–55).

DENTURE BASE WAX-UP

The contour, position, and color of the denture base influences the esthetics and function of the final prosthesis. Lingual and facial contours can affect the movement of food, the actions of tongue and cheek, and the contour of the face (Figs. 20–56 and 20–57). The shape of

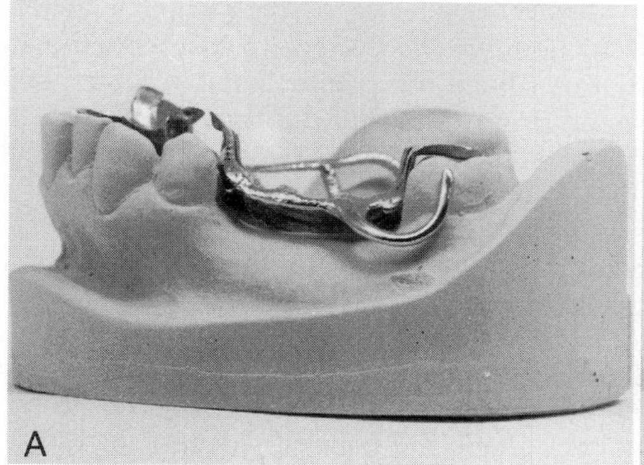

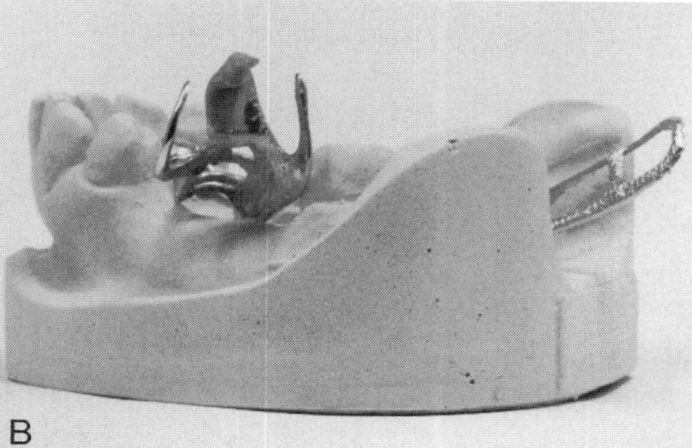

Figure 20–51 ■ *A*, The casting is seated on the master cast until resistance is encountered. Do not use force. *B*, Areas of contact are located and metal relieved. These areas are identified by presence of stone particles or by using a disclosing medium.

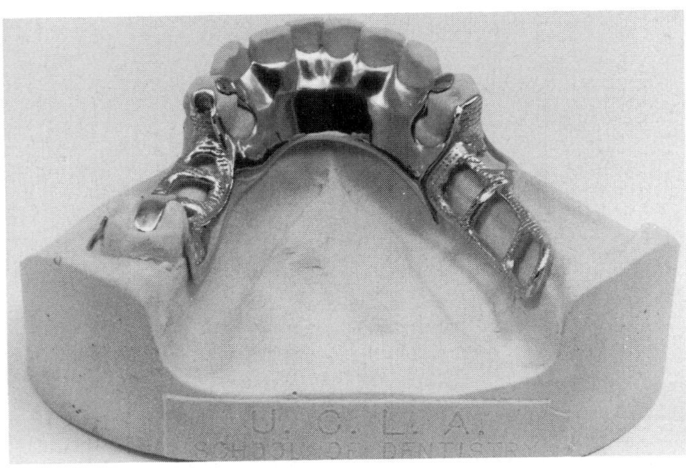

Figure 20–52 ■ The fitting steps are repeated until the metal casting slips on the master cast with minimal force.

the denture base at the cervical and interproximal areas of the teeth has a profound effect on the mold and size of the teeth. This is especially evident when teeth are *overwaxed* or overcovered with the denture base, making them appear short and small and not compatible with adjacent natural teeth.

Procedure

1. The contours should be a continuation of those in adjacent dentulous areas; there should be no abrupt changes (Fig. 20–58).
2. The cervical and interproximal height of the gingiva is at an equal level between natural and prosthetic teeth.
3. The use of a donor cast of a complete arch of natural teeth is useful as a guide for wax-up.

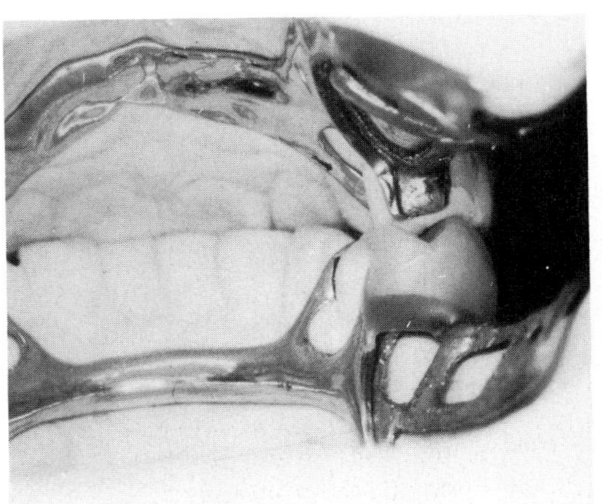

Figure 20–53 ■ The first prosthetic tooth is placed for proper cusp-fossa relationship with the remaining natural teeth, and the occlusion is adjusted for compatibility in centric and eccentric positions.

4. A natural, stippled appearance of the gums is produced by softening the surface of the wax and then lightly tapping it with the denture brush.
5. Remove all excess wax from tooth surfaces.
6. When the waxing is completed, check the occlusion for possible tooth movement in all positions (Fig. 20–59).

FLASKING OF THE PROSTHESIS

The primary objectives of flasking the partial dentures are to

1. Form a core to hold the exact position of the denture teeth in relation to the metal casting when the wax is removed.
2. Preserve the wax contours of the denture base.

Procedure

1. Remove the waxed-up cast from the articulator. (Place the plaster base in water before separating the partial denture stone base from the plaster mounting base).
2. Place a thin coat of petroleum jelly on *all* exposed stone areas of the cast, including remount keys, *or* cover the stone base with aluminum foil.
3. Coat the inner surfaces of the denture flask with petroleum jelly (Fig. 20–60). Prepare dental plaster (100 gr of stone to 30 ml of water). Place the base of the cast in the lower portion of the flask up *to the wax, covering all portions of the metal casting.* The plaster is trimmed and shaped while in a soft state to

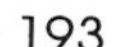

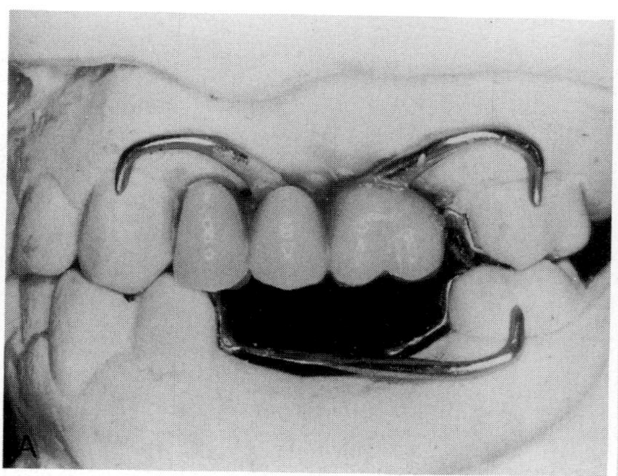

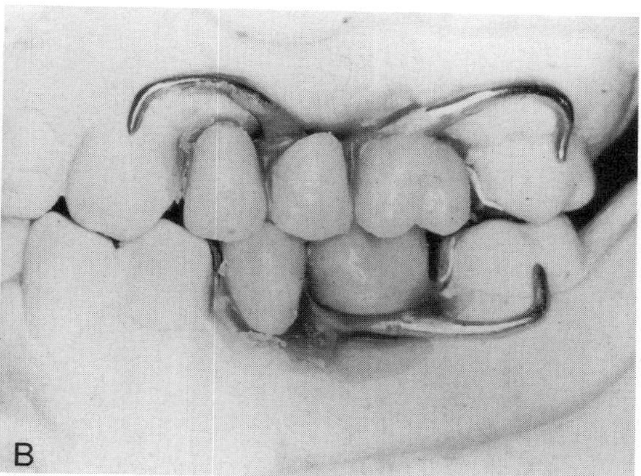

Figure 20–54 ■ *A*, When developing occlusion, one arch is placed in an ideal position and then fixed in position by cooling the wax. *B*, Opposing teeth are then placed in centric occlusion and adjusted to remove interference in excursions.

remove all undercuts. The *larger* the *angle of draw* the fewer the *separation difficulties* (Fig. 20–61).

4. Coat all surfaces of the exposed plaster liberally with petroleum jelly.
5. Place the top half of the metal flask in position. Ensure intimate adaptation of the two parts.
6. Coat all exposed surfaces of the denture teeth and the wax with a thin layer of silicone material or with dental stone (Fig. 20–62). (The silicone material such as Dent-Kote makes separation of the flask easier, with less potential of cast fracture.)
7. Pour the plaster into the top half of the flask, level with the occlusal surfaces of the denture teeth. The occlusal surfaces remain exposed.
8. When the plaster is set, apply a thin layer of petroleum jelly to all exposed surfaces, fill with plaster, and close the flask lid.

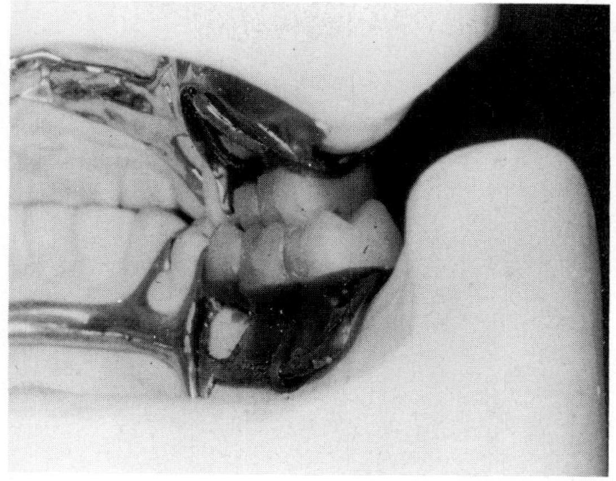

Figure 20–55 ■ Although the technician may have arranged the tooth placement, it is the doctor's responsibility to evaluate and alter it as necessary at insertion.

WAX REMOVAL

The objective of this procedure is to remove the wax used to form the denture base from the flask with minimum liquefaction of the wax. Excess heat

1. Forces the wax into the stone and makes elimination difficult.
2. Weakens the investing stone.
3. Interferes with the application and effectiveness of the separating medium.

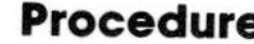

Procedure

1. When the plaster is completely set, place the flask in hot water for 5 min.
2. Remove it from water and *carefully* separate the two halves of the flask (Fig. 20–63).
3. Remove the wax (it should be in a softened but *not* liquid state).
4. Wash out the remaining wax under hot water (Fig. 20–64). (Excessive washing under hot water will erode the dental stone.)
5. Allow the flask to dry and cool. Brush a thin coat of separating material onto the stone surfaces of *both halves* of the flask.
6. Allow to dry for 10 min or more, and apply a second thin coat of separating material (Fig. 20–65).

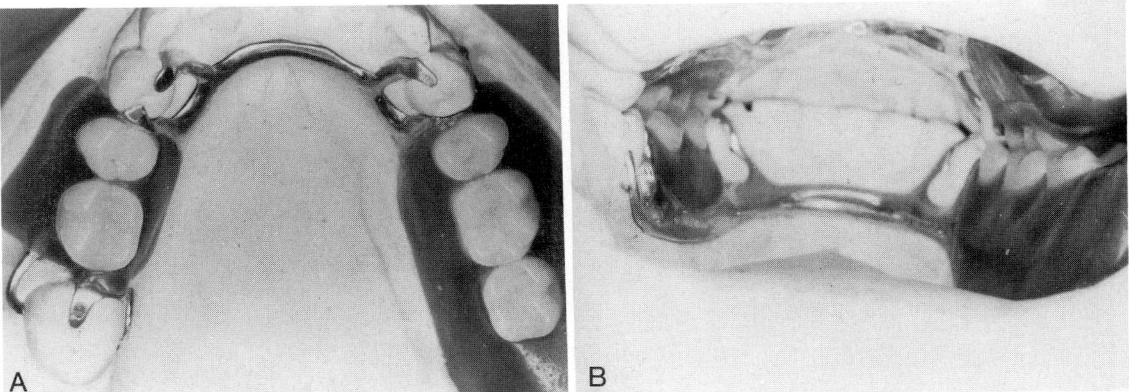

Figure 20–56 ■ *A*, Denture base areas are contoured to reproduce the original structures and to make a smooth transition between prosthesis and remaining tissues. *B*, Lingual surfaces of the denture base are contoured so that the lateral surface of the tongue can help to hold the prosthesis in place on the ridge.

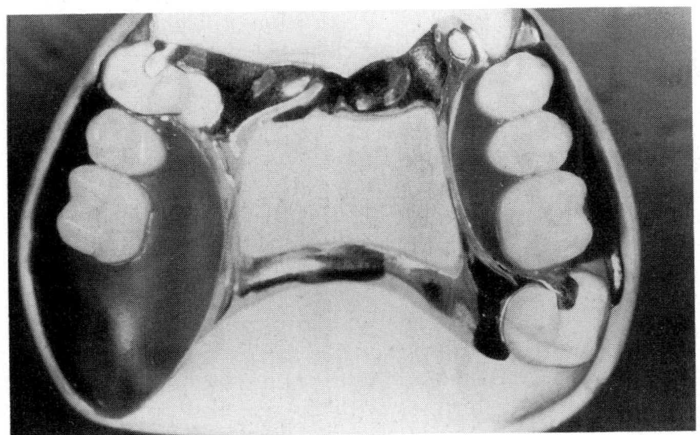

Figure 20–57 ■ Junction or union of tooth and denture base reproduces former anatomy.

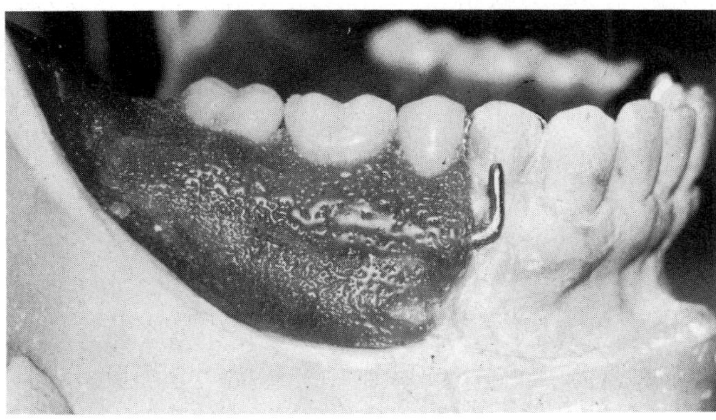

Figure 20–58 ■ The denture base is sculptured to form a natural continuation of existing anatomy.

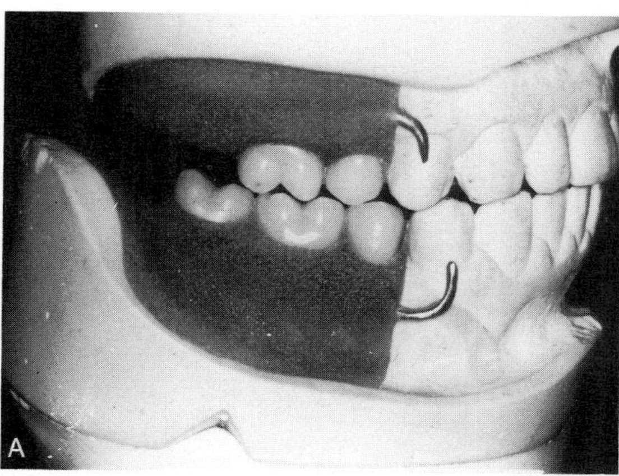

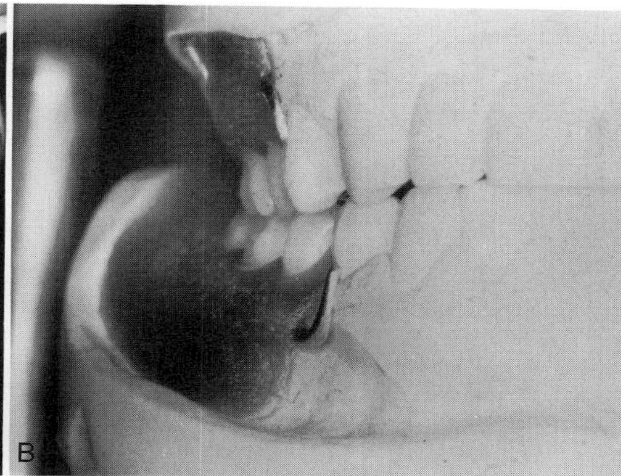

Figure 20–59 ■ *A*, Check occlusion in excursions after waxing is completed to ensure that no tooth movement has occurred. *B*, A final check for good centric contacts is essential.

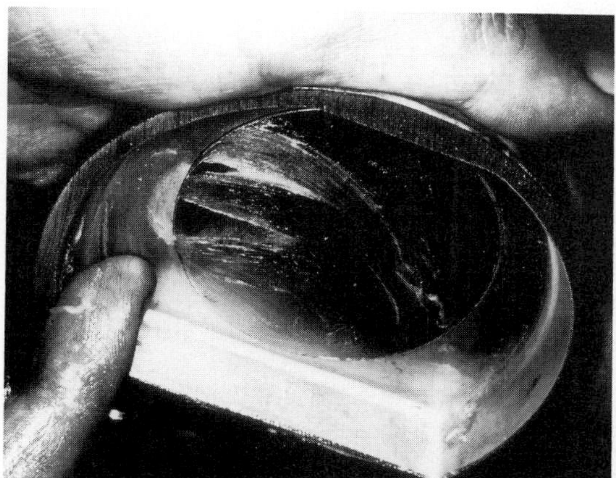

Figure 20–60 ■ Lubrication of the interior surfaces of the denture flask ensures easy, nontraumatic removal of the prosthesis after processing and also preserves the flask.

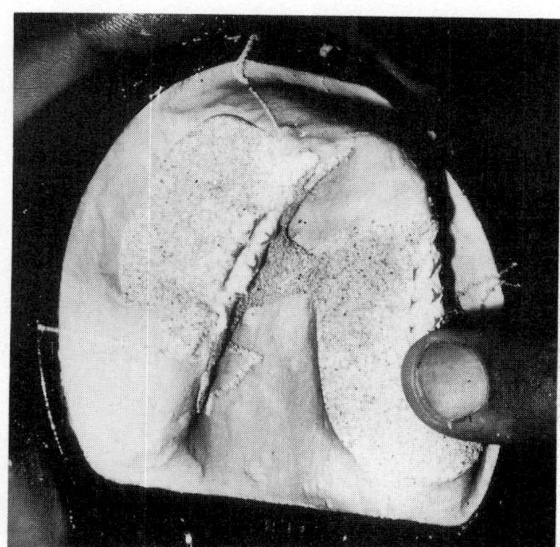

Figure 20–62 ■ Silicone material is painted on the teeth and wax, and the surface is sprinkled with crushed walnut shell for adherence to the overcoat of plaster. The silicone provides easy separation in deflasking.

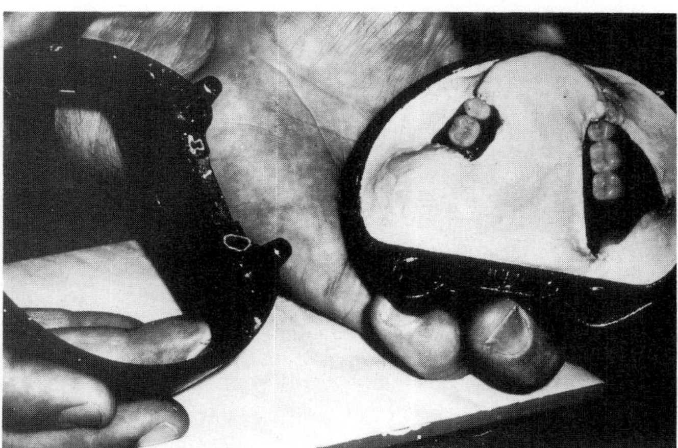

Figure 20–61 ■ The waxed prosthesis is embedded in plaster in the lower half of the flask with only prosthetic teeth and wax exposed. The plaster is shaped so that no undercuts are present in the plaster.

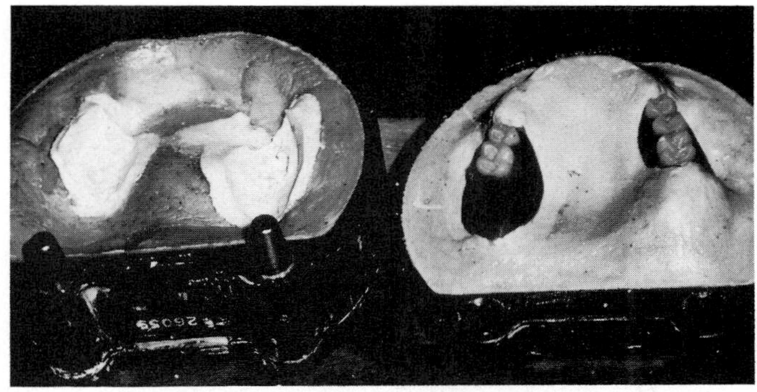

Figure 20–63 ■ The top half of the flask is filled with plaster and allowed to set, then placed in hot water and separated. The softened wax is removed.

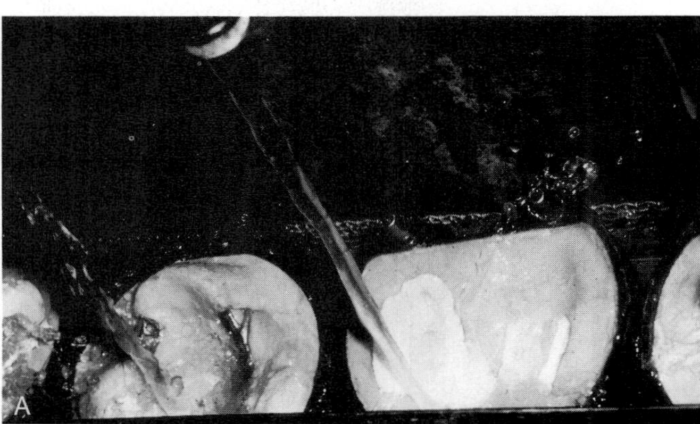

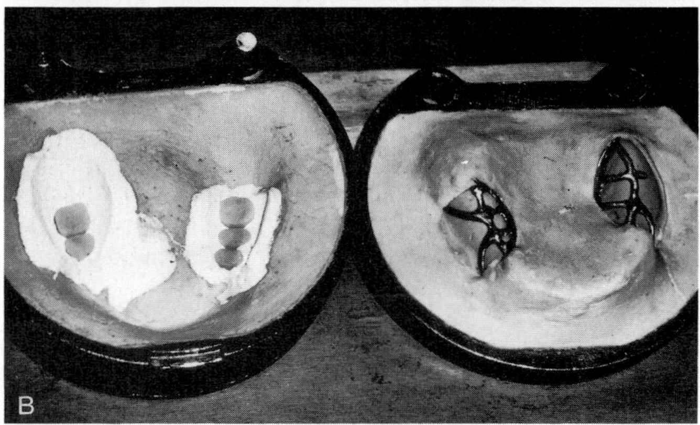

Figure 20–64 ■ *A*, The residual wax is removed with boiling water. *B*, The separated halves of the flask are allowed to dry and cool.

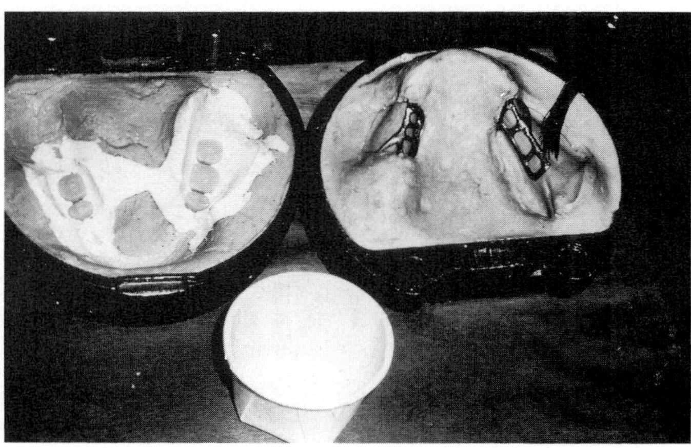

Figure 20–65 ■ A thin coat of separating medium is brushed on the stone edentulous area and allowed to dry, and a second thin coat is applied.

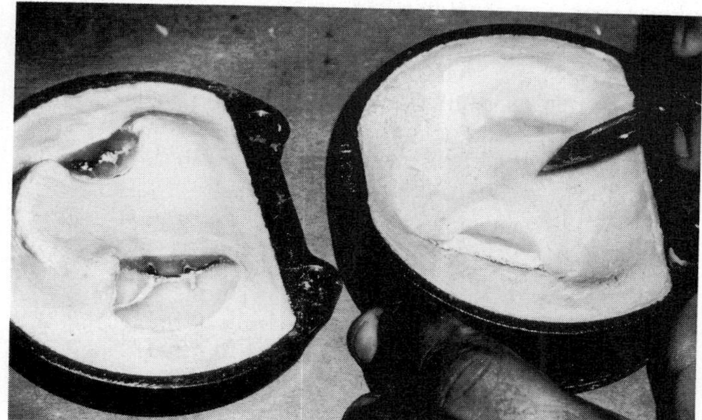

Figure 20–66 ■ Acrylic is placed on both halves of the flask, a plastic sheet is positioned between the halves, and the flask is placed in the press. The flask is separated, and excess acrylic is removed by cutting.

PACKING THE ACRYLIC INTO THE FLASK

The objectives of this laboratory procedure are to

1. Replace the denture base wax contours with acrylic.
2. Unite the denture teeth to the metal casting.
3. Form the tissue surface over the edentulous area.

Procedure

1. Measure the acrylic portions of the prescribed type and color (1 part liquid to 3 parts powder). Mix and allow to set in a covered container until it is no longer sticky. The container can be cooled, which prolongs the working time available before it hardens.
2. A small portion of auto-curing acrylic is placed between the most distal part of the metal denture base retention area and the stone cast. The purpose is to prevent bending of the metal during packing.
3. Place the acrylic in *both* halves of the flask sufficient to *overfill* the area by one third. Form into the approximate shape of the existing space.
4. *Place separating plastic* between the two flask halves and carefully close them.
5. Close the press gently, allowing the acrylic time to flow. Excess pressure will break the stone, move the teeth, and bend the metal casting.
6. Separate the flask, remove excess acrylic from all surfaces (Fig. 20–66), replace the separating plastic, and repeat the process until *no* excess material is expressed.
7. *Remove the separating plastic,* coat the opposing surfaces of the acrylic with liquid monomer, and close the flask and place it in a processing clamp.

Other methods of investing and packing are injection and pouring procedures that accomplish the same objectives with other methods and materials.

CURING THE ACRYLIC

The objective when curing acrylic is to bring the two constituents of acrylic (the polymer powder and the monomer liquid) up to the curing temperature, at which point a reaction takes place between the two materials that is then self-perpetuating. When the reaction begins, excess heat is given off that can be detrimental to the acrylic; therefore, it is desirable to prevent a rise in temperature beyond the temperature of polymerization.

Procedure

1. Secure the flask in the curing press, which is placed in cold water.
2. Bring the water temperature to 158°F, and hold it there for 8 hr.
3. Bring the water temperature to 165°F, and hold it there for 1 hr.
4. Allow the flask to bench cool to room temperature.

Step 2 brings the acrylic to the reaction temperature, and then the water acts as a cooling agent to suppress the temperature. The elevation of the temperature in Step 3 is a measure to ensure that the temperature does rise to the reaction point.

DEFLASKING THE DENTURE

Care must be exercised not to damage or distort the prosthesis, the stone casts, or the remount indexes on the base, so that the casts with the processed prosthesis can be mounted, intact, back on the articulator.

Procedure

1. Remove the lid and the entire bulk of the stone intact from the flask. (If the entire inner surface of the flask has been coated with petroleum jelly, this procedure can be easily accomplished.)
2. Remove the top of the final pour of stone.
3. Make a series of cuts into the stone on all sides, taking care not to involve the prosthesis.
4. Carefully separate the cuts until the basic stone cast, with the prosthesis in place, remains.
5. Do not damage or destroy the index grooves on the cast base.
6. Remove all investing stone.

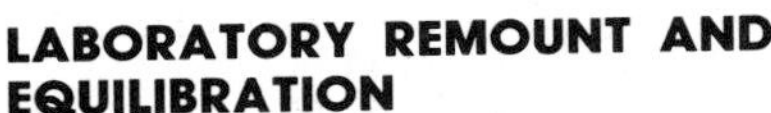

LABORATORY REMOUNT AND EQUILIBRATION

The objective of this procedure is to correct any dimensional or positional discrepancies that may have occurred during the wax-up, flasking, or processing procedures.

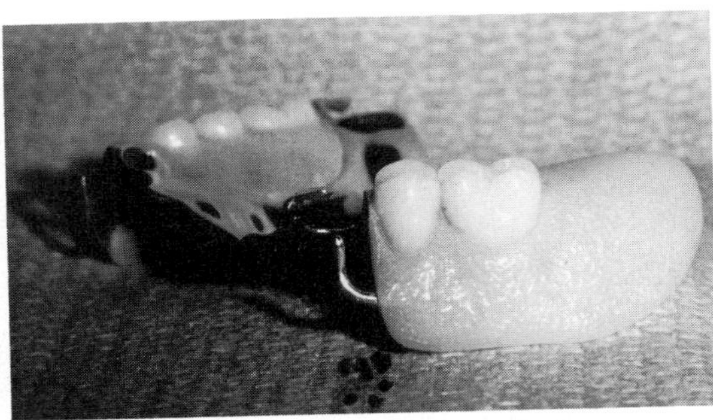

Figure 20–68 ■ The prosthesis is removed from the master cast, then trimmed and polished.

Procedure

1. Reposition the casts with the processed prosthesis in place back on the articulator (Fig. 20–67).
2. The index of the cast and the articulator mounting must be *completely seated.*
3. Secure the cast to the articulator mounting with sticky wax or plaster.
4. Check the articulator for proper adjustments.
5. Reestablish centric occlusion, marking contacts with red articulating ribbon. Restore the original vertical dimension of occlusion.
6. Equilibrate the occlusal surfaces in lateral and protrusive position, using blue articulating ribbon. *Do not remove centric area markings in red.*

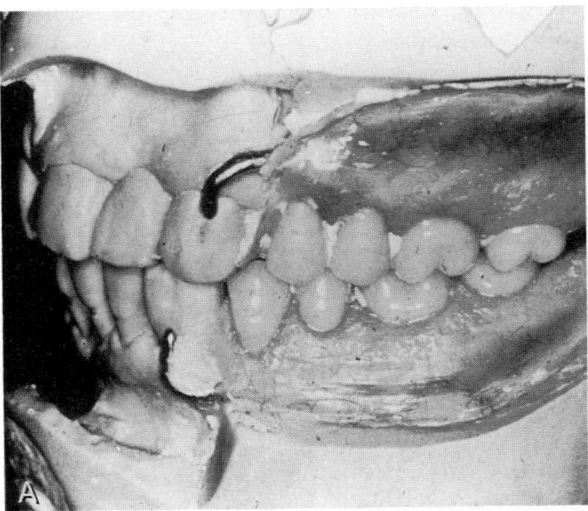

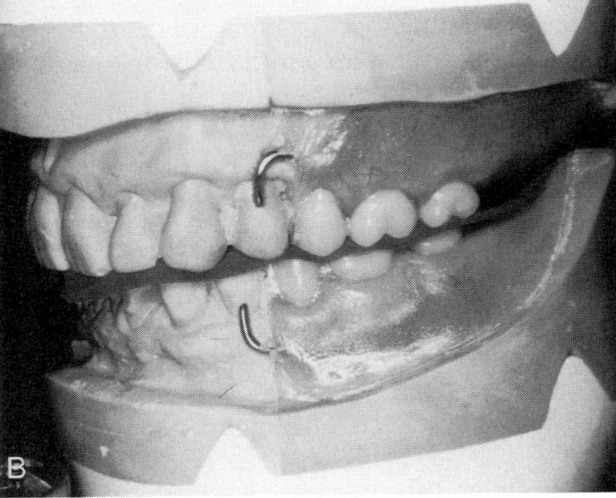

Figure 20–67 ■ After they are processed, the stone casts with the cured prostheses in place are remounted on the articulator. *B*, The prostheses are adjusted to the original vertical dimension established on the articulator by equilibration of the teeth, using articulating ribbon and stones. Eccentric interferences are removed.

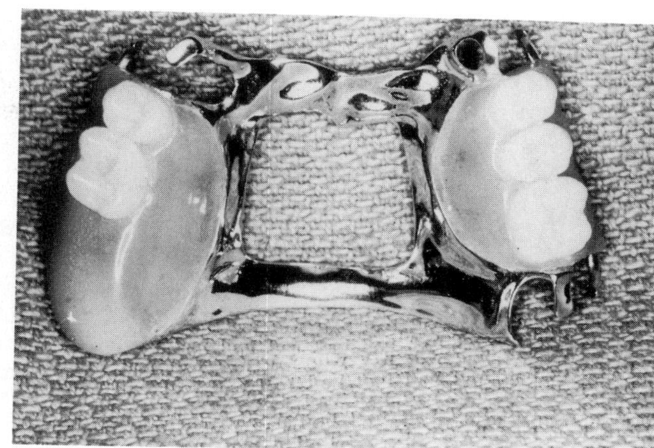

Figure 20–69 ■ The junction of acrylic and metal is shaped and smoothed with a soft rubber wheel.

The occlusal contacts that control the relationship of the maxillary arch to the mandibular arch have now been restored to the same position they occupied on the articulator prior to flasking and processing.

FINISHING THE PROSTHESIS

Procedure

1. A series of cuts are made with the plaster saw around the base of the cast.
2. The cuts are separated carefully to remove portions of the stone cast without deforming the prosthesis.
3. Excess acrylic is removed and contoured if necessary (Fig. 20–68).
4. Excess acrylic *next to metal* is removed, using a rubber wheel (Fig. 20–69).

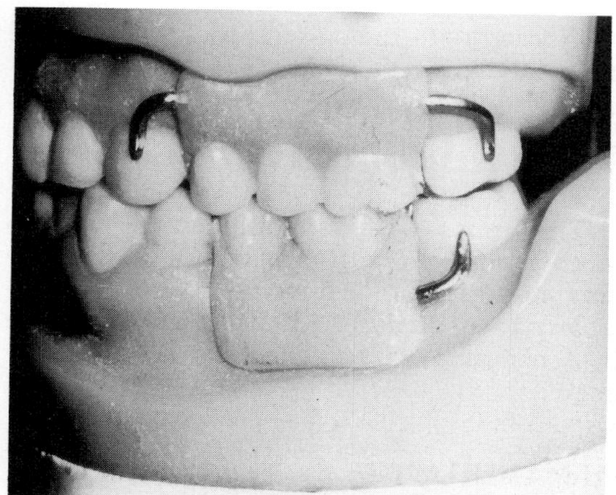

Figure 20–70 ■ The adjusted occlusal surfaces of the porcelain teeth are soothed with procelain polishing wheels.

5. Use brushes *only* for polishing. Use coarse pumice, fine pumice, and whiting, in that order.
6. Polish the occlusal surfaces of porcelain teeth with porcelain polish wheels (Fig. 20–70).
7. Store the prosthesis in water.

REFERENCES

References for Laboratory Procedures

Beck HO: Alloys for removable partial dentures. Dent Clin North Am November:591–596, 1960.

Bolouri A, Hilger TC, and Gowrylok MD: Modified flasking technique for removable partial dentures. J Prosthet Dent 34:221–223, 1975.

Dirkson LC and Campagna SJ: Mat surface and rugae reproduction for upper partial denture castings. J Prosthet Dent 4:67–72, 1954.

Dootz ER, Craig RG, and Peyton FA: Influence of investments and duplicating procedures on the accuracy of partial denture castings. J Prosthet Dent 15:679–690, 1965.

Dootz ER, Craig RG, and Peyton FA: Aqueous acrylamide gel duplicating material. J Prosthet Dent 17:570–577, 1967.

Gronewald AH, Paffenbarger GC, and Dickson G: The effect of molding processes on some properties of denture resins. J Am Dent Assoc 44:269–284, 1952.

Johnson HB: Technique for packing and staining complete or partial denture bases. J Prosthet Dent 6:154–159, 1956.

Perry CK: Transfer base for removable partial dentures. J Prosthet Dent 31:582–584, 1974.

Peyton FA: Cast chromium alloys. Dent Clin North Am November:759–771, 1958.

Peyton FA and Anthony DH: Evaluation of dentures processed by different techniques. J Prosthet Dent 13:269–281, 1963.

Rudd KD, Eissman HF, and Morrow RM: Dental laboratory procedures: Removable Partial Dentures, Vol. III. St Louis, CV Mosby Co, 1981.

Tuccillo JJ and Nielsen JP: Compatibility of alginate impression materials and dental stones. J Prosthet Dent 25:556–566, 1971.

See also references for Chapter 10 and Chapter 17.

CLINICAL PROCEDURES

First Appointment

For a partially edentulous patient who requires a removable prosthesis, diagnostic casts are mounted on the articulator for treatment planning. Impressions for use in fabricating these diagnostic casts are made at the first appointment.

ARMAMENTARIUM

Mouth mirror
Explorer
Radiographs if available
Impression trays
Periphery wax strips
Alginate
4 × 4 gauze squares
Forms as required

CLINICAL PROCEDURE

1. Proceed with history-taking and diagnostic examination; fill out the necessary records.
2. Prior to taking diagnostic cast impressions, a basic prophylaxis with rubber cup and pumice is performed, so that better diagnostic impressions can be made.
3. Take a face bow record.
4. Make a centric relation record.
5. Mount the diagnostic casts for study.
6. Order radiographs as necessary.

DIAGNOSTIC PROCEDURE

1. Evaluate all information obtained: clinical information, history, diagnostic casts, and radiographs.
2. Plan your recommended treatment procedure. Outline the steps on paper and on the diagnostic casts. If necessary, discuss your proposed treatment with consultants prior to the second appointment with the patient.
3. Request consultations with specialists if necessary.

Second Appointment

The purpose of this appointment is to present a final treatment plan for approval by the patient and the doctor.

ARMAMENTARIUM

Radiographs
Mounted diagnostic casts
Treatment plan
History records and laboratory tests as required

CLINICAL PROCEDURE

1. Show and explain to the patient the situations that exist in the mouth. Use the diagnostic casts for training aids.
2. Obtain consultation from all specialists involved in the treatment. *Write down or enclose* their proposed treatment in your records.
3. Formulate the final treatment plan.
4. Upon completion of the treatment plan, all steps must be outlined in the patient's record.
5. Draw the final partial denture design on the diagnostic casts prior to beginning restorative procedures. The partial design often influences the size and contour of the restorations.

When treatment plan and diagnosis are completed, a case presentation is made to the patient. Explain in detail and be sure that the patient is informed of the cost. It is always desirable to have the treatment plan and cost in writing.

Proceed with the surgical, periodontal, and restorative procedures.

Third Appointment

The purpose of this appointment is to accomplish the final mouth preparation and to take final impressions for fabrication of the removable partial denture. All necessary operative and periodontal procedures have been completed.

ARMAMENTARIUM

Diamond stones
Number 6 round burs
Burlew rubber wheels
Sandpaper disks
Pumice
Rubber cups
Alginate and trays
4 × 4 gauze squares

CLINICAL PROCEDURE

1. Refer to your diagnostic cast, which indicates where parallel guiding planes must be prepared. Make these guiding surfaces parallel first with a diamond stone, and then smooth with sandpaper disks and rubber wheels.

2. Alter other tooth surfaces as preplanned where necessary. Prepare rests with a number 6 or 8 round bur or diamond for posterior teeth. *Do not* leave sharp edges or parallel sides. They must be smoothly rounded with 1 mm of space provided for the metal rest.

3. Check anterior rests, which have been placed in inlays or crowns to make sure that they have positive, rounded rest seats. Recontour and polish them if necessary. Prepare anterior rests on natural tooth surfaces as planned.

4. Cleanse the mouth well before taking final impressions. Make two final impressions with alginate in a stock tray.

5. Pour these impressions *immediately* in vacuumed stone.

6. Make an occlusal index for proving the accuracy of the master cast(s). Use a tray acrylic matrix or a metal plate. Place the registration paste on one surface of the matrix in the shape of the arch. Place it in position in the mouth to record all occlusal and incisal surfaces.

LABORATORY PROCEDURE

1. Inspect the casts closely for defects such as bubbles. Select the better one to be the master cast.

2. Finalize the design on the *design cast.*

3. Tripod and mark the master cast.

4. Fill out the laboratory prescription form in duplicate.

5. Submit both casts to the laboratory with the occlusal index and the prescriptions.

Fourth Appointment

The basic objectives of this appointment are to

1. Try-in the casting and to make physiologic adjustments.

2. Alter the cast impression if necessary.

3. Obtain maxillomandibular registrations for transferring a duplication of the patient's oral anatomy to a laboratory situation upon an articulator.

ARMAMENTARIUM

Gold rouge	Face bow
Chloroform	Articulator
Brush	Carbide burs

For altered cast procedures add

Base plate wax	Zinc oxide impression paste
Acrylic tray material	A water bath
Gray stick modeling composition	

CLINICAL PROCEDURE

1. Coat the guiding planes and the rests of the casting with gold rouge and chloroform. Dry with air. Place in the patient's mouth and check for positive seating of the rests. If the rests are not seating or if the casting binds, inspect the gold rouged areas for interferences. Adjust with a high speed fissure bur where indicated.
2. In extension cases, coat the guide planes with gold rouge, and produce extension movement of the casting in the patient's mouth. Relieve the binding areas as disclosed by the gold rouge until the castings move freely.
3. In extension cases requiring altering of the master cast, proceed as outlined.
4. In a toothborne case, proceed with the following:
   a. A face bow record.
   b. Mount the maxillary cast on the articulator.
   c. A centric relation record.
   d. Mount the mandibular cast on the articulator.
   e. Verify the centric relation records with a second set of records.
   f. Make a protrusive record, and adjust the articulator.
   g. Select teeth.
5. In a toothborne case, proceed with the laboratory fabrication of the prosthesis.
6. In extension situations, see the fifth appointment, discussed next.

Fifth Appointment

The basic objectives of this appointment are to obtain maxillomandibular registrations and to transfer a duplication of the patient situation to a laboratory situation upon an articulator. Specific details and instructions are found in Chapter 16.

This appointment is necessary *for extension prostheses only.*

ARMAMENTARIUM

Face bow
Record materials, such as quick set plaster, modeling composition, or registration paste
Articulator

CLINICAL PROCEDURE

1. An altered cast impression has been used to alter the master cast by repouring the edentulous area. Upon this refined master cast a sprinkle-on acrylic record base has been adapted to the edentulous area to provide a stable base for records.
2. Mount the maxillary cast on the articulator with the face bow record.
3. Evaluate and mark the vertical dimension of occlusion.
4. Adjust the plastic occlusion rim to allow space for the interocclusal record.
5. Make the centric record.
6. Mount the mandibular cast on the instrument.
7. Verify the articulator mounting with a second centric record.
8. Make the protrusive record.
9. Adjust the instrument.

When anterior teeth are involved or if there are esthetic considerations, an additional appointment is necessary.

LABORATORY PROCEDURE

1. Refine occlusion on the articulator.
2. Set up the teeth.
3. Process and finish the prosthesis.

Sixth Appointment

The insertion appointment requires final adaptation of

1. The casting to the remaining teeth.
2. The denture base to the edentulous areas.
3. Refinement of occlusion by a patient-articulator remount procedure.

ARMAMENTARIUM

Pressure indicator paste
Periphery paste
Impression trays
Alginate
Low-fusing metal and a ladle
Quick-set plaster, registration paste, or modeling composition for records
Articulating ribbon
Occlusion adjustment stones

PROCEDURE

Refer to Chapter 18, Insertion Principles and Procedures.

Complete the remount procedure and equilibrate the occlusion.

Give the patient a removable partial denture instruction sheet (see Chapter 19).

Give 24-hr and 1-week postinsertion appointments.

Index

Note: Numbers in *italics* refer to figures.